APHASIOLOGY

Volume 21 Number 10/11 October/November 2007

CONTENTS

APHASIOLOGY

SUBSCRIPTION INFORMATION

Subscription rates to Volume 21, 2007 (12 issues) are as follows:
Institutional subscriptions: £1175.00(UK); $1940.00 (Rest of the world).
An Institutional subscription to the print edition also includes free access to the online edition for any number of concurrent users across a local area network.
There is also a personal (print only) rate available which is strictly for personal, non-commercial use only. The reselling of personal subscriptions is strictly prohibited. Personal subcriptions must be purchased with a personal cheque or credit card and must be received at a personal (private) address. Personal subscribers may purchase a maximum of 4 subscriptions. Proof of personal status may be requested. For full information please visit the Journal's homepage.
Individual subscriptions: £494.00 (UK); $817.00 (Rest of the world).
A subscription to the print edition includes free access for any number of concurrent users across a local area network to the online edition, ISSN 1464-5041.
Print subscriptions are also available to individual members of the British Aphasiology Society (BAS), on application to the Society.

For a complete and up-to-date guide to Taylor & Francis's journals and books publishing programmes, visit the Taylor and Francis website: http://www.tandf.co.uk/

Aphasiology (USPS permit number 001413) is published monthly. The 2007 US Institutional subscription price is $1940.00. Periodicals Postage Paid at Jamaica, NY by US Mailing Agent Air Business Ltd, c/o Priority Airfreight NY Ltd, 147-29 182nd Street, Jamaica, NY 11413, USA. **US Postmaster**: Please send address changes to Air Business Ltd, c/o Priority Airfreight NY Ltd, 147-29 182nd Street, Jamaica, NY 11413, USA.
Dollar rates apply to subscribers in all countries except the UK and the Republic of Ireland where the pound sterling price applies. All subscriptions are payable in advance and all rates include postage. Journals are sent by air to the USA, Canada, Mexico, India, Japan and Australasia. Subscriptions are entered on an annual basis, i.e., from January to December. Payment may be made by sterling cheque, dollar cheque, international money order, National Giro, or credit card (AMEX, VISA, Mastercard).

Orders originating in the following territories should be sent direct to the local distributor.
India: Universal Subscription Agency Pvt. Ltd, 101–102 Community Centre, Malviya Nagar Extn, Post Bag No. 8, Saket, New Delhi 110017.
Japan: Kinokuniya Company Ltd, Journal Department, PO Box 55, Chitose, Tokyo 156.
USA, Canada and Mexico: Psychology Press, a member of Taylor & Francis, 325 Chestnut St, Philadelphia, PA 19106, USA
UK and other territories: Psychology Press, c/o T&F Customer Services, Informa UK Ltd, Sheepen Place, Colchester, Essex, CO3 3LP, Tel: +44 (0)20 7017 5544; Fax: +44 (0)20 7017 5198; UK.
E-mail: tf.enquiries@tfinforma.com

Typeset by H. Charlesworth & Co. Ltd., Wakefield, UK, and printed by Hobbs the Printers Ltd., Totton, Hants, UK. The online edition can be reached via the journal's website: http://www.psypress.com/aphasiology

Back issues: Taylor & Francis retains a three-year back issue stock of journals. Older volumes are held by our official stockists: Periodicals Service Company, 11 Main Street, Germantown, NY 12526, USA, to whom all orders and enquiries should be addressed. Tel: +1 518 537 4700; Fax: +1 518 537 5899;
E-mail: psc@periodicals.com; URL: http://www.periodicals.com/tandf.html

---

APHASIOLOGY, 2007, 21 (10/11), 911–915

Psychology Press
Taylor & Francis Group

Preface to this special issue on verbal perseveration

Jacqueline Stark
Austrian Academy of Sciences, Vienna

> "Pathological conditions with perseveratory tendencies are mainly of a transitory nature and, for that reason, seldom provide the opportunity for continuous observation. Also, the phenomena are either too simple, and then not informative enough, or too complex and often less transparent. For this reason I grasp the opportunity to publish observations which exhibit these imperfections to a lesser extent and therefore present themselves as particularly suited and instructive; in particular the longer duration allowed me to make statements which, to date, had not been possible to present in this manner.
>
> The aim I am pursuing with this publication is, first of all, the continuation of my attempts to determine the stage of the event on which the process, in this case perseveration, is active.
>
> A further goal of this publication is the delineation of the relationship of perseveratory processes to the remainder of the psychological processes, as this has not received sufficient acknowledgement to date. This presentation is meant to demonstrate how perseveration, or the triggered processes, which I call 'perseverates', just as they themselves experience such influences from the other psychological processes, do not only stand ineffectively between them, but rather, under specific circumstances, are able to exert intense influence on all the other processes."
>
> Pick, 1921, p. 94.[1]

It seems highly appropriate to begin this special issue of *Aphasiology* with a quote from Arnold Pick's 1921 article on perseveration: *"Motor" and "static" perseveration; at the same time a contribution to the teaching on catatonic phenomena*. From 1883 to approximately 1934, Pick, Hughlings Jackson, Gairdner, Heilbronner, Kleist, Lissauer, Liepmann and other colleagues in Germany, England, France, etc. were involved in a lively debate about perseveration and verbal perseveration in particular. The issues cited by Pick, namely the "stage of the event", are still relevant and open to further debate. Various definitions and taxonomies are alluded to in these classic publications.

Considering the prevalence and pervasive influence of perseveration in the diagnosis and even more so in the treatment of clients with severely impaired oral language production (global, Wernicke's, transcortical sensory aphasia, etc.), the topic of perseveration is, surprisingly, not well documented in textbooks and introductions to aphasia. With regard to therapy issues, notable exceptions are Helm Estabrooks' *Treatment of Aphasic Perseveration* (TAP) therapy programme (Helm Estabrooks, Emery, & Albert 1987), the work of Basso (2004), and therapy studies presently being carried out.

http://www.psypress.com/aphasiology DOI: 10.1080/02687030701198197

In a study specifically addressing the occurrence of perseveration in aphasic patients performing various tasks, Allison and Hurwitz (1967) observed perseveration in 16 out of 24 people; that is, in nearly 70% of the cases. These authors stress two points—That none of the 16 people with aphasia perseverated on each and all of the tests given, and that in all but five instances, perseveration was confined to tasks requiring the use of speech and language. Albert and Sandson (1986) report that 72% of the aphasic patients in their study perseverated at least once on the confrontation-naming task (mean ratio of perseveration total responses: 14.3).

However, the relevance of perseveration as a topic of investigation is documented by the publication of an issue of *Seminars in Speech and Language* in November 2004 entitled *Perseveration in Neurogenic Communication Disorders* and edited by Hugh Buckingham and Sarah Christman. In this recently published *Seminars* issue, perseveration is elucidated in seven papers spanning the topics of the neuropharmacology of verbal perseveration to connectionist approaches, etc. The topics of the papers in this special issue of *Aphasiology* demonstrate a continuation of this revival of interest in perseveration.

Research on verbal perseveration in aphasia follows three main strategies. The first involves reports based on actual protocols (routine clinical testing) from individuals presenting with a specific pattern of perseverative responses. The aims of these studies have been to arrive at an understanding of the underlying mechanisms of the impaired language or cognitive, nonverbal performance that have resulted in perseverative responses. According to the second strategy, perseverative language data produced under experimental test conditions are analysed or an attempt is made to elicit perseverative responses by altering the variables including the test conditions and/or the structure of the stimuli; for instance, the rate of presentation or the semantic difficulty, i.e., relatedness of the stimuli. This strategy follows the same goals.

In recent years another strategy has been adopted, namely that of modelling patterns of breakdown. Computational modelling studies have been carried out in which specific variables of the model are manipulated in order to observe the ramifications of the adjustments on the hypothetical performance. These investigations extend the limitations set by individual single cases and allow analysis of numerous factors that might potentially affect performance in actual cases. As interesting as simulated responses and patterns of hypothetical performance can be, analysis of verbal perseverations actually produced by brain-damaged persons provide *real* language data which can be used to account for the circumscribed deficits in language processing, and in particular the phenomenon of "perseveration".

Despite their methodological differences, all strategies applied in this research domain share a common goal, namely to understand the origin of the phenomenon of "perseveration" in healthy participants and clients with brain damage. The first two strategies are primarily represented in this special issue of *Aphasiology*. An overriding claim throughout the papers is the specific nature of the phenomenon of perseveration—namely that perseveration reflects the client's primary language-processing deficits.

The first three papers in this issue are introductory in nature, in that they provide an overview of topics relating to perseveration. In the first, Buckingham addresses very innovative issues in discussing when perseveration happens to an aphasic client. In his description of a client with conduction aphasia, DW, whom he has been studying longitudinally, Buckingham uses the term "qualia" to refer to his client's feeling of sensing things. "Qualia" refers to the inner contents of the "feel" of sensing things. According to Buckingham, when perseveration happens to clients and they are startled by their perseverative response, they find themselves at "the nexus of the conscious and the unconsciousness". The specific nature of the perseverative responses produced by DW is also emphasised by Buckingham.

In the second paper, Stark provides a survey predominantly of the German classical aphasiological literature. The aim of the paper is to summarise the stimulating peer discussions of the classical researchers—Heilbronner, Liepmann, Lissauer, Kleist, Pick, Von Soelder, etc.—on clients exhibiting verbal perseveration, and peer debates on the origin of perseveratory phenomena. Attention is drawn to similarities among the classical accounts of verbal perseveration and more recent proposals, with the conclusion that the classical accounts are actually quite up to date.

In the third paper, Moses, Nickels, and Sheard provide a review of the research on recurrent perseveration in speech production, focusing on various theoretical accounts. They compare issues addressed in the non-language-impaired population and in aphasia in their discussion of two theories: (1) breakdown in the underlying levels of language processing and (2) impaired inhibition of recent memory traces. They conclude that in the most recent studies on aphasic clients, a systematic link exists between the pattern of perseverative responses and the underlying levels of language-processing breakdown.

In the following paper, Moses, Sheard, and Nickels examine recurrent perseverative errors produced by five aphasic clients in repetition, reading aloud, and picture naming, using a case series approach. The occurrence of different types of recurrent perseverative errors was found to be influenced by the processing demands of the administered tasks, relative to each client's language-processing deficits. The authors stress the necessity of analysing both whole-word and phoneme perseverative responses to gain understanding of the relationships that hold between perseveration and language-processing impairments. In accounting for the observed errors, these authors suggest that the recurrent perseverative errors are a direct result of the underlying processing breakdown.

Martin and Dell's paper on common mechanisms underlying perseverative and non-perseverative sound and word substitutions provides evidence that perseveration errors are generated by the same mechanisms as non-perseverative errors, namely weak activation of the intended word in the context of a competition from other activated words. Based on data collected from individuals with aphasia, they show that whole-word perseverative and non-perseverative errors are associated with weak spreading of activation between semantics and the target word form, whereas perseverative and non-perseverative sound errors are associated with word retrieval impairment profiles characterised by weak spreading of activation between the target word form and its corresponding sounds.

Ackerman and Ellis address the question of where aphasic perseverations come from in their case MM, who showed a substantial semantic impairment as well as phonological and orthographic deficits. This client produced numerous perseverations in naming, reading, and repetition. They provide a detailed analysis of the errors in the various modalities, applying the theory put forward by Martin and Dell (in this issue) and also Cohen and Dehaene's model (1998). MM's pattern of performance revealed differences among naming, reading, and repetition.

Whole-word perseverations predominated in the object-naming task and the perseverative responses for this task were predominantly unrelated to the target items. Regarding the causes of these perseverations, Ackerman and Ellis suggest for MM that a temporary de-afferentation struck at random times and this periodically deprived his semantic and phonological system of input.

In their study on the phenomenon of conversational perseveration in traumatic brain injury, Frankel and Penn examine the hypothesis that deficient inhibitory control, accompanied by unique disruptions of specific self-regulatory functions as defined by Barkley (1998), can account for various manifestations of perseveration in two individuals with TBI. Furthermore, these discrete profiles provide an explanatory basis for conversational characteristics. The occurrence of recurrent and stuck in set perseveration, respectively, is demonstrated with reference to two case studies. The response of the identified perseverative behaviours, in both neuropsychological and conversational data, to pharmacotherapy is examined.

Analysis of verbal perseveratory responses, which were the initial symptoms in a case of Creutzfeld-Jakob disease, is the topic of investigation in the paper by Stark, Kristoferitsch, Graf, Gelpi, and Budka. The pervasive nature of perseveration—they constituted up to 95% of the overall errors—is considered to reflect the magnitude of the language-processing deficits at the time of testing. The nature of verbal perseverative behaviour in this patient and the rapid deterioration of language functions are discussed with regard to the need for documentation of the language deficits in progressive degenerative diseases.

In the final paper, Stark interprets intricate examples of verbal perseveration produced by a client with transcortical sensory aphasia, MH, who showed dissociation between syntax and semantics. She documents the complex interactions of the perseveratory errors and illustrates that, although semantic processing—production and monitoring of utterances—is impaired, syntactic abilities are relatively spared as judged by the grammatically correct production of semantically anomalous responses. MH's language performance is interpreted with reference to intact and impaired components of Levelt's (1993) model of language production and comprehension.

All of the papers were peer reviewed by internal reviewers (contributors to this issue) and the following external reviewers (in alphabetical order):

Wolfgang Dressler (University of Vienna)
Jean K. Gordon (University of Iowa)
Desmond O'Neill (Adelaide and Meath Hospital)
Rebecca Sowman (Adelaide and Meath Hospital)
Gloria Streit Olness (University of Texas Dallas, Northern Texas University)
Diana van Lancker Sidtis (New York University)
Claus-W. Wallesch (Medical University of Magdeburg)

I thank them for their willingness to review the papers and for their constructive comments to the individual authors. My special thanks go to Nadine Martin, as well as to my colleagues Christiane Pons, Leena Martin, Karin Geisler, Maura Bayer, Lotti Viola, and Heinz-Karl Stark, for their assistance and feedback at various stages of the project. I am very grateful to Chris Code and his *Aphasiology* team for their support.

Last but not least—without perseverating—I would like to thank all the contributors for their papers on perseveration and for their patience, and I would like to apologise for the long gestation period.

NOTE

[1] Pick's original text in German (Pick, 1921, p. 4): *Pathologische Zustände mit perseveratorischer Tendenz sind meist transitorischer Art und bieten deshalb selten Gelegenheit zu länger anhaltender Beobachtung; auch sind die Erscheinungen entweder zu einfach und dann nicht genügend aufschlußgebend oder zu kompliziert und oft wenig durchsichtig; deshalb ergreife ich die Gelegenheit zur Mitteilung von Beobachtungen, die diese Mängel weniger aufweisen und aus diesem Grund sich als besonders geeignet und lehrreich darstellten; insbesondere die längere Dauer ermöglichte es, Feststellungen zu machen, die bisher in dieser Weise nicht gelungen waren.*

Der Zweck, den ich mit dieser Mitteilung verfolge, ist zunächst die Fortsetzung meiner Versuche, festzulegen, in welcher Station des Geschehens der Vorgang wirksam ist, der sich uns schließlich als Perseveration darstellt.

Einen weiteren Zweck verfolgt die Mitteilung durch die Klarlegung des Verhältnisses der perseveratorischen Vorgänge zu dem übrigen psychischen Geschehen. Man hat das bisher kaum genügend gewürdigt. Die Darstellung hier ist nun bestimm, zu zeigen, wie die Perseveration, bzw. Die durch dieselbe ausgelösten Vorgänge, die von mir sog. Perseverate, ebenso wie sie selbst solche Einwirkungen von diesen erfahren, nicht bloß wie ein Fremdkörper wirkungslos zwischen den anderen psychischen Vorgängen stehe, vielmehr unter bestimmten Bedingungen ganz intensive Einwirkungen auf alle übrigen auszuüben imstande sind.

REFERENCES

Albert, M. L., & Sandson, J. (1986). Perseveration in aphasia. *Cortex*, *22*, 103–115.

Allison, R. S., & Hurwitz, L. J. (1967). On perseveration in aphasics. *Brain*, *90*, 429–448.

Barkley, R. A. (1997). Behavioural inhibition, sustained attention and executive functions: Constructing a unifying theory of ADHD. *Psychological Bulletin*, *121*, 65–94.

Basso, A. (2004). Perseveration or the Tower of Babel. *Seminars in Speech and Language*, *25*(4), 375–389.

Buckingham, H. W., & Christman, S. (Eds.). (2004). Perseveration in neurogenic communication disorders [special issue]. *Seminars in Speech and Language*, *25*(4).

Cohen, L., & Dehaene, S. (1998). Competition between past and present assessment and interpretation of verbal perseverations. *Brain*, *121*, 1641–1650.

Helm Estabrooks, N., Emery, P., & Albert, M. L. (1987). Treatment of Aphasic Perseveration (TAP) Program: A new approach to aphasia therapy. *Archives of Neurology*, *44*, 1253–1255.

Levelt, W. J. M. (1993). Language use in normal speakers and its disorders. In G. Blanken, J. Dittman, H. Grimm, J. C. Marshall, & C.-W. Wallesch (Eds.), *Linguistic disorders and pathologies: An international handbook* (pp. 1–15). Berlin: Walter de Gruyter.

Pick, A. (1921). "Motorische" und "statische" Perseveration, zugleich ein Beitrag zur Lehre von den katatonen Erscheinungen. *Abhandlungen aus der Neurologie, Psychiatrie, Psychologie und ihren Grenzbgebieten, Heft 13* (pp. 94–141). Berlin: Karger.

APHASIOLOGY, 2007, 21 (10/11), 916–927

Psychology Press
Taylor & Francis Group

Introductory essay: Perseveration happens!

Hugh W. Buckingham

Louisiana State University, Baton Rouge, LA, USA

Patients with recurrent perseveration as part of a fluent left temporal lobe aphasia often consciously intend to produce a requested target on confrontation testing in the clinic. However, suddenly and quite unexpectedly, they will have a perseveration happen to them. Being focused on the task at hand, and having no discernable attention deficit, the modular and automatic utterance of a whole-word perseverate will startle patients, leaving them puzzled and at a loss to explain such a blunder. In this paper the claim is made that, in a sense, these patients have found themselves at the nexus of the conscious and the unconscious. This phenomenon is discussed based on data from a longitudinal study of a patient who has classical conduction aphasia with severe word-finding deficits, but intact comprehension and attention. He perseverates only in the response modes that have been compromised by his brain damage.

Damage to the cerebral cortex often results in perseveration of one sort or another. Frontal lobe lesions often lead to "stuck-in-set" perseveration, where patients have difficulty shifting attention from one form of responding to another. Right hemisphere damage often leads to a "continuous" perseveration, where once some activity begins it tends to continue in a loop-trapped action that is serially repeated. Temporal lobe lesions that result in fluent aphasia will often have "recurrent" perseveration as a sequela. Recurrent perseveration involves the inappropriate production of an action (or the production of words or segments) that has been previously activated, only to be produced again at some later point not too far down-line, but where correct responses may well have intervened. Various factors seem to be involved that trigger the recurrent perseveration.

This essay will concentrate on the recurrent perseveration of the whole-word "predilection" form /peɪpər/ "paper", together with slightly altered forms, most of which were the phonological alternate /pɛpər/ "pepper", itself a word in English. There is no semantic relation between these words, but they are close associates phonologically. Both are two syllable trochaic items that share all but the initial nucleus. There were other nonword productions such as /sleɪpər/, most of which were formed by a phonemic carryover from a close-order word with an /sl-/ onset. Interactive blendings in this patient have been reported previously in Buckingham and Christman (2004). This patient, DW, was right-handed, and had a single stroke that affected the left temporal lobe in such a fashion that he tested as having a conduction aphasia on the Boston Aphasia Exam. He presented with severe

Address correspondence to: Hugh W. Buckingham, Louisiana State University, Baton Rouge, LA 70803, USA. E-mail: hbuck@lsu.edu

http://www.psypress.com/aphasiology DOI: 10.1080/02687030701198205

word-finding deficits and produced marked phonemic paraphasia when repeating and reading orally. His comprehension was well within normal limits; he had full control of his limbs and had no ambulatory difficulties at all. His syntactic constructions were of the paragrammatic form, where the automaticity was reflected in the production of matrices held together by the well-placed functional morphemes, both free and bound; intonation was quite natural. It was clear that this patient only perseverated when undergoing confrontation naming with objects, pictures of objects, or larger depictions of scenes. That is to say, this patient's perseverative behaviour was tied to his responses within the deafferented system of lexical access. Nevertheless, when operating within this response domain, the patient appeared focused on the task and in control of the search activity—at least he "felt" that way until the utterance act happened to him.

The present paper will concentrate on the verbal descriptions that the patient offers of his startled "qualia", and how it "felt" for him to have intended wilfully and with conscious control to produce a target word, but where instead a recurrent perseveration happened to him – quite out of control, rapid, encapsulated and "automatic".[1] I will try to relate to the startled reaction of surprise, which must have an eerie twinge to it for the patient since it happened within a cognitive surround of voluntary activity. That is, the patient was not encumbered by diminished attention or focus, the horizontal faculties that are intact during conscious and controlled wilful activity. I will consider some philosophical aspects of the qualia of agency, where the normal person will have the "feeling" of conscious existence during a volitional movement such as raising the arm to an internal command to raise the arm. An external command to raise the arm may bring on other complicating factors, which I will not pursue here, since failure on movement to verbal command is possibly indicative of an apraxia of sorts—verbal or limb. In any event, I will make an attempt to interpret the feeling of surprise of the patient who perseverates recurrently as a result of straddling the border of the automatic and the wilful. I will conclude by considering the need to evaluate the patient with perseveration in more depth, concentrating on "the whole patient". I also call for more elicitations of the verbal descriptions by these patients as to just how they "feel" when the perseverations happen to them. In a sense, we are attempting to "get into the mind" of the patient who makes these types of responses. Furthermore, at least as concerns the patient described here, it appears that the whole-word recurrent perseveration startles the most. Nonword productions of perseverates that are

[1] "Qualia" refers to the inner contents of the "feel" of sensing things. What it is to "see" a red object as red must somehow be characterised and the rather nebulous notion must at least have a label, so that whatever it may turn out to be, it can at least be subject to scientific and philosophical consideration. In psycho-physical parallelism or identity theory, the claim is often that the physiological activity stimulated by the physical characteristics of the red object run in parallel with or can be identified with the perceiver's qualia of "seeing red" (Buckingham, 1986). The qualia would be quite different in an agnosic who "perceives" but does not realise he/she perceives or is unaware—he/she simply can make no sense of the object "seen". Jason Brown's (personal communication) model of microgenesis does not restrict qualia to the individual self; rather he links qualia with subjectivity and claims that subjectivity is limited by the world. I will continue to incorporate the term "qualia", but I will be referring to inner "feels" of the human and the occasionally offered self-reports of these states-of-mind "feels". It would be an interesting project to inquire more deeply into perseveration through the lenses of Brown's microgenesis of cognition, where the intransitive verb "to feel" is paramount in describing mentality at multiple levels of processing.

formed, say, by phonemic carryover do not seem to "catch the mind" of the speaker as clearly as the whole-word perseverate, and perhaps especially whole-word perseverates that bear no association at all with the target. I am also unaware of any studies or mere observations of startle qualia on the heels of the production of non-perseverated paraphasias in the fluent patient.

VERBAL DESCRIPTIONS OF THE QUALIA OF SURPRISE BY PATIENT DW

(1) Describing a scene picture of a barbershop:

D.W. "...a man cutting paper...pet pepper...um...paper pape"
H.B. "Paper keeps coming out."
D.W. (quizzical) "I know, I know."
H.B: "It just keeps popping up."
D.W. "No, it's just...I don't know why it comes out."

(2) Repetition:

glasses → glakis...lakis
razor → razor
pencil → paper
" → paper
" → slaper
" → slippers ... slips .... slippers ....slip
.
.
.
.
newspaper → paper...pepper ...pepper
tap → təpeɪ .... peɪpər
dub → klupper.....klubber
keep → kweep....kwip ..... kwipper
big → keep..... kipper.....kwipper
good → klapper
HB: (Asking DW about his perseveration) "Tell me about it...you get something on your mind...
DW: "Uh, no." (puzzled) "It's just right there. It just comes out. That's it, You know....exactly what it is."

(3) Picture naming:

toothbrush → kerrer
" → pepper...pupper
HB: (cueing pt.) "Is that paper?"
DW: "No"
HB: "Is that pepper?"
DW: "No"
HB: "Is that a TV?"
DW: "No"

HB: "Is that a toothbrush?"
DW: "You got it. That's it."
HB: "What is it?"
DW: "pepper....pepper.... No! I did it again." (puzzled, frustrated)

(4) On non-verbal apraxia testing and pointing:

HB: "Stick out your tongue and move it side to side. [correct response]
"Close your eyes" [correct response]
"Wave goodbye" [correct response]
"Pretend like you're angry" [correct response]
"Blow out your cheeks" [correct response]
"Salute" [no response]
"Show me how you brush your teeth" [correct response]
HB: "Point to the ceiling" [correct response]
HB: "Point to the floor" [delayed response] Pt beginning to tire.... "Oh, down There." [more delay] "Pepper....there we go again." Pt was quite puzzled, especially since this was a non-verbal response task.

(5) Functional description of objects:

HB: "Tell me what you do with a book"?
DW: "Look, or whatever I can get out of it."
HB: "What do you do with a pen"?
DW: "uh......pepper. There we go again." (puzzled)
HB: "What do you do with a door"?
DW: "Pepper, uh...duce...pepper, oh Lord. Here we go again with that.

Several aspects of this patient's responses should be mentioned. DW produced the predilection recurrent perseverate "paper" and its many phonologically similar trochaic associates such as the nonwords "papper" and "pupper", or the sound-related noun "pepper". Moreover, there were numerous blended cluster onsets of phonemic carryovers, such as "kwipper" and "klapper" (Buckingham & Christman, 2004). These perseverations and paraphasias continued to occur well into the acute stages of DW's aphasia over a period of testing that stretched for roughly a year or so.

There is always some puzzlement over just how, when, and why the predilection forms take hold of the patient. In the first session, DW's clinical therapist and I were talking with the patient about the news, and we asked him what he read for that. Several minutes went by as he struggled for the word "newspaper". After much directed search, his frustration led to tears; we went to something else. This episode seemed to have caused the patient some degree of anxiety, for which some investigators have suggested at least a partial causative role in perseveration (e.g., Allison, 1966). The discussion topic with DW remained on the news of the day, and in a less confrontational conversation he then indeed uttered "newspaper" with no struggle at all. He became a bit shaken and began to assure us that he did much better "at home", when there was no confrontational clinical command/request to do things such as say, read, and repeat words. I mention this here only to point to the initiation of the productions of his predilection form "paper". I have no other account of why he may have been subject to the recurrent production of that high-frequency trochee. Furthermore, various contiguity associates of the predilection form would appear, for instance when DW was asked to repeat "newspaper" or "pencil", the predilection form would most often appear, and quite rapidly post stimulus.

Note, too, that in dialogue #1 above, DW produced "paper" and not the target "hair", since the scene picture was of a barbershop. Contiguity associates are formed through the frequent co-occurrences of verbs and their highly typical arguments, and so it is quite natural to expect that "cut hair" may trigger the production of "cut paper". Clearly, in associative terms this is association by collocation and not by similarity. The semantics here relate to argument structure and linguistic patterns of selectional restriction, which are nevertheless ordered contiguously in utterance inputs and outputs.

DW, however, suffered from conduction aphasia, and accordingly his paraphasias were for the most part phonological. Buckingham and Christman (2004) suggested that perhaps a metrical foot template could be subject to perseveration as well. We pointed to the large class of whole-word-like or real-word productions of trochaic forms, most of which were either "paper" or carryover perseverative blends, such as "playper", "klubber", "slayper"—all strong/weak trochaic forms. There is a clear lexical effect here because, without a doubt, the highest-frequency two-syllable words are the trochees. This should not be difficult for the connectionists to simulate.

Another extremely important point is that, on repetition, DW claims he "loses" the word to be repeated or, he claims, "It's right there, then gone". On the other hand, he could easily point to the correct picture in a group when he was provided the spoken name by the examiner. He could delay his response, but upon showing him the picture subsequently, he had no trouble pointing to the correct one. This caused us to reassess our original suspicion that he had a generalised short-term memory span disruption. It is more likely that his articulatory attempts on repetition served to erase the original acoustic/phonological stimulus from the operating buffer. This "…it just goes; I lose it…" may not have occurred in the passive, non-articulatory pointing to pictures of spoken words, even after some degree of time delay. We note that he never perseverated on the pointing task. It is likely that DW could hold on to the semantics of the picture for later pointing, but could not hold on to the phonological elements in order to repeat them well. A modular phonological operating memory suggests itself here.[2] Although he could not read printed words aloud, and perseverated often on oral reading, he could easily match pictures with printed words. He could distinguish minimal phonemic pair pictures, such as "bee" and "pea" or "mail" and "pail". Nowhere on this task did DW produce recurrent perseveration.

THE "FEEL" OF THE QUALIA WHEN PERSEVERATION HAPPENS TO A PATIENT

I am not aware of any collection of self-reports for each kind of perseveration, but I would suspect that, at least for continuous perseveration, clonic perseveration, and

[2] I thank Nadine Martin for reminding me of this time-worn distinction. It also accords with the fact that the deafferented phonological buffer memory predicted all the recurrent perseveration and that there was no perseveration at all on the nonverbal, passive pointing task, which pressed the operating memory for semantics only.

other more motoric recurrent utterances, there would be less instantaneous puzzlement at having such non-planned forms come to utterance. The recurrent and repetitive nature of clonic and continuous perseveration seems not to give the patient the time to startle although, as mentioned above, we are in uncharted territory in terms of qualia and their possible variations due to *type* of perseveration. Moreover, I have not teased apart whether semantic inappropriateness may exacerbate the startle, and thus I do not know if degree of semantic relatedness might correlate with degree of surprise. It may turn out that whole-word perseverates that are semantically associated in some way with the target do not jolt the patient as would a phonological associate or, worse yet, when the perseverate bears absolutely no association with the target.

Jennifer Sandson and Martin Albert (1984) argued that an attention deficit may underlie continuous perseveration, but this is certainly not the case with DW's recurrent perseveration. A lack of startle would logically correlate with an attested attention deficit, for if there were no attention then it would be unlikely the patient would be focused enough to realise the inappropriateness of the perseverate. The literature on "stuck-in-set" perseveration has pointed to failures in switching focus or attention from one to another task domain. Perhaps there is something cognitively unique in the patient with recurrent perseveration that allows it to happen to the patient, when the patient can nonetheless focus, attend, and shift these normally. Perhaps it is that continuous perseveration is simply a motor loop phenomenon and that stuck-in-set is not primarily a lexical access disruption at all, but simply one of focus shift to a different attention set. Attention would allow for recognition of incongruity, whereas an attentional deficit would not allow for recognition of inappropriateness. At least for one of her recurrent perseveration patients, Basso (2004) argued that attention was not the cause of the perseveration. She writes, "TS1 (treated subject #1) was unable to stop his perseverative verbal behavior even when he was aware of the perseverations and attempted to stop it" (2004, p. 388). Attention was not an issue.

In any event, it would be interesting to inquire in some way about the patient's qualia with these two forms of perseveration. Qualia, again, is the philosopher's term for how it "feels" to be in a conscious mental state. They ask "how does it feel" to see red, hear a noise, smell a rose; to which I would add "to feel you are in charge, in control". This is the essence of what some call consciousness, and a primary "feel" here is one of agency.

Jason Brown (1988, 1996, 2005) has developed a microgenetic model of the unfolding of cognitions of all kinds. He attempts to characterise the role of the self in terms of distinct "feels" experienced as processing proceeds. One reads much of these self-feels through Brown's descriptions of the microgenesis of cognition. There has still been no final word by Brown on the issue of qualia and the perseverating patient, but there have been many occasions where he has touched ground with what I am briefly outlining here. In past papers, Brown has focused on certain of the frontal lobe perseveration types of A. R. Luria, many of which turn on one or another type of "stuck-in-set" perseveration, which seem to be caused by lesions of the meso-limbic connections from frontal cortex that involve dopaminergic systems. In Brown (1988) he discusses frontal lobe perseveration cases where "...the patient is aware and can describe inappropriate performances but cannot correct them" (p. 327). He discusses their attentive verbal descriptions of their failures to perform on tests like the Wisconsin Card Sorting Test, which is the classic measurement of one's ability to NOT get "stuck in sets". He goes on to say: "The presence of error awareness and an ability to describe the correct activity without being able to alter it has been observed by many authors" (p. 327).

I am claiming that we need to collect and take a serious look at these self-reports for a fuller understanding of the individual patient in each case. Degree of awareness is a very difficult item to measure, but Brown would claim that the temporal lobe patient would tend to have less degree of awareness than the frontal patient, when he writes that this frontal lobe patient may have an additional temporal lobe dysfunction since even he suffers from some degree of unawareness. Nevertheless, Brown ploughs the cognitive field of consciousness through internal "feels" that reflect the patient's (he says, "the self") self-reports of their derailments. Brown's descriptions of typical left temporal lobe patients with aphasia and paraphasia are that "Such patients may have little insight into their paraphasic errors" (p. 328). At least DW maintains a good degree of awareness of the fact that he is perseverating—but only post utterance.

In his chapter on "Autonomy and agent causation" Brown (1996) once again traces a person's awareness "feels" of being in control—or "agency". Without overly simplifying Brown's complex mental-physical microgenesis, I have been trying to account for DW's puzzled and startled reactions to his perseverations as a kind of cognitive/consciousness garden-path jolt, where the typical "feel" of agency is abruptly cut off when the consciously and attentively searched-for target is replaced by the automatic deliverance of the recurrent perseverate—it just happens. For Brown, there are several components of agent causation, among which is "... the feeling of spontaneity in decision-making [and] the feeling that the self as a cause and the action as an effect are distinct occurrences" (1996, p. 104). Brown goes on to write that "... agency requires a self in consciousness in a particular context" (p. 106). In the context of the recurrent whole-word perseveration in DW, the sudden withdrawal from the feeling of agency in the patient who can at least instantaneously monitor post-articulatory perseverates, would seem to be disconcerting to the extent of puzzlement.

In a series of new publications on "process thought" Brown (2005) places his microgenetic model into a much fuller scheme of human individual lives and values, where he again interprets most of what we do in the world and what happens to us in terms of our inner selves. Quite often, it is the "feel of things"—what I have rather loosely related to qualia. Here again, his sections on "agency and recipience" and "feeling and intentionality" are germane. He writes (2005, p. 83) that:

> We feel that we are thinking things up even if the effort of thinking does not help in their production. ... We search for and actively generate images and concepts. Linguistic objects are the obvious tools of agency. For the feeling of self-generated activity, the self must be in opposition to objects, in the mind and in the world. Indeed, the voluntary action of a limb is bridge to that world.

CONTROLLED VERSUS AUTOMATIC PROCESSING AND THE ABILITY TO MONITOR

Stark (1988) wrote at length on the monitoring of post-production and the monitoring of pre-production; the two are distinct. Pre-production monitoring is often labelled as "prepair". Stark cites the work of Karmiloff-Smith, who focuses on pre-conscious access as a modular metaprocedure, where "prepair" refers to the more recondite notion of operations within encapsulated and fast cognitive reflex systems of automatic spreading activation; it is "incipient" cognition and is not computed by the sentient/conscious self. The "prepairs" are a production of the cognitive pre-conscious modular system, which, because they are reflex-like and automatic, are considered to be "dumb"—but as a sine qua non of our cognition they are truly not so dumb. We just can't help them along. Many simply claim that both types of repair are "self-repairs", but they occur at different processing levels. It could very well be that the automatic prepairs are in reality the structural constraints built into the system as a result of the architectures of the language inputs to the system, which are induced by that system as language is acquired. These are the constraints we study in "optimality theory" (Prince & Smolensky, 2004), and that are simulated in connectionist work, such as Wheeler and Touretzky (1997), and discussed in den Ouden and Bastiaanse (2005). For Stark (personal communication), a prepair would occur when the patient was asked to name a cigarette and would say, "No, not a cigar," and then would name the cigarette correctly. In this case, the would-be error was caught, as indicated by the "no ... not a ...". What must have happened for this to occur is that somehow the speaker, before uttering, penetrated the modular processes. On the face of it, this would seem strange. The speaker became consciously aware of the reflex that activated "cigar", in which case the automatic process somehow was accessed, only to be instantaneously ruled out by the speaker. Again, how were the modular processes penetrated to the pre-production point of awareness?

Post-utterance monitoring is quite different, but if some plan-external item escapes from the metaprocedures that does not meet with the conscious intentions of the self, one would expect some startle reaction—in Freud's office it might be an embarrassment. The pre-production processing represents one of the most complex situations for the clinician when it comes to rehabilitating the recurrent perseverations of a patient. Of this there can be no doubt.

All of the above is intertwined with the distinction between "controlled" and automatic processing, e.g., in Stark (1988) where she makes it clear that conscious access is not to be equated totally with controlled processing. DW can be said to have conscious access without controlled processing. The perseveration is again delivered up by the reflex processing of metaprocedural control; his feel is one of surprise. His conscious access had led him down the garden path. All psycholinguists are aware of what happens to those who are led down garden paths: they are startled. In parsing theory, the modular processing begins its patterned top-down parse in the mind of the hearer, but when expectancies in the string being parsed are not met the startle appears, and the parse has to begin again. This slows down comprehension as experimentation has shown but, like DW, what is ultimately uttered does not match the expected. Brown, too, writes of automatic vs conscious control (1988, p. 329). In Luria's work on perseveration, Brown claims that:

> ... it is not altogether clear whether control of action is a conscious or unconscious effect. On the one hand, there is the directive function of language and the presumed role of inner speech. This entails conscious mediation. On the other hand, there is an early decisional element that seems to require a conceptual or linguistic organization

appearing in the preliminary action plan. There are studies that indicate that actions are programmed prior to an awareness of the decision to act.

So, deliberate and automatic processing are operationally independent, as Stark (1988) emphasises. However, performance in any given task must necessarily require an interaction of both. Therefore, an automatic production of the plan-external perseverate would necessarily cause a mental state of startle; the recurrent perseverate is incongruous.

The automatic perseveration may very well come wrapped within overall controlled/strategic processing, and it would evoke a conscious feeling of helplessness, placing the patient for an instant at the border, so to speak, of consciousness and unconsciousness—a mixed feeling of agency and non-agency, having a will then losing it. How strange when perseveration happens to a patient!

Stark (1988) discusses the patients with fluent aphasia who, in agreement with the current typology of perseveration, most often present with recurrent perseveration—the left temporal lobe lesioned patient. Albert and Sandson (1986) claim that it is recurrent perseveration that is most often part of an aphasia, and there they believe it to be an integral part of the symptom complex. And Martin and Dell (2007, this issue) have shown just how similar in nature recurrent perseverations are to paraphasias. They are subject to semantic, lexical, and phonological factors. Any linguistic analysis of recurrent perseveration will reveal and has revealed very similar architecture and form constraints regarding both. It is also likely that for the three types of perseveration, distinct neuropharmacological systems or mixes of them are involved. But the neurochemical accounts must still await further behavioural analyses of the perseverating patient.

Three candidates for explanation have been offered for recurrent perseveration: disruptions of inhibition of post-activated elements and faulty memory recall. A second is where the onus is placed on a lethargy of post-activation decay rates, where what goes awry is an overly slow rate of return to resting states. Another explanation is gaining strong support of late. It claims no inhibition problem, nor any lethargy in decay rates. Rather the new accounts place the onus squarely on what the lesion does directly to neuropsychological domains of action and perception. Each symptom complex will affect certain domains of cognition and leave others unharmed. The perseveration will only be observed in the responses elicited in the damaged components. The weakened connectivity in the affected domains will be such that decay rates of post-activated elements gain the upper hand by fiat, allowing for the non-intended plan-external elements to appear once again. Both semantic and phonological associations become involved as well, because they can up the activation rate of a previously uttered word, boosting it accordingly into post-articulatory action. If, for whatever reason, the symptom complex improves and the patient recovers to one degree or another, the perseveration will diminish accordingly without being tampered with by the clinician at all.

Taking off her neurolinguistic hat and putting on her clinical garb, Stark (1988, p. 206) discusses the difficulty that faces the therapist regarding recurrent perseveration. First, somehow the solipsistic metaprocedural system must be penetrated so that pre-articulatory tendencies towards perseveration might be monitored and repaired. We have already discussed the unlikelihood of this ever happening. Stark (1988, p. 296) claims that this penetration of the modular processing would be exacerbated by any increase in the rate of production.

Patients with jargon aphasia have often been observed to speak with a somewhat enhanced rate. In any event, Stark is correct to point out that the paragrammatic matrices of the adult with fluent aphasia are often replete with typical paraphasias and recurrent perseverates (see Buckingham, 1985, for examples of this). Clearly, however, the automaticity of the perseverations is a tough clinical nut to crack.

WHEN PERSEVERATION HAPPENS IN THE CLINIC

In recent years there has been a marked increase in focus on the individual person with aphasia and its sequelae—the client as a whole person dealing with his/her disabilities inside the home, outside the home, at work, at play, and in the rehabilitation unit. More is being made of the ecological aspects of stroke, TBI, and the dementias, and more ethnographic research is being done on the multifarious settings of aphasic patients. The client is being approached as a complete individual, normal in all respects except communication. I would hope that part of this trend would be more attention paid to their self-reports and introspections on their problems—even while they suffer from the aphasia, as opposed to after recovery.

Recent publications are indicative of this increased attention to the individual with aphasia and quality of life (Byng, Duchan, & Pound, 2006; Byng, Pound, & Swinburn, 1999; Worrell & Holland, 2003) Along with these there have been some recent attempts to penetrate some degree of automaticity and unconscious control, "... to bring perseverative behavior to patients' level of awareness and help them suppress perseverative responses and produce non-perseverative, correct naming responses" (Helm-Estabrooks & Albert, 2004, p. 203). Hopefully, the foregoing points in this essay will serve to warn the reader that this is not an easy thing to bring about—it forces the patient to steer between the Scylla of the automatic and the Charybdis of the conscious. The border between is worthy of a Borges short story. Helm-Estabrooks and Albert (2004, p. 201) write that the best candidates for their TAP (Treatment for Aphasic Perseveration) should be:

> Fully alert with at least moderately preserved auditory comprehension and good memory skills, as indicated by formal test scores (and they should have) some confrontation naming ability but moderate to severe perseveration in the form of recurrent perseveration, as determined by the procedure described in the TAP methodology section.

It is not the point of this paper to give any details of this programme or its success, which have been notable.

The other issue that is not without interest is broached by Basso (2004) and elsewhere. She feels that the new theoretical accounts for perseveration render unnecessary any direct management of the recurrent perseveration. Others from time to time have felt that the perseveration was perhaps more a sequela to the damaged response mechanism, due to the nature, extent, and location of the lesion, than a direct result of it. Nevertheless, it would appear that most investigators and clinicians have accounted for perseveration in terms of disrupted cortical neurodynamics of inhibition and activation, or that something was awry with the processes whereby activated elements are deactivated so they can return to their original resting states; i.e., decay rate. The claim was that the decay procedure was slowed down to the point of exacerbating the reappearance of a previously produced element—it was often called disrupted recall memory or the like. Stemming from the novel work of Dell, Burger, and Svec (1997), and of Cohen and Dehaene (1998), Gotts, della Rocchetta, and Cipolotti (2002), and more recently Gotts and Plaut (2004), the pathological onus has been placed squarely on disrupted neuropsychological abilities of different domains depending on the nature of the infarct, its extent and location. The weakened nature of these disrupted systems produces such weak activations of new stimuli that previous ones, still in the deactivation mode with only mild normal boosts from the semantic and or phonological noise, will activate once again, causing the perseveration to happen to the speaker. Therefore, by fiat, the perseveration is a natural outcome of the "deafferented" neuropsychological stimulus–response modalities. The support for this explanation is twofold. First, recurrent perseveration only appears when the patient is confronting stimulus–response tasks in the damaged domain. Other tasks do not reveal the perseveration. Second, as Basso (2004) has shown, there is a marked fall-off of perseveration, not because it receives any rehabilitative management, but because the intervention focuses on the disrupted neuropsychological behaviours themselves; as they improve, the perseveration wanes. The final word is not out on all of this competing theory and rehabilitation practice, but the simulations of this scenario are powerful and were part and parcel of the renewed accounts put forth for recurrent perseveration.

CONCLUDING REMARKS

I have tried to demonstrate the usefulness of self-description and introspective reports by patients with aphasia who perseverate. Aside from the inherently interesting commentary by patients in the course of straddling different levels of conscious control and pre-conscious cognitive reflex processing, it helps to sensitise us to the individual tragedy witnessed by a person struggling with the shards of brain damage and coming to grips with the sometimes bizarre ways that the mind and body interact as a consequence. It can also help us to gain deeper insight into the individual's altered microgenesis as well guiding us in our inquiry about how the systems cooperate in normality. The papers in the present special issue of *Aphasiology* will shed further light on the clinical-pathological and linguistic nature of perseveration, and the various ways in which it disrupts communication when it happens to patients with aphasia.

REFERENCES

Albert, M., & Sandson, J. (1986). Perseveration in aphasia. *Cortex*, *22*, 103–115.

Allison, R. (1966). Perseveration as a sign of diffuse and focal brain damage. *British Medical Journal*, *2*, 1095–1101.

Basso, A. (2004). Perseveration or the tower of Babel. *Seminars in Speech and Language*, *25*, 375–389.

Brown, J. (1988). *The life of the mind: Selected papers*. Hillsdale, NJ: Lawrence Erlbaum Associates Inc.

Brown, J. (1996). *Time, will, and mental process*. New York: Plenum Press.

Brown, J. (2005). *Process and the authentic life: Toward a psychology of value*. Lancaster, UK: Ontos Verlag.

Buckingham, H. (1985). Perseveration in aphasia. In S. Newman & R. Epstein (Eds.), *Current perspectives in dysphasia*. Edinburgh, UK: Churchill Livingstone.

Buckingham, H. (1986). Language, the mind, and psychophysical parallelism. In I. Gopnik & M. Gopnik (Eds.), *From models to modules: Studies in cognitive science from the McGill workshops* (pp. 209–228). Norwood, NJ: Ablex Publishing Corp.

Buckingham, H., & Christman, S. (2004). Phonemic carryover perseveration: Word blends. *Seminars in Speech and Language, 25*, 363–373.

Byng, S., Duchan, J. F., & Pound, C. (Eds.). (2006). *Aphasia therapy file* (Vol. 2). Hove, UK: Psychology Press.

Byng, S., Pound, C., & Swinburn, K. (Eds.). (1999). *Aphasia therapy file* (Vol. 1). Hove, UK: Psychology Press.

Cohen, L., & Dehaene, S. (1998). Competition between past and present: Assessment and interpretation of verbal perseverations. *Brain, 121*, 1641–1659.

Dell, G. S., Burger, L. K., & Svec, W. R. (1997). Language production and serial order: A functional analysis and a model. *Psychological Review, 104*, 123–147.

Den Ouden, D.-B., & Bastiaanse, R. (2005). Phonological encoding and conduction aphasia. In R. J. Hartsuiker, R. Bastiaanse, A. Postma, & F. Wijnen (Eds.), *Phonological encoding and monitoring in normal and pathological speech* (pp. 86–101). Hove, UK: Psychology Press.

Gotts, S. J., della Rocchetta A., I., & Cipolotti, L. (2002). Mechanisms underlying perseveration in aphasia: Evidence from a single case study. *Neuropsychologia, 40*, 1930–1947.

Gotts, S. J., & Plaut, D. C. (2004). Connectionist approaches to understanding aphasic perseveration. *Seminars in Speech and Language, 25*, 323–334.

Helm-Estabrooks, N., & Albert, M. L. (2004). *Manual of aphasia and aphasia therapy* (2nd ed.). Austin, TX: Pro-Ed.

Martin, N., & Dell, G. S. (2007). Common mechanisms underlying perseverative and non-perseverative sound and word substitutions [special issue on perseveration]. *Aphasiology, 21*, 1002–1017.

Prince, A., & Smolensky, P. (2004). *Optimality theory: Constraint interaction in generative grammar*. Malden, MA: Blackwell.

Sandson, J., & Albert, M. (1984). Varieties of perseveration. *Neuropsychologia, 19*, 591–594.

Stark, J. A. (1988). Aspects of automatic versus controlled processing, monitoring, metalinguistic tasks, and related phenomena in aphasia. In W. U. Dressler & J. A. Stark (Eds.), *Linguistic analyses of aphasic language* (pp. 179–223). New York: Springer-Verlag.

Wheeler, D. W., & Touretzky, D. S. (1997). A parallel licensing model of normal slips and phonemic paraphasias. *Brain and Language, 59*, 147–201.

Worrall, L., & Holland, A. (Eds.). (2003). Quality of life in aphasia [special issue]. *Aphasiology, 17*(4).

APHASIOLOGY, 2007, 21 (10/11), 928–959

Psychology Press
Taylor & Francis Group

Review Article

A review of classical accounts of verbal perseveration and their modern-day relevance

Jacqueline Stark
Austrian Academy of Sciences, Vienna

Background: Although the topic of perseveration—in particular, verbal perseveration—is crucial for understanding various aspects of language and other cognitive functions, it has only recently begun to receive the attention it deserves. However, reports on the history of perseveration remain highly selective in their scope. This is due in part to a language barrier. Numerous relevant publications from the "classical" aphasiological period were published in German, leaving them inaccessible for interested colleagues.
Aims: The aim of this paper is to provide an overview of the historical development of publications on the phenomenon of perseveration, and thus to draw attention and give credit to the classical clinicians and researchers who participated in vigorous debates on the topic.
Main Contribution: A survey is given of the main points discussed in publications on perseveration dating back to 1866. Particular attention is paid to the German classical literature. An attempt is made to graphically portray the hypothetical mechanisms that constitute the three classical accounts of perseveration.
Conclusions: Concepts put forward in the classical studies on the origin of perseveration are in many ways comparable to modern accounts of the phenomena. The predictions of the three classical accounts—(1) deficit account, (2) overactivation account, and (3) underactivation or weak activation account—as well as other "old" ideas on perseveration expressed in the classical publications are relevant for a comprehensive understanding of recent accounts of perseveratory phenomena. Therefore, they should be considered when interpreting perseveratory and/or paraphasic errors produced by aphasic clients.

Modern-day accounts of verbal perseveration are often selective in their citation of classic historical accounts and references. Highly relevant papers on perseveration are often not cited, or are referred to indirectly, i.e., without a complete citation to the original source. There are two reasons for this restriction in citation of classic references on the topic. First, several of the significant publications have not been

Address correspondence to: Jacqueline Stark PhD, Department of Linguistics and Communication Research, Austrian Academy of Sciences, Kegelgasse 27/3rd Floor, A – 1030 Vienna, Austria. E-mail: jacqueline-ann.stark@univie.ac.at

Particular thanks go to Emanuel Wenger of the Department of Visualisation of the Austrian Academy of Sciences for his realisation of the various theories on perseveration in diagram form. I would also like to thank Christiane Pons, Maura Bayer, Caroline Brew, Karin Geisler, Lotti Viola, and the reviewers of this paper for their constructive comments.

http://www.psypress.com/aphasiology DOI: 10.1080/02687030701198239

available in English.[1] Second, the original papers on the topic or comments therein have only been alluded to in older, original classical papers on the topic. One example is J. Hughlings Jackson's article published in *Brain* (1880, and as a reprint in 1915) entitled "On affections of speech from disease of the brain", in which reference is made to W. T. Gairdner's terminology of "barrel-organism" (pp. 335, 355–356; see later text and also Buckingham, 1985).[2] In this and other instances the original papers cannot be accessed, resulting in inaccurate citation and evaluation of the concepts referred to by Jackson. As another example, Pick (1892) notes that he was unable to obtain a copy of Gairdner's paper in the book trade, so that he is "... not in a position to determine, whether Gairdner himself realized the importance of the phenomenon in a broader context" (p. 900, footnote).

The aim of this paper is to draw attention to several key publications on the origin of perseveration which serve as a basis for our present-day understanding of verbal perseveration, and to relate them to current approaches. As is the case for aphasia in general, and agrammatism in particular, the German classical literature on perseveration between 1890 and 1931 abounds with discussions relating to the ongoing debates taking place among the then-renowned clinicians and aphasiologists, including Lissauer, Neisser, Liepmann, Heilbronner, Pick, Kleist, von Soelder, and Rosenberg, *inter alia*. By providing descriptions of the classical interpretations of verbal perseveration and discussions of the issues that were relevant to the classical aphasiologists, due credit can be given to those authors. In turn, ideas put forward in more recent proposals can be evaluated more completely with regard to the merits and shortcomings of the earlier literature and what the classical accounts of perseveration have in common with the more recent ones. For the sake of not misinterpreting specific ideas or opinions of the classical authors on perseveration in general, in a variety of neurological disorders and verbal perseveration in particular, excerpts from the original German and French texts are also provided in numerous cases. Moreover, reference will be made to related ideas in more recent publications, subsequent to discussing the classical literature, when they apply.

HISTORICAL PERSPECTIVE

In this review, perseveration in general is addressed with the ultimate goal of better understanding verbal perseveration in particular. The earliest direct use of the term "perseveration" is by Neisser (1894, printed in 1895). Historically speaking, however, several other authors address relevant points prior to Neisser's coinage of the term. Rogers (1935) notes that "... perseveration in mental activity is by no means a new idea. Wynn Jones discerns a suggestion of it in Aristotle, and Spearman

[1] A notable exception is Jason Brown's translation of Arnold Pick's handbook article on aphasia, which was published posthumously by R. Thiele (see Brown, 1973). A few German classical papers on agrammatism and paragrammatism have also been translated into English, e.g., DeBleser, 1987; Howard, 1985; Stark and Dressler, 1990, etc. Stark (1984) presents an overview of the historical accounts of perseveration in German.

[2] Sir William Tennant Gairdner (1824–1907) was a professor of medicine at the medical faculty of the University of Glasgow. In 1866 he gave a talk to the Philosophical Society in Glasgow entitled: "On the function of articulate speech, and on its connection with the mind and the bodily organs". Only a French version of that talk (in an abbreviated form) was available as a primary source. Dr Jules Falret (1866) translated the talk and wrote a preamble to the text. The title is "De la fonction de langage articulé avec une observation d'aphasie". See later text for further explanation.

quotes from Plato" (p. 138; see also Jasper, 1931). Hughlings-Jackson (1880) refers to the pathological phenomenon of "barrel-organism", which he considers to be a "temporary recurring utterance" in contrast to a more permanent recurring utterance. This analogy with a barrel organ[3] stems from the above-mentioned W. T. Gairdner. Hughlings-Jackson refers to Gairdner's term as follows: "The patient gets the word or phrase on his barrel-organ. It becomes a temporary recurring utterance; the permanent recurring utterance in loss of speech may be called permanent barrel-organism" (1880, p. 306, or 1915, p. 166). In a French translation by Falret of a paper by Gairdner (1866), reference is made to patients described by Trousseau, one of whom repeatedly used the jargon production "cousisi" as a unit and only in that combination: "His ability was absolutely reduced to that of a parakeet producing those syllables in that order *like the tone of an organ pipe when this pipe has once been put in place and the movement is initiated*"[4] (pp. 17–18 of the French manuscript).[5]

In 1890 Lissauer presents a case of "Seelenblindheit" (Eng.: "mind blindness"), i.e., optic agnosia, in which the "law of getting stuck" (Ger.: "Haftenbleiben") applies to the patient's deficits. Following a detailed description of patient data, Lissauer (1890, p. 268) puts forward three categories of errors observed in his case study regarding failures to recognise the objects presented (Ger.: "Verkennungen"), the second of which is most relevant for the current review:

> The second category refers to false recognitions [Ger.: "Verkennungen"] in which every bridge between the object and the used term is missing, and in pursuance of which first of all makes an arbitrary, incomprehensible impression. Some of the errors in this category could be categorized in the first category, because hidden or partial similarities play a role of which the client is not even aware; for the most part of these recognition errors in this category, a completely different relation appears to be the case, a relation, in which one could discover a specific law - *the law of getting stuck on concepts or ideas [Ger.: "Vorstellungen] which were once activated.*[6]

Lissauer's case study produced a substantial number of exemplars from the second category, which he describes (1890, p. 268) as follows:

[3] Using the barrel organ or barrel-organism with reference to temporary perseveration is a visual and dynamic analogy: the spoken output gets caught on the revolving cylinder with studded pegs and is repeated temporarily.

[4] Italics are used to highlight the relevant portion of the original citation.

[5] See also footnote 3. Original French text: "Il était de même du malade qui répétait constamment cousisi et qui ne pouvait jamais arriver à dire séparément coucou ou sisi; sa capacité de perroquet était absolument réduite à ces syllabes cousisi dans leur ordre déterminé, comme *le son d'un tuyau d'orgue quand ce tuyau a été une fois mis en place et que le mouvement est commencé*" (pp. 17–18 of the French manuscript).

[6] Lissauer's original German text: "Die 2. Kategorie betrifft Verkennungen, bei denen jede Brücke zwischen Objekt und dem darauf angewandten Begriff vermisst wird, und welche in Folge dessen zunächst einen willkürlichen, unbegreiflichen Eindruck machen. Ein Teil dieser anscheinend willkürlichen, Verkennungen mag tatsächlich der ersten Kategorie zugehören, indem verborgene Ähnlichkeiten, bes. partielle Ähnlichkeiten, die dem Patienten selbst nicht zu vollen Bewusstsein kommen, mitspielen; für ein beträchtliches Kontingent dieser Verkennungen stellt sich jedoch ein ganz anderer Zusammenhang heraus, ein Zusammenhang, in dem man *ein besonderes Gesetz – das Gesetz des Haftenbleibens der einmal lebendig gewordenen Vorstellungen* – erblicken könnte" (1890, p. 268).

> Namely, when a specific, concrete term actively appeared in the patient's consciousness and dominated it a while, there is a striking tendency, to carry over this term for all sorts of different objects, which the patient, as a consequence of his mind blindness, is not capable of recognizing. Very often we are confronted with the situation that after the patient has correctly recognized an object ***a*** by means of vision, touch, suggestion or in some other way, the following objects ***b*** and ***c*** which are shown to him/her are also assigned the term ***a***. Numerous examples of this type are found in the patient's test protocol, and precisely the most absurd errors of failure of recognition come about by this means – e.g. an umbrella as a flower pot, a clothes brush as a cat. This entire phenomenon, which by the way has its analogue in certain occurrences in aphasia, is so strange, because the patient has just seen object ***a***, thus, since he does not momentarily forget visual impressions, he should exactly know, that the objects ***b*** and ***c*** are different from ***a***.[7]

In considering the origin of the errors, Lissauer puts forward a deficit account: "Whether the psychological genesis of the failures of recognition are this or that, so much is certain, *that they are the result of a deficit and that this deficit is to be sought in the loss of associations in a specific sense sphere*" (1890, p. 270).[8]

In referring to Lissauer's case, Pick (1892) describes a client who reveals the same symptoms, but in spontaneous speech, naming, and reading-aloud tasks. Pick terms these deficits "pseudo-apraxia". The main feature he is referring to is the "sticking" to earlier functions. He stresses that these symptoms are not apractic in nature, rather they are "pseudo-apractic".

As noted earlier, the term "perseveration" was first coined by Neisser in 1894 in a discussion of a case presented by Heilbronner at the 65th meeting of the members of the East German Psychiatrists in Breslau (published in 1895, pp. 1014–1016). Neisser commented on a remark made by Pick in response to Heilbronner's presentation of a case of "asymbolia". Pick addressed the symptom of "getting stuck on the impressions"[9] (Ger.: "Haftenbleiben an den Eindrücken") which he had observed in a client with aphasia, and which he had described as "pseudo-apraxia". In his remark, Neisser suggested that the phenomenon Pick called "pseudo-apraxia" was very appropriate for the particular case in question. Neisser, however, pointed out that this symptom was found in very different conditions. For this reason, he asserted that it is necessary to have a term that can be applied to all the conditions; namely, "perseveratory response" or "perseveration". Due to the impact of Neisser's

---

[7] Lissauer's original German text: "Ist nämlich im Bewusstsein des Kranken einmal ein bestimmter, konkreter Begriff lebhaft aufgetaucht und hat eine Zeit lang das Bewusstsein beherrscht, so zeigt sich die auffallende Neigung, diesen Begriff auf alle möglichen sinnlichen Objekte zu übertragen, welche der Patient in Folge der Seelenblindheit nicht zu erkennen vermag. Besonders häufig begegnet uns diese Tatsache in der Form, dass der Kranke, nachdem er den Gegenstand ***a*** durch Gesicht, Tastsinn, durch Suggestion oder sonst auf irgend einem Wege richtig erkannt hat, nun die ihm weiterhin vorgezeigten Objekte ***b*** oder ***c*** ebenfalls dem Begriffe ***a*** zurechnet" (1890, p. 268).

[8] Lissauer's original German text: "Sei nun die psychologische Genese der Verkennungen diese oder jene, soviel steht fest, *dass dieselben auf dem Boden eines Defectes erwachsen sind und dass dieser Defect im Ausfall von Associationen einer bestimmten Sinnessphäre zu suchen ist*" (p. 1890, p. 270).

[9] Several German psychological terms are difficult to translate into English. One reason for this difficulty is that the concepts are theory dependent and/or are ambiguous in the original text. For example, for the German word "Vorstellung (Pl. –en)" the English translations include: concept, idea, mental image, association, imagination, etc. Other terms that are difficult to translate include "Vorstellungsablauf", "Erinnerungsbild", "Eindruecke".

comments on all my later discussions of perseveration, I would like to provide a translation of the original text (1895, p. 1016):[10]

> The term "pseudo-apraxia" was very appropriate for Pick's case. However, the symptom can be found in very different states, in cases of psychosis as well as in localized lesions of the brain and, to be sure, it can be found in every type of action. For example, he observed how a delirious patient, whose pupil response was tested several times by moving a finger towards and away from the subject's eye, afterwards displayed many spontaneous convergence movements of the pupil (Bulbi - dilations of the pupil). *It is necessary to have a term which is applicable to all instances of the symptom. The term perseveratory reaction or simply perseveration offers itself as such. To date this symptom has not been sufficiently considered and theoretically it has not been studied at all. Yet it plays a significant role.* In pure form perseveration is often observed in written language performance. In terms of differential diagnosis, verbigeration in written language and amnestic agraphia (Freund) are to be considered. By chance Neisser is able to demonstrate such an example.

Since this discussion among Heilbronner, Pick, and Neisser, Neisser's term has been adopted. However, it has been defined differently by several authors.

PERSEVERATION DEFINED

Before discussing the mechanisms put forward in the classical publications, a working definition of "perseveration" based on the features addressed by the classical authors is warranted:

> Perseveration is a phenomenon whereby the subject unintentionally produces or gets stuck on an information unit, a particular linguistic form or action unit, which he/she has previously produced or at some level has heard, i.e., auditorily processed, or seen, i.e., visually processed.

Extending the definition to cover ideas and thoughts or language units that are *unintentionally* processed, whatever the input modality, is motivated by discussions by Pick and von Soelder. In a discussion of one of Pick's cases, von Soelder (1899) stresses that the patient not only produced wrong words, which *he himself had not previously produced*, but also ones that he had only *heard* before: "… also such words pushed themselves into the utterances of the patient, which were spoken totally by chance by persons next to him and to which he did not actively attend" (p. 481).

[10] Neisser's original German text of the discussion that took place at the Breslau meeting in 1894: "Herr *Neisser*: Die Bezeichnung 'Pseudoapraxie' sei in dem Falle von *Pick* sehr wohl zutreffend gewesen. Das Symptom findet sich aber bei sehr verschiedenartigen Zuständen, sowohl bei Psychosen als auch bei Hererkrankungen des Gehirns und zwar kann es bei jeder Art von Bethätigung zu Tage treten. So habe er z.B. gesehen, wie ein deliranter Patient, bei welchem soeben die Pupillenreaction bei Annäherung eines Fingers an das Auge geprüft worden war, danach viele Male spontane Convergenzbewegungen der Bulbi ausgeführt habe. *Es sei nothwendig einen Terminus zu haben, welcher bei allen Erscheinungsformen des Symptoms brauchbar ist. Als solcher empfehle sich perseveratorische Reaktion oder schlechtweg Perseveration. Dies Symptom sei bis jetzt bei den Descriptionen nicht genügend beachtet und theoretisch noch gar nicht studiert worden.* Dasselbe spiele eine große Rolle. Besonders rein tritt die Perseveration oft in schriftlichen Productionen zu Tage. Differential-diagnostisch kommt dann die schriftliche Verbigeration und die amnestische Agraphie (Freund) in Betracht. *N.* ist zufällig in der Lage ein bezügliches Schriftstück demonstrieren zu können" (Neisser, 1895, p. 1016).

Moreover, von Soelder states that single examples demonstrate that ideas (Ger.: "Vorstellungen") can also be perseverated, even if they are only activated by inner association and are not produced orally, i.e., spoken (p. 491).[11] The latter exist, although they are difficult to ascertain. Buckingham (1985) also refers to such examples in his discussion of a client with neologistic jargon (J.T.), when he cautions that it is difficult to be certain whether what is perseverated is the idea or thought—in this case, of children—as opposed to the actual phonological form (p. 123). Regarding one source of perseveration he maintains: "The intentional perseverate as a competing plan is something that locks itself in on the mind, begins to take part in the inner workings of consciousness and imposes itself ultimately on the output to the extent that it cannot be inhibited" (p. 151).

Based on data from single cases, Pick (1906) describes complex interactions and repercussions of perseveration on subsequent thoughts. In agreement with Pick's overall view (1914, 1931) that "... the individual mechanisms which constitute the path from thinking to speaking can also be separately affected by perseveration" (1914, p. 418),[12] the resulting complexity of examples of perseveration can vary from clear-cut "simple" cases to highly intricate "complex" cases extending in length and temporal duration. Simple and complex refer to the overall structure of the perseverates—i.e., the input for the perseveration and the produced perseveration—with regard to how deducible the perseverated unit is in the language sample. Examples of two simple cases are (a) a blend of the target item and the previous response

such as in example (1):

(1) "Blind man's bluff" ("blind cow") (Ger.: "**Bl**inde K**u**h" → "**Bl**inde **Bl**uhe" and then the immediate additional attempt at correcting the first response: "Bl**u**nde Kuh"

or (b) the production of the entire previous target item as in example (2), taken from a visual confrontation naming task as an example from an oral confrontation task of pictured objects:

(2) (a) table → "table"

(b) book → "table"

Complex cases of verbal perseveration alluded to by Pick are also documented in the aphasia literature. An example of a complex case is the following, which is taken from language data produced by a transcortical sensory aphasic (MH) in response to consecutive items from the Story Completion Test (SCT) (Goodglass, Gleason, Bernholtz, & Hyde, 1972, pp. 197–199). This task requires the participant to complete various syntactic structures to orally presented scenarios (1a to 14b). The following and other German language examples from MH's language data are discussed in more detail in this special issue:

[11] Von Soelder's original German text: "Es lehren einzelne Beispiele, dass Vorstellungen auch dann perseverieren können, wenn sie rein durch innere Assoziation geweckt wurden und keinen Ausdruck nach außen finden" (von Soelder, 1899, p. 491).

[12] Pick's original German text: "... dass die einzelnen, den Weg vom Denken um Sprechen ausmachenden Mechanismen auch die einzeln perseveratorisch gestört sein können" (Pick, 1914, p. 418).

Task Item MH's Response

6a)	Did you call me?	(correct response)
6b)	Did you really brush your teeth?	(correct response)

(7a) Target response: Where did you put my shoes?)

7a)	*Did you* put *your* shoes anywhere?
7b)	How did you repair the toy? (correct response)

(8a) Target response: He (=Peter) will work again

8a)	He asks: *Where did you put Peter's toy?*

(8a) Target response: He will work again (item repeated)

(Item 8a repeated)	It will be the case that *he asks Peter:*
	Where did you put Peter's toy?
(8a)	Ger.: "*Wo hast Du Peters Spielzeug hingestellt?*"
	Eng.: *Where have you Peter's toy put?)*
SCT item:	7a 8a 7b 7a

The last response "Wo hast Du Peters Spielzeug hingestellt?" consists of words perseverated from three test items from the story completion task. The resulting complex perseveratory response is syntactically correct, albeit semantically inadequate. Reference will be made to simple and complex examples of perseveration in the classical explanations discussed in the following sections of this paper.

In addition to simple and complex cases of perseveration, other types of perseveration are also introduced in the classical literature. Rosenberg (1912) introduces the term "generic" perseveration to describe a pattern of performance elicited from a patient by means of presenting different kinds of stimuli in a specific order. He states that "... perseveratory responses could be evoked by further presentation of the stimuli with a certain degree of regularity, which were congeneric with the actual object" (1912, pp. 127–128). He explains the generic perseveration with respect to a "generic feeling" one has when something is not completely forgotten, rather some aspect of a produced word is still active and for that reason a related term is perseverated. The activated generic idea creates an obstacle for anything else to be produced and becomes overpowering. For this reason a similar type, i.e., a generic perseveration, is produced instead of a completely unrelated other word.

DIMENSIONS CHARACTERISING THE OCCURRENCE OF PERSEVERATION

Perseveration has been considered with reference to several issues including the difficulty of determining when to consider a response perseveratory, how long a perseveration can "last", whether perseverations can actually be elicited by altering specific stimulus features, etc.

In his analysis of apractic responses, Liepmann (1905, pp. 104–105) addresses the crucial issue of determining whether a particular response is perseveratory in nature:

> The interpretation of a single response will naturally involve a certain amount of latitude; what at first glance appears to be a totally "structureless" aggregate of movements can, upon closer examination, turn out to be a throwing together or fusion of parts of differentiable purposeful movement parts (namely when perseveration plays a role). But a more extensive examination should lead to a decision.

In the case of single errors, the main difficulty in determining whether a response is perseveratory in nature or "only" a paraphasia relates to a lack of extensive language data from the ongoing language production of a single client. Gloning (1975) alluded to the misclassification of aphasic responses as paraphasic errors, when they were actually perseveratory. This applies in particular to the error types random paraphasia and "wild paraphasic misnaming".[13] Related to the context in which a perseveratory response is found, another feature is the appropriateness of the "exciting stimulus" (McNalty, 1961, in the *British Medical Dictionary*).[14] The degree of overlap and similarity among the target, paraphasia, and/or perseveratory response is also alluded to in this context (see Heilbronner, 1906, pp. 306–307).

In terms of the temporal aspects of duration—i.e. for how long perseveration can be considered to be discernible—the longer the temporal interval between two responses, the more difficult it will be to definitively consider a response to be a perseveration. Examples of perseveration extending over days are discussed in Heilbronner (1906, p. 306) (see also Stark, 2007 this issue, Cohen & Dehaene, 1998, and Moen, 1993).

With regard to whether, after a certain time interval, a response is indeed a perseveration, von Soelder states that an important criterion for making a decision is that "... the recurring idea (Ger.: "Vorstellung") is without motivation in its new combination" (p. 503). In this context the temporal dimension—i.e., the amount of time between utterances—is not crucial in interpreting the response, but rather the fact that in between perseveratory responses either correct or incorrect non-perseveratory responses are made (see discussion in Cohen & Dehaene, 1998).

MANIPULATING THE TASK DEMANDS OR DEAFFERENTING CERTAIN LANGUAGE RESPONSE DOMAINS RESULTING IN PERSEVERATORY RESPONSES

Several classical authors refer to the possibility of inducing, eliciting, and regulating the occurrence of perseveration by means of task, task difficulty, item selection, and/or order of item presentation (e.g., Heilbronner, 1906, p. 306; Lissauer, 1890; Pick, 1914; Rosenberg, 1912; von Soelder, 1899). In general the classical aphasiologists

[13] "Wild paraphasic misnaming" or "random paraphasia" (Ger.: "zufällige") refer to types of paraphasic error where the produced response shows no relations or similarities to the target and are thus considered to be "wild" paraphasic errors. These types of paraphasic errors are discussed in Gloning (1975), Poeck (1978), and Goodglass and Kaplan (1983).

[14] McNalty's (1961) definition of perseveration: "The continuation or recurrence of an experience or activity without the appropriate exciting stimulus" (*British Medical Dictionary*).

were very well informed in the area of contemporary psychology. For this reason, tasks and task features were taken over and employed by various authors in their examination of their patients, based on the psychological investigations being carried out with healthy control subjects by the contemporary psychologists including, e.g., Müller and Pilzecker (1900) and their study of the "perseveratory tendency". With regard to the discussion of aphasic perseveratory responses as a pathological increase of a physiologically active tendency, Heilbronner (1906, p. 307) remarks that if the examples from healthy controls tell us something about the genesis of perseveration, then it would be necessary not only to address the issue of why the error took the form it did, but also to raise the preliminary question of why the incorrect response, i.e., slip of the tongue, was produced in the first place.

In describing the perseveratory responses produced by one of his patients, Rosenberg (1912) states that "... it is a matter of an experiment with the game of perseveration, which is triggered by the examiner by means of displaying the objects or asking specific questions" (p. 124). He found that by ordering the stimuli in a certain manner he could elicit perseverations in a regular fashion.[15] Von Soelder (1899, p. 503) points out that Lissauer was able to influence his client's responses by the order of stimulus presentation, and von Soelder also observed the same phenomenon with his clients. Heilbronner (1897) describes in great detail differential task difficulty and how, in an examination, the test stimulus order can affect performance in different clinical populations. For example, he refers to the differential effect of concrete versus abstract nouns with regard to their processing in a word association task.

Although several classical authors refer to the possibility of "inducing" specific perseveratory responses by presenting the stimuli in a particular order or array, Heilbronner (1906) discusses very fundamental issues pertaining to obtaining perseveratory responses according to a specific test protocol; i.e., being able to evoke and analyse perseveratory responses according to a fixed schema. He maintains that what makes perseveration such a fascinating phenomenon to analyse is that it is not possible to set up an experimental design and for each test item be able to predict that a perseveration will be produced for that specific item. That is, it is not possible to predict exactly when a perseveration will occur—i.e., be produced. Heilbronner (1906, p. 313) stresses that in order to be able to give an adequate answer to why a perseveration is produced as a response to a particular task item, one would have to know all the contributing factors and also be able to vary them arbitrarily:

> At the present time, with regard to this last point, we are dependent on one component, namely the level of complexity of the task. For this reason, as required theoretically, one can in fact, predict and determine in certain cases with a degree of certainty, whether a correct or perseveratory response will occur. The examiner is, however – as far as my knowledge and experience are concerned – not able to prophesy which of the concepts will be perseverated.

[15] Rosenberg's original German text: "Es handelt sich um ein Experiment mit dem Spiel der Perseveration, welche vom Untersucher durch das Vorzeigen von Gegenständen oder das Stellen bestimmter Fragen erzeugt wurden" (Rosenberg, 1912, p. 124). It should be noted that he is referring to a client who had suffered two CVAs and showed signs of dementia.

Heilbronner (1906) comments on examples from epileptic clients in which, after a series of perseveratory responses are produced, an easy item is presented and correctly answered. According to Heilbronner, this finding speaks against von Soelder's account based on the predominance (Ger.: "Überwertigkeit") of the perseveratory image or concept or idea. The same holds true for cases in which a very difficult item is presented, since the chances that the client can produce the response are minimal from the start. Heilbronner maintains that if perseveration is brought about by a particularly intensive active preponderance of the perseverating idea or concept or image, then the type of question or task—i.e. the greater or lesser difficulty of the required task performance—should not influence the performance in any way. If, on the other hand, the perseveration occurs subsidiarily, because the correct response to an item is impossible, then the difficulty of the task should play a role in the frequency of the perseveratory responses (1906, pp. 308–309). With reference to one of his cases at hand, Heilbronner maintains that perseveration parallels the complexity of the respective task and a close connection exists between them (1906, p. 312).

Heilbronner continues his discussion of methodological design issues by referring to examinations carried out with psychotic patients: The number of cases for which perseveratory responses are produced in an initial test series and then later correctly named was substantial. In discussion of other language test data, Heilbronner (1906, p. 311, see also Sommer, 1893) raises the following question:

> Why in the case of two of the tasks an incorrect response is unexpectedly produced, and, on the other hand, why the item "fish" is correctly named in both series right from the start, cannot be explained. Such attempts, and thus also the possibility of carrying out mass examinations and reporting the findings numerically in table form fail due to the complexity of the conditions/circumstances which have to be considered for every single response.[16]

RELATED PHENOMENA

In numerous classical publications the authors debate the various terms and discuss the differential diagnosis of the symptom of perseveration in contrast to related phenomena including verbigeration,[17] echolalia, logorrhoea, paraphasia, word repetitions produced by clients with phobias and compulsive disorders (see Kleist, 1934; Neisser, 1865; Pick, 1931; von Mayendorf, 1911; von Soelder, 1899). Rosenberg (1912) counters von Mayendorf's assertion that echolalia, logorrhoea, and perseveration derive from the same source—that they are the reflection of right hemisphere functions. Von Mayendorf offers as support for his claim, that the three

[16] Heilbronner's original German text: "Warum bei zweien der Aufgaben wider Erwarten eine Falschbenennung erfolgt, warum andererseits gerade der Fisch in beiden Versuchsreihen von Beginn an richtig bezeichnet wird, lässt sich nicht erklären. Derartige Versuche damit aber auch die Möglichkeit, Massenprüfungen anzustellen und den Befunden einen Zahlenmäßigen Ausdruck in Tabellenform zu geben, scheitern an der Kompliziertheit der bei jeder Einzelreaktion in Betracht kommenden Verhältnisse" (Heilbronner, 1906, p. 311).

[17] Verbigeration, also referred to as catalogia, is the incoherent repetition of meaningless words and sentences.

symptoms share an automatic character. For Rosenberg, perseveration is to be differentiated and does not belong to this trio of symptoms.

OTHER CHARACTERISATIONS OF PERSEVERATION

Without considering each issue in detail, there are other characterisations of perseveration in the classical aphasiological literature stress, for example:

(a) The normal versus pathological nature of its occurrence (e.g., Heilbronner, 1906; Rosenberg, 1912; von Soelder, 1899).
(b) The voluntary or involuntary, automatic nature of the phenomenon (e.g., Rosenberg, 1912; von Mayendorf, 1911).
(c) Cortical dynamics, i.e., the state of activation/inhibition of neurons[18] (see Jasper, 1931); persistence, after-functioning (Ger. "Nachfunktion"), secondary function (see Gross, 1902); equalisation process (see Goldstein, 1948).
(d) The role of fatigue (e.g., Goldstein, 1948; Heilbronner, 1906; Pick, 1892, 1903, *inter alia*; von Soelder, 1899).
(e) The relationship to memory processes (e.g., von Soelder, 1899), attention (Kleist, 1934; Rosenberg, 1912), and self-monitoring (Heilbronner, 1906; von Soelder, 1899).
(f) The localising value of the phenomenon (e.g., Heilbronner, 1897; Kleist, 1934; Pick, 1914).
(g) The occurrence of perseveration as a protective mechanism to avoid catastrophic conditions (see Goldstein, 1948).

CLASSICAL EXPLANATIONS

With the above-mentioned introductory comments in mind, the classical explanations of perseveration put forward by Heilbronner, Lissauer, Pick, von Soelder, Liepmann, Sommer, and Rosenberg are discussed here.

Figures 1 to 4 attempt to capture the essence of the classical accounts pertaining to the origin of perseveration of various linguistic units. The simple cases portrayed in Figures 1, 2a, 3a, and 4 can be illustrated with reference to an oral confrontation-naming task, in which the production of one single-word response following another is required. Complex cases illustrated in Figures 2b and 3b can be illustrated with reference to responses exceeding the single-word level. These figures refer to hypothetical units (indicated by X, O, and N in the figures) ranging from perseveration of distinctive features such as the presence or absence of voicing contrasts, phonemes, morphemes, lexical items, semantic features, syntactic constructions to ideational or conceptual features.

Hypothetical normal situation

As a starting point, the normal or average situation—i.e. one in which there is no perseveration—is presented in Figure 1. For example, in an oral confrontation-naming task it is assumed that after the correct response is produced, the level of

[18] More recent publications by Azcoaga (1963) and Luria (1974) address the issue of cortical dynamics.

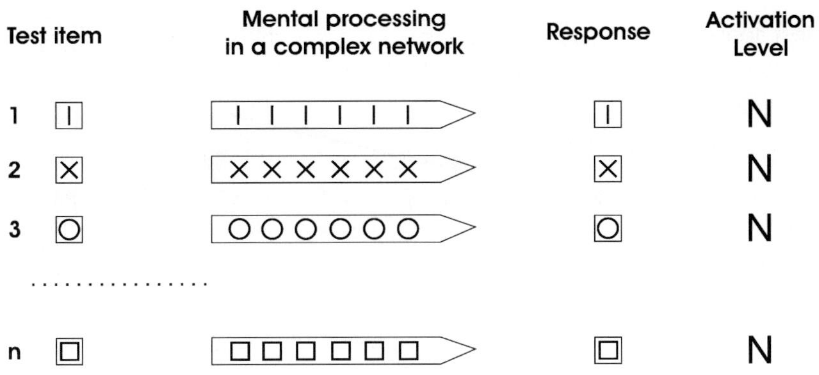

Figure 1. Hypothetical normal case.

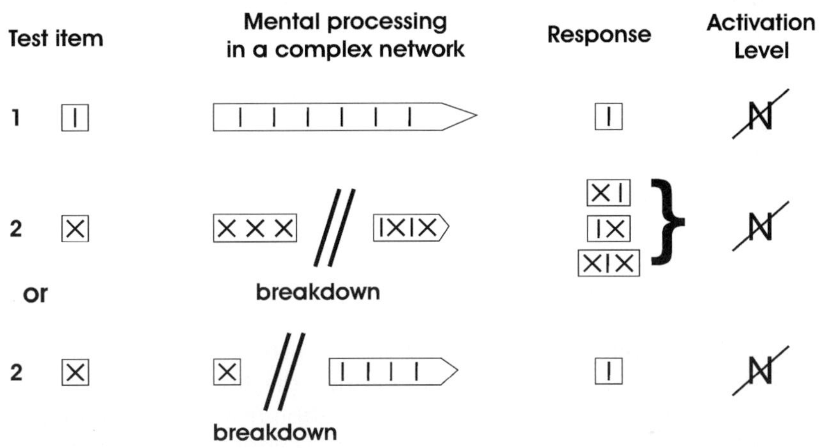

Figure 2a. Heilbronner's and Lissauer's account of the origin of perseveratory responses for a simple case.

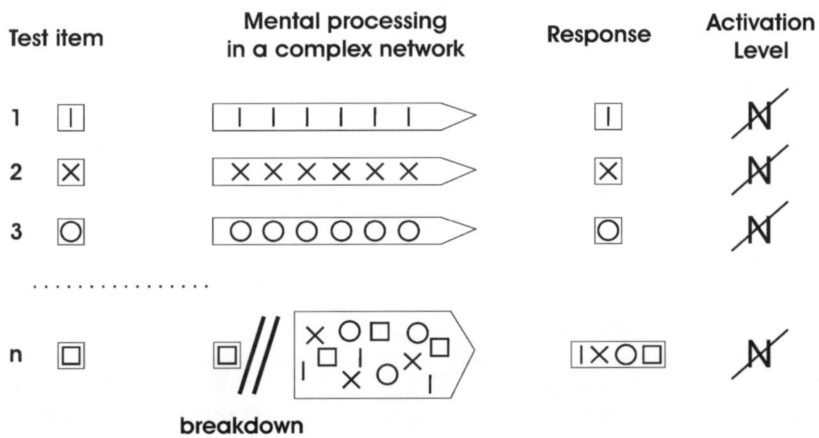

Figure 2b. Heilbronner's and Lissauer's account of the origin of perseveratory responses for a complex case.

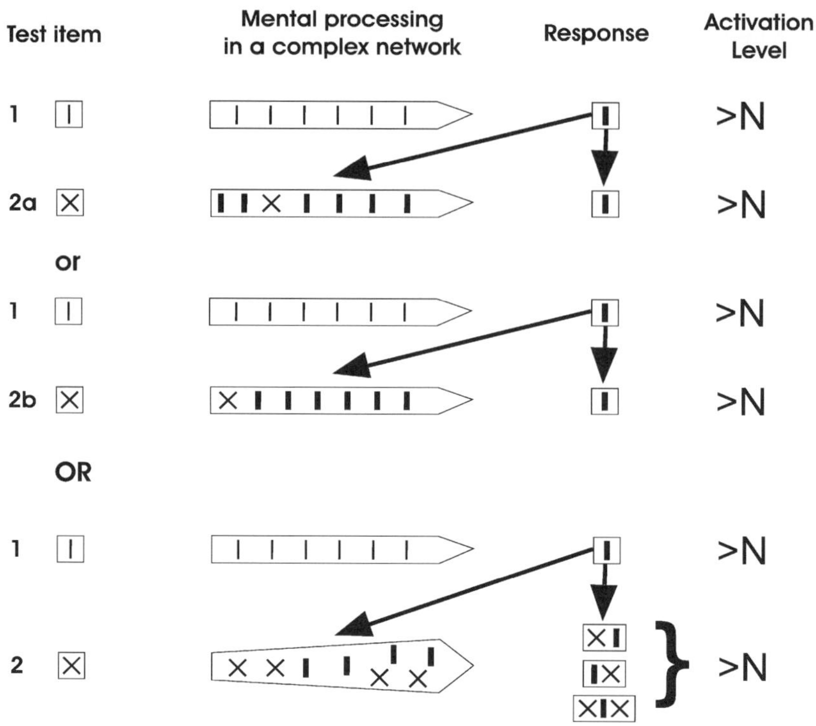

Figure 3a. Von Soelder's account of the origin of perseveratory responses for a simple case.

activation returns roughly to its pre-response "normal" resting state (N) rather quickly. However, in carrying out tasks in which the production of one response after another is required, a minimal residual activation from one response to the next is assumed to remain. It is further assumed that in an unimpaired state—e.g. in tasks carried out with a healthy control person—the level of activation is considered to be normal (N).

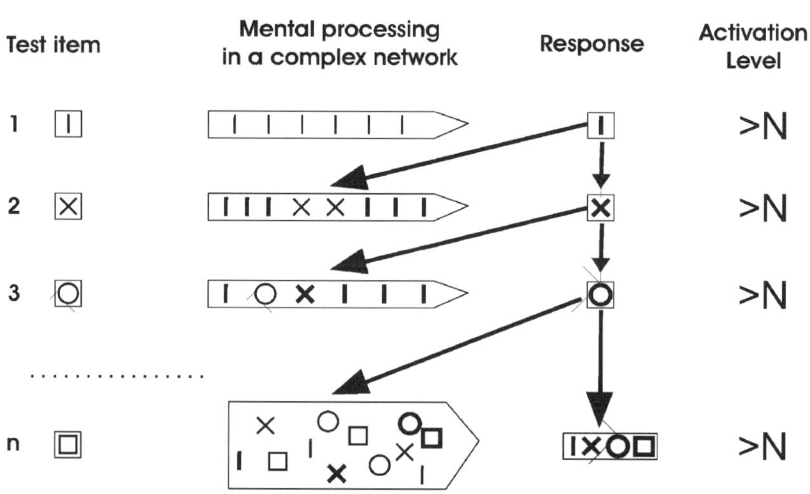

Figure 3b. Von Soelder's account of the origin of perseveratory responses for a complex case.

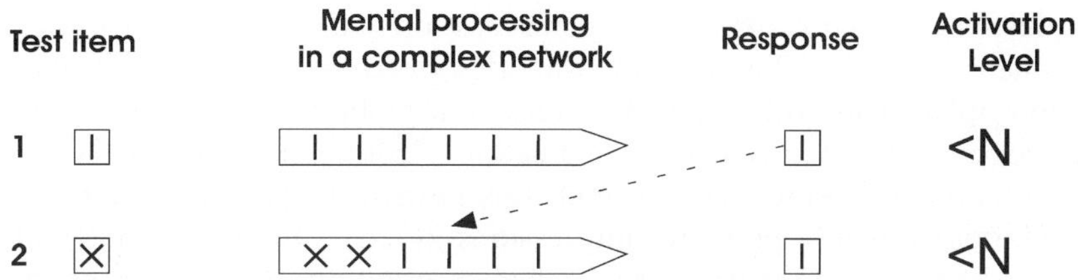

Figure 4. Pick's account of the origin of perseveratory responses.

In contrast, in a pathological state following brain damage (Figures 2a through 4, see later), the classical accounts refer either to a continuous/ongoing state of underactivation (characterised as <N), or of overactivation or persisting activation (characterised as >N), or the level of activation is not normal (represented in the figures by a crossed-out N). In all figures, one or two hypothetical cases (sequences of test item with responses that illustrate perseveration) are portrayed. Other hypothetical response patterns are also possible. It must be stressed that these do not account for the exact internal processing assumed to be going on, which can only be estimated even if it is illustrated in such a simplified manner.

Three classical accounts of perseveration

Three accounts can be differentiated in the classical literature. Starting with the earliest publication (1890), these accounts can be summarised by the following key words:

1. *Deficit account*: perseveration as a secondary symptom, the primary one being another (Heilbronner, 1895, 1897, 1906; Lissauer, 1890) (illustrated in Figures 2a and 2b).
2. *Overactivation account*: perseveration as primary symptom—active preponderance of perseverated form (Von Soelder, 1895, 1899) (illustrated as >N in Figures 3a and 3b).
3. *Underactivation or weak activation account*: passive preponderance—weakness of other processes perseveration as a secondary symptom (Pick, 1892, 1900, 1902, 1903, 1906, etc.) (illustrated as <N in Figure 4).

The first and third accounts are related to a certain extent; however, they merit separate discussion. They mainly share the secondary nature of the phenomenon in contrast to von Soelder's account of perseveration as a primary symptom. Each of these will be discussed and illustrated in the following paragraphs.

Deficit account (Heilbronner/Lissauer)

Von Soelder (1899) cites Heilbronner's publication "On asymbolia" from 1897 as the first theoretical treatise on the origin of perseveration. In this publication, Heilbronner bases his theoretical treatise on asymbolia on data from three clients with asymbolia. Each patient—the first patient to a greater degree—responded with a perseveratory reaction which expressed itself as follows: "... when shown an object for example, he responded as he had correctly done so for the previously shown object or should have responded" (1897, p. 55). One of the clients discussed in the 1897 paper is the case that was presented at the 1894 East German Meeting to which

Neisser responded with his term "perseveration" or "perseveratory reaction" (Heilbronner, 1895).[19] This patient was described as having an almost pure conduction aphasia in addition to his sensory asymbolic symptoms. In summary, Heilbronner considered his client to be a case of "conduction asymbolia". Over the two-and-a-half-year period during which this patient was studied, he perseverated (Ger.: "Haftenbleiben") previous impressions (Ger.: "Eindrücke"). Heilbronner characterised his behaviour as follows: when responding, the movements appeared to be initiated correctly, but by the end of producing the particular response they were incorrect.

Heilbronner reserves the German term "Haftenbleiben" for pathological instances of perseveration, in contrast to the more general term "perseveration" which is also used to describe physiological processes in a broader sense. Heilbronner refers to Lissauer's (1890) case study and agrees with his account that perseveration is an independent symptom, which arises in the context of a breakdown in processing. In the 1897 and 1906 publications, Heilbronner refers to a law put forward more by Rieger (*On normal and cataleptic movements*, 1882) to explain simple reflexes and also more complex cortical/brain reflexes. Rieger's statement regarding the situation in which the pathways from the central nervous system to a muscle that is paretic are interrupted, forms the basis for Heilbronner's account of perseveration: "Furthermore, we now know from our everyday experience and also from the experiments on reflex movements, that innervation processes, which for some reason do not reach their goal and for that reason cannot be accomplished, strike different paths, which make it possible to reach that goal" (Heilbronner, 1897, p. 55).[20] Heilbronner takes this assumption a step further and maintains that innervation processes, which advance in the normal manner, can also take the byways, when minimal resistance is present in these byways. In that case the false byways would be taken, which allow perseveration to come about. The course of an excitation or excitatory process (Ger.: "Ablauf eines Erregungsvorganges") between two nerve centres leaves behind, as a residue, a facilitated receptiveness (Ger.: "erleichterte Anspruchsfähigkeit") in the circumscribed area (Heilbronner, 1906, p. 343).

In his later publication entitled: "On perseveration (Ger.: "Haftenbleiben") and stereotypy", Heilbronner (1906) addresses two questions at length, the first of which will be addressed here: Is perseveration a primary symptom, independent of other elementary disorders, i.e. does the perseveratory idea [Ger.: "Vorstellung"] (idea in its broadest sense) play a dominant role out of its own power, or does it arise only secondarily out of—regardless of the reason—the regression of other ones?

For Heilbronner (1897, 1906) and also Lissauer (1890), the patient's deficit—i.e. particular language-processing difficulty—is the primary cause of perseveration. Both authors stress that perseveration occurs when the correct response is not available for the patient. A perseveratory response is thus a secondary symptom, which is produced in place of the expected target item. The gap caused by the primary deficit, e.g., the inability to retrieve a lexical item, allows perseveration to

[19] Neisser's original quote and translation are provided in the previous section.

[20] Rieger's original German text: "Nun wissen wir aber ferner als eine alltägliche Erfahrungstatsache und ebenso aus den Experimenten über Reflexbewegungen, dass Innervationsvorgänge, die aus irgend welchem Grunde nicht zu ihrem Ziel gelangen und nicht zum Ausdruck kommen können, andere Bahnen einschlagen, auf denen ihnen dies möglich ist" (Rieger, 1882, p. 449).

come into play and fill a gap. It is not a primary symptom that suppresses or inhibits the correct production of a particular item. A perseveratory response is just one way of responding incorrectly.

A graphic representation of the ideas put forward by Heilbronner and Lissauer is given in Figures 2a and 2b for the previously discussed simple and complex cases respectively. Heilbronner discusses the aforementioned simple and complex types of perseveration. As previously stated, after a particular form is produced the activation level should return to a "normal" level (N). In the case of a patient with a specific language-processing deficit, e.g., word-finding difficulties, the activation level remains higher and thus increases the chance of producing a previous target item, when a gap or processing difficulty arises. Heilbronner's deficit account is less articulate about the level of activation. He refers to a reduction in the number of functioning elements. The N is crossed out to indicate that the level of activation is not normal. The main feature in both cases—simple and complex examples—is the primary deficit or breakdown in processing, which is illustrated in Figures 2a and 2b for test item 2 by the double slashes. Several hypothetical perseveratory responses are possible and these are listed under the response heading for item two. In Figure 2b the breakdown in processing hypothetically occurs for item n and the result is a perseveration consisting of elements from the first three test items.

Overactivation account (Von Soelder)

Von Soelder's account stands in disagreement with Heilbronner's and Lissauer's primary deficit account. For von Soelder (1895, 1899) individual concepts (Ger.: "Vorstellungen") or groups of ideas or mental images are aroused, either by means of external impressions (Ger.: "Eindrücke"), or by means of inner associations, and it is these that enter into the immediately following associations, in place of those ideas or mental images that would normally be expected (1899, p. 492). It can even occur that an entire stream of ideas (Ger.: "Vorstellungsablauf") can be interrupted or almost every logical development of associations can come to a halt. Thus, for von Soelder, perseveration represents "... a formal disturbance in the flow of ideas, which expresses itself in that a once aroused idea recurs in following complexes of ideas in a senseless combination" (1899, p. 501).[21]

According to von Soelder's view, perseveration is caused by a greater intensity or higher level of activation of the previous response than the next response which reduces the chance that the next response will be correctly produced.[22] However, in addition, the necessary inhibitory potential essential for the retrieval of the next items is also reduced or destroyed in the area of single functions. Perseveration is thus the result of a pathological persistence in activation of the previously produced unit: "The patient is not forced to take a different 'route' due to the impassability of the correct route, rather he gets into the wrong route because this one is particularly

[21] Von Soelder's original German text: "Perseveration ist eine bei Gehirnerkrankungen verschiedener Art auftretende formale Störung im Vorstellungsablaufe, die sich darin äußert, dass eine einmal geweckte Vorstellung in den unmittelbar nachfolgenden Vorstellungsreihen in sinnloser Verbindung wiederkehrt" (von Soelder, 1899, p. 501).

[22] Von Soelder's original German text: "... die besondere Intensität, mit der sich die perseverierende Vorstellung aufdrängt und das Zustandekommen der richtigen Reaktion verhindert" (von Soelder, 1899, p. 519).

accessible" (1899, p. 519). Von Soelder also differentiates between simple and complex cases of perseveration with regard to the units underlying the perseverations. Figures 3a (simple case) and 3b (complex case) represent an attempt to depict von Soelder's ideas on the origin of perseveration for the simple and complex cases respectively. The increased level of activation (>N), which leads to the perseveratory response, is crucial in von Soelder's account. Single concepts (Ger.: "Vorstellungen"), single complex units, and short strings (Ger.: "Reihen") can be affected.[23] The hypothetical responses for a possible simple case in response to item 2 are illustrated in Figure 3a. With regard to longer and more complex processes or units, larger or smaller fragments tend to recur, as depicted in Figure 3b for the hypothetical test item n.

The tendency for newly activated concepts (Ger.: "Vorstellungen") to suppress later ones is greater the more they are activated. According to von Soelder, the type and extent of the perseveratory response depends on the locus of the impairment: "The clinical appearance of the symptom takes on the form according to the area, to which the perseverating function is associated and according to the way in which the underlying image/concept is activated" (1899, p. 504).[24]

Based on data from five of his cases and the available data on patients described in the contemporary publications, von Soelder provides an overview of the forms perseverated, which are listed below:

1) Perseveration of spoken words:
   a) one or more words are perseverated in their unchanged form (response for test item 2a and 2b in Figure 3a);
   b) the perseverated word is produced next to the correct word (the first two hypothetical responses [XI and IX] in lines one and two for test item 2 in Figure 3a);
   c) the perseverated word is a blend of the target and the perseverated word (the last hypothetical response for test item 2 [XIX] in Figure 3a);
   d) the perseverated word is altered with regard to its formal structure (Ger.: "Das perseverierte Wort wird im Sinne des augenblicklichen Vorstellungsinhaltes umgemodelt").
2) Perseveration of words only heard by the client.
3) Perseveration in writing (e.g., of whole words, syllables, single letters).
4) Perseveration of read words (e.g., of the same types as for spoken words, usually a blend is the result.
5) Perseveration of movements (e.g., after being asked to close his/her eyes, instead of giving someone his/her hand, the client closes his/her eyes).
6) Perseveration of semantic concepts or associations (Ger.: "begriffliche Vorstellungen").

[23] Von Soelder's original German text: "Immer sind es nur isolierte Vorstellungen, einfache Komplexe oder kurze Reihen, welche die Erscheinung des Perseverierens zeigen; aus längeren und komplizierteren Processen pflegen nur größere oder kleinere Fragmente wiederzukehren" (von Soelder, 1899, p. 502).

[24] Von Soelder's original German text: "Die klinische Erscheinung des Symptoms gestaltet sich verschieden je nach dem Gebiete, dem die perseverierende Funktion angehört und nach der Art, in der die zu Grunde liegende Vorstellung geweckt worden ist" (von Soelder, 1899, p. 504).

With regard to self-correcting a perseveratory response, von Soelder maintains that if the perseveration affects a single word, a client will be more able to detect the perseveration and produce a self-correction. However, if the perseveratory response (1899, p. 503) encompasses a longer and more complex response, the perseveration is likely to remain undetected by the client.

Von Soelder stresses that other "laws" that pertain to paraphasia do not hold for perseveration. These include that the phonological and semantic (content) relations between the displacing, i.e. perseverated, word and the suppressed target word apply in the production of a paraphasia.

Underactivation or weak activation account (Pick)

Pick is one of the leading classical aphasiologists. Thus his ideas, which were presented in numerous publications (1892, 1900, 1902, 1903, 1906, 1914, 1921, 1931; also Thiele, 1931, and Brown, 1973, etc.), are crucial for a comprehensive treatment of the topic of perseveration. Over time Pick also modified his views in light of discussions with his colleagues and additional evidence from his own single-case studies and cases from contemporary colleagues. Pick (1906) sought to characterise the impact and retroactive influence of perseveration on the development of thoughts and ideas. Pick also investigated the role of perseveration and other mechanisms as the source of agrammatic phenomena; i.e., grammatical errors in written and oral language production. For both Pick (1903) and von Soelder (1899) perseveration is considered to originate in the context of fatigue. Regarding the diagnostic relevance of perseveration, in his 1914 paper Pick agrees with Heilbronner that it "...represents the first symptom of a focal lesion" (p. 418).

In his handbook article on aphasia (1931, p. 1460, posthumous publication by Rudolf Thiele; Brown, 1973), Pick also discusses perseveration:

> One assumes that it [=perseveration] is a matter of an increase in an otherwise normal symptom, that for example a produced word continues to be active in the course of producing a sentence or it even reappears (demonstrated in the occurrences of normal slips of the tongue). Pathological perseveration emerges exactly in this form especially in the context of the herein discussed deficits: in word amnesia as an intruding, often multiple repetition of the same error affecting the whole word, only a syllable or a letter, in the same way with the paraphasia as a repetition of the same distortion of a word or malapropism, as the continuing effect of an earlier used sentence construction or word inflection in the incorrect place and thus sometimes simulating agrammatism; as a counterpart to it/thereto the correct grammatical construction in which perseverated words, perseverated false accentuation of a correct words, as evidence that the impairment affects only one unit/part in an otherwise correct ongoing process.[25]

[25] Pick's original German text: "Man nimmt an, dass es sich um eine Steigerung der der Norm zu entnehmenden Erscheinung handelt, dass z.B. ein gebrauchtes Wort auch weiterhin im Zuge des Satzes nachwirkt oder selbst neuerlich auftritt (nachzuweisen in den Erscheinungen des normalen Versprechens). Gerade in dieser Form tritt die pathologische Perseveration im Rahmen der hier besprochenen Störungen besonders hervor: bei der Wortamnesie als sich aufdrängende, oft mehrfache Wiederholung der gleichen Fehlleistung, das ganze Wort oder nur eine Silbe, einen Buchstaben betreffend, in gleicher Weise bei den Paraphasien als Wiederholung derselben Wortentstellung oder Wortverwechslung, als Fortwirken einer früher gebrauchten Satzkonstruktion oder Wortbiegung an unrichtiger Stelle und dadurch gelegentlich Agrammatismus vortäuschend; als Gegenstück dazu die richtige grammatische Konstruktion an dem perseverierenden Worte, perseverierende falsche Betonung eines richtigen Wortes, zum Beweise, dass die Störung nur ein Stück in einem sonst korrekt ablaufenden Vorgange betrifft" (Pick, 1931, p. 1460).

Pick attributes the origin of perseveration to a weakening in the activation level or intensity of activation, whereby the required response—i.e., the target for test item 2—does not receive enough activation to be produced. Pick (1892, 1903) speaks of a "passive weight(iness)" of the already produced hypothetical response for test item 1 in Figure 4, so the new target does not, so to speak, push the target out of the way because of its force. This is consistent with von Soelder's account. According to Pick (1903), the new or next target item (e.g., for test item 2 in Figure 4) is too weakly activated and has less chance of being retrieved and produced: "... the perseveration of a specific representation originates due to passive preponderance. In short, I attribute the increase in intensity of the perseverated ideas to the decrease in intensity of the other representations due to fatigue" ... "the passive preponderance of the perseverated ideas is due to the erasure of the other ideas" (1903, p. 10).[26] Pick's ideas, which stress a weakened level of activation characterised as <N, are depicted in Figure 4.

The preponderance of a particular concept (Ger.: "Vorstellung") arises out of the adynamia or weakness (Ger.: "Schwäche") of the main associations. Thus, the perseverated item owes its strength to the weakness of the other mental processes (Pick, 1931, pp. 1460–1461):

> Its nature [=perseveration] is not with certainty clarified; that while at least for a part of the cases with regard to the norm, the assumption is valid (von Soelder), that due to the particular attention, interest, the added effort is the reason for the heightened after-effect, in the pathological cases it appears to be the case that the inferiority of the other performance or output (Ger.: "Leistungen") due to fatigue, reduced level of awareness or consciousness, which gives rise to the increased emergence of the just now perseverated.[27]

In a later paper, Pick (Thiele, 1931) describes the causes of perseveration and verbal paraphasia in the following manner: In the case of verbal paraphasia, there is a weakening of coherence (within the lexical network) and the otherwise strict determining tendency that leads to the production of the correct item is weakened. His discussions of verbal perseveration and also paraphasia support the specificity of the processing difficulties, in that "... the deficit affects a particular aspect/part of an ongoing otherwise correct production/process" (1931, p. 1460).[28]

---

[26] Pick (1903): "... j'estime que la persévération d'une représentation déterminée naît par voie de prépondérance passive. En un mot, j'attribue l'augmentation de l'intensité de la représentation persévérante à la diminution de l'intensité des autres représentations par suite de l'épuisement".... "...de la prépondérance passive que prennent les idées persévérantes, en raison de l'effacement des autres representations" (Pick, 1903, p. 10 of reprint copy of the original publication).

[27] Pick's original German text: "Ihre Natur ist nicht mit Sicherheit klargelegt, während von der Norm her, wenigstens für einen Teil der Fälle, die Annahme (von Soelder) berechtigt ist, dass etwa die durch besondere Aufmerksamkeit, Interesse, verstärkte Leistung der Grund ihres verstärkten Nachwirkens ist, scheint es in den pathologischen Fällen die Minderwertigkeit der übrigen Leistungen infolge der Ermüdung, herabgesetzter Bewusstseinshöhe zu sein, die das verstärkte Hervortreten der eben perseverierenden zur Folge hat" (Pick, 1931, p. 1461).

[28] Pick's original German text: "... dass die Störung nur ein Stück in einem sonst korrekt ablaufenden Vorgange betrifft" (Pick, 1931, p. 1460).

For Pick, the opposition between activation and inhibition must always be considered in any explanatory account.[29] Depending on the stage or the point in processing when disinhibition comes into play, different types of errors are to be expected.[30] Disinhibition plays a decisive role in Pick's characterisation of both paraphasia and perseveration (Pick, 1931, p. 1455):

> The explanation of the respective impairments from disinhibition results from the separation of its effects on word substitution (=verbal paraphasia) and word distortion/deformation (Ger.: "Wortentstellung" (=phonological paraphasia), which make it probable from the start, that the difference is due to the setting in of the impairment in different stages of the language production process.[31]

In terms of degree of activation and/or disinhibition, for Pick a perseveratory response occurs in the context of mild disinhibition, whereas a paraphasic response is produced in the context of greater disinhibition[32] (see Pick, 1931, p. 1461). In characterising the relationship among echolalia, logorrhoea, and paraphasia, Pick maintains that the differentiation of the various forms supports the view that the point where inhibition is lacking must be a different one for each form.

The aforementioned distinction between simple and complex cases of perseveration is related to task demands. Pick comments that the overall difficulty of the word-finding task should be considered in the case of both perseveratory and paraphasic errors: "It is certainly not a coincidence that in the case of the loosening of (the) coherence leads to such disinhibition in word-finding; the relative difficulty of the required task to be performed plays a role" (Pick, 1931, p. 1461).[33]

DEBATED ISSUES REGARDING THE MECHANISMS RESPONSIBLE FOR PERSEVERATION

In addition to Heilbronner, Lissauer, von Soelder, and Pick, other classical authors such as Sommer (1893), and Liepmann (1905) stress that one cannot decide among the accounts put forward on the mechanisms responsible for perseveration. In his analysis of dyslexic errors in his progressive paralytic client, for instance, Sommer differentiated among three symptoms the third of which relates to perseveration: (1)

[29] The neurophysiologist Jung (1953) maintained that both activation and inhibition are not absolute opposites, but rather both complement each other in the coordination of the nervous system. Order is only possible through selection of separate processes with inhibition of all competing ones. A balancing is necessary. Every inhibition has to follow an activation. Others authors stress cortical dynamics, in particular the role of inhibition or lack of it, in their discussions of aphasia and perseveration, e.g., Azcoaga (1963), Luria (1974), etc.

[30] In Figures 1 to 4 reference is made to activation level as N, <N, >N, and crossed-out N. However, exact definitions are not supplied by the authors for the terms activation, inhibition, and disinhibition.

[31] Pick's original German text: "Die Erklärung der entsprechenden Störungen aus Enthemmung geht aus von der Scheidung ihrer Effekte in Wortverwechslung und Wortentstellung, die es von vornherein wahrscheinlich macht, dass diese Differenz durch das Einsetzen der Störung in differenten Stadien des Sprachvorganges gegeben ist" (Pick, 1931, p. 1455).

[32] Pick's original German text: "Als ein letztes Argument ist noch zu erwähnen ein gewisses Verhältnis zur Intensität der in Betracht kommenden Enthemmung: Perseveration bei leichter, Paraphasie bei stärkerer Enthemmung" (Pick, 1931, p. 1461).

[33] Pick's original German text: "Es ist gewiss kein Zufall, dass in beiden Fällen gerade bei der Wortfindung die Lockerung der Kohärenz zu so deutlicher Enthemmung führt; es wird dabei gewiss die relative Schwierigkeit der Leistung eine Rolle spielen" (Pick, 1931, p. 1461).

dyslexic errors, (2) uninhibited word associations resulting in paraphasias, and (3) abnormal persisting effect, which presented itself as a repetition of words and parts of words in reading and naming objects. He concludes (1893, p. 683) that an intermediate stand is necessary: "... the phenomenon of sticking to a once produced sound entity, which played such a role in the reading examples, is also present in naming objects". Further, for Sommer it cannot be decided "whether the phenomenon of psychical after-effect is the primary one. In that case the preference/prevalence of a phoneme/sound form to a certain degree//quasi hinders the retrieval of the correct name. Or, is it the case that a periodically arising inability to name objects is the primary deficit and the psychical after-effect only incidentally joins in."[34]

Kleist (1934, p. 1339) further emphasises a combination of two factors playing a role in the occurrence perseveration: increased decay rate and a delayed activation rate. He states that:

> ... the fundamental process of perseveration presents itself not only as a delayed decaying – as an enormously long lasting readiness of a once activated memory (Ger.: "Erinnerungsbild") to resurface – rather also as a delayed and exacerbated hint and emergence of new ideas or images. Perseveration is the reverse of the aggravated emergence of new ideas or images. Both, the delayed excitation (Ger.: "Weckung") of the forthcoming and the deferred delay of (out-)going ideas, are equal/equivalent sides of the same basic process; both sides can be subsumed under the mutual concept of an impediment in changing ideas.[35]

In an attempt to explain the construct "generic" perseveration, Rosenberg (1912) compares von Soelder's active preponderance account of perseveration with Pick's relative preponderance due to the weakening of other processes, and he suggests that Pick's ideas are to be preferred for two reasons: (1) the weakening of the other processes can be demonstrated and (2) his interpretation can be applied to normal psychology in that the pathological phenomena can be viewed as only excessively distorted with regard to the normal.

As a way of summing up the classical accounts on perseveration published mainly in German on perseveration, Liepmann (1905) provides a comprehensive list of relevant questions in his discussion of intentional perseveration in apraxia—i.e., perseveration of actions (Ger. "handeln") and components of actions. Liepmann's long list of questions and comments is quoted in full to portray the intensity of the debate on perseveration and demonstrate the issues that were relevant in the classical accounts (Liepmann, 1905, pp. 122–123):

---

[34] Sommer's original German text: "Ob nun das Phänomen des psychischen Nachwirkung das Primäre ist, derartig, dass vermöge der Prävalenz eines Lautgebildes gewissermaßen die Entstehung des richtigen Namens gehindert wird, oder ob eine periodisch auftretende Unfähigkeit, Gegenstände zu benennen, das Primäre dabei ist und die psychische Nachwirkung nur nebensächlich hinzutritt, lasse ich vorläufig unentschieden" (Sommer, 1893, p. 683).

[35] Kleist's original German text: "Der Grundvorgang der Perseveration stellt sich aber nicht nur als ein verzögertes Abklingen – als eine abnorm lange nachdauernde Bereitschaft zum Wiederauftauchen eines einmal aktivierten Erinnerungsbildes – dar, sondern auch als ein verzögertes und erschwertes Anklingen und Auftauchen von neuen Vorstellungen. Die Perseveration ist die Kehrseite neuer Vorstellungen. Beides, die verzögerte Weckung der kommenden und die verzögerte Dämpfung der gehenden Vorstellungen, sind gleichwertige Seiten desselben Grundvorgangs; beide Seiten aber lassen sich unter den gemeinsamen Begriff einer Erschwerung des Vorstellungswechsels bringen" (Kleist, 1934, p. 1339).

Is the (intentional, which I always refer to in the following unless otherwise stated) *perseveration the actual cause of disrupted action, or result? That is, is the new innervation not brought about, because the old one persists abnormally long, or does the old one persist, because the new intended one finds an obstacle and the stream now flows in the old bed? More strongly formulated: Does the perseverating [item] have a longer duration than normal, so that the abnormally long duration of an arousal/excitation hinders the realization of other ones? Or, does a normally longer lasting arousal substitute only for a new arousal, which does not come about due to obstacles in the pathway?*

Does then the pathology consist *primarily of a slight damping of nervous elements*, just previously operating or of the interruption of many other pathways? Apparently the latter. It would be inconsistent to assume that a lesion would primarily place the intact [function] in a state of greater tenacity, instead of making the impaired [function] less able to operate. Normally the just previously operating nervous substance retains a certain responsiveness.

That a mental image or idea (Ger.: "Vorstellung") possesses a certain extended duration beyond the time, in which it is explicitly and clearly present in one's mind, is known to psychologists (cf. also Gross, "secondary function"). If then for reasons still to be discussed, obstacles are put in the way of a new intention, it is understandable, that the excitation betakes to the elements which are still in the state of heightened receptiveness. (cf. Heilbronner, Asymbolia.) It is very probable that secondarily, as a consequence of the impassibility of many pathways, the extended duration of excitation existing at one point will be abnormally long. Thus, it is to be assumed that impassibility of certain pathways and the corresponding functional disorder is primary, and that due to this the extended duration of certain excitations will be amplified and thus the earlier once again roused excitation takes the place of the actually not materializing intended excitation. Accordingly we must look for *the real cause of the perseveration in the area in which the path is damaged, not there where the perseverating innervation ultimately comes about.*[36]

[36] Liepmann"s original German text: "Ist die (intentionelle, die ich ohne weiteren Zusatz jetzt immer im Auge habe) Perseveration selbständige Ursache gestörten Handelns, oder Folge? D.h., wird die neue Innervation nicht zustande gebracht, weil die alte abnorm persistiert, oder persistiert die alte, weil die neu intendierte ein Hindernis findet und nun der Strom in das alte Bett geht? Schärfer gefasst: Hat das Perseverierende eine größere Nachdauer als normalerweise, so, dass das abnorm lange Nachdauern einer Erregung das Zustandekommen anderer behindert? Oder substituiert sich eine normalerweise nachdauernde Erregung nur der durch Hindernisse in der Leitung nicht erreichten neuen Erregung? Besteht also das Krankhafte in einer primär geringeren Dämpfung eben in Funktion gewesener Nervenelemente, oder in der Unterbrechung vieler anderer Bahnen? Offenbar das letztere. Es wäre ja ungereimt, anzunehmen, dass ein Herd in erster Linie das Erhaltene in einen Zustand größerer Haftfähigkeit setzte, statt, dass er das Lädierte weniger leistungsfähig macht. Es behält normalerweise die in Funktion gewesene nervöse Substanz eine gewisse Ansprechbarkeit. Dass eine Vorstellung eine gewisse Nachdauer hat über die Zeit hinaus, in der sie deutlich und klar bewusst ist, ist den Psychologen bekannt (Vergl. auch Gross, Sekundärfunktion.) Wenn nun aus zu erörternden Gründen einer neuen Intention sich Hindernisse in den Weg stellen, so ist es verständlich, dass sich die Erregung in die noch im Zustande erhöhter Ansprechbarkeit befindlichen Elemente begibt. (Vergl. Heilbronner, Asymbolie.) Dass sekundär, infolge der Unwegsamkeit vieler Bahnen, die Nachdauer einmal bestehender Erregung abnorm lange wird, ist dabei sehr wahrscheinlich. Jedenfalls ist also anzunehmen, dass Unwegsamkeit gewisser Bahnen und die entsprechende Funktionsstörung das Primäre ist, dass dadurch die Nachdauer gewesener Erregungen verstärkt wird und nun an Stelle der ausfallenden intendierten, die wiederwachgerufene frühere Erregung tritt. Hiernach müssen wir die eigentliche Ursache der Perseveration in dem Gebiet suchen, in dem die Leitung geschädigt ist; nicht da, wo schliesslich die persevererierende Innervation zustande kommt" (Liepmann, 1905, pp. 122–123).

PERSEVERATION AS A FOCAL OR GENERAL SYMPTOM

In addition to the difficulty of deciding among the accounts put forward by the classical aphasiologists, several authors differentiate between types of perseveration based on whether they represent a focal or a general symptom. Kleist (1934), for example, makes reference to two types of perseveration in his discussion of perseveration observed in clients suffering from missile wounds of the brain due to war injuries:

1. Sticking to sensory, language, action, recognition, and thought engrams due to deficits of cortical function, whereby perseveration is strongest in that domain where the focal symptoms are present.
2. A general symptom due to a brain stem lesion. In this case it is comparable to so-called other general symptoms including unconsciousness, somnolence, etc.

He stresses that in spite of the first type of tendency of perseveration, there can be substantial differences in the degree of perseveration in the various areas. This is not due to the effect of the general tendency to perseverate stemming from brain stem lesions, rather it depends on the particular occurrence due to the respective cortical lesions (Kleist, 1934, p. 1337):

> If such are present, it is understandable that they will here or there create a locus of reduced resistance, apparently a functional gap - be it in the linguistic, or action (Ger.: "Handelndem") or in the realm of thoughts - in which the general tendency to perseverate pushes forward more strongly than in other undamaged cortical areas. Possibly, under certain circumstances the influence of a minimal tendency for perseveration can be so reduced, that it only becomes apparent in the locus of an impaired cortical function.[37]

In this case, for instance, an isolated literal perseveration is observed in cited cases. Von Soelder (1899) also differentiates two groups of cases in which perseveration is observed: (1) circumscribed deficits of simple associative functions and (2) diffuse organic brain damage.

It is interesting to note that Allison (1966a, 1966b) also refers to perseveration as a sign of diffuse and focal brain damage. In the first case it is associated with states of disturbed consciousness. Allison asserts that it may pass unnoticed in the context of other symptoms associated with cloudiness of consciousness, including disorientation in time and place, delirium, impairment of recent memory, etc. It is also present in patients recovering from carbon monoxide poisoning, and it shows up as an early sign of dissolution in Alzheimer's and Pick's disease. In contrast to perseveration in relation to general disturbances of brain function, perseveration is also observed in patients with focal brain lesions with aphasia and is linked "… not only with speech and language but with the actual disabilities found, and to that extent it is thought to have focal significance" (Allison, 1966b, p. 1101).

[37] Kleist's original German text: "Wenn solche vorhanden sind, so leuchtet es ein, dass sie da oder dort einen Ort verminderten Widerstandes schaffen, gewissermaßen eine Funktionslücke – sei es auf handelnden oder auf gedanklichem Feld – in der sich die allgemeine Perseverationstendenz stärker vordrängt als an andern unversehrten Rindenleistungen" (Kleit, 1934, p. 1337).

INTEGRATION WITH MORE RECENT ACCOUNTS

Perseveration was considered by classical German neurologists to be an important albeit complex symptom in focal brain damage. This review of the classical accounts of perseveration has thus far aimed at covering the relevant issues discussed by those renowned clinicians and researchers, in greater or lesser detail. In this section the issues and classical accounts regarding perseveratory phenomena will be related to more recent accounts.

Based on the classical literature, the following interrelated questions emerge:

1. What can we learn from the aforementioned studies regarding the origin of perseveration?
2. What do the classical accounts have in common with those put forward in "more recent" analyses of perseveration?
3. What are the merits and shortcomings of the discussed classical accounts?

Foremost, it is striking that the classical authors produced such intellectually vigorous literature on the topic of perseveration, which addresses numerous relevant issues that are still open to debate. Their profound interest in perseveration, and their in-depth descriptions of the various aspects contributing to the complexity of the perseveratory phenomena, are commendable. This can be considered one of the merits of the classical studies.

Of the classical accounts of perseveration, the deficit account put forward by Heilbronner and Lissauer captures what can be considered to be a central issue: A person with aphasia perseverates (and/or produces paraphasic responses) in accordance with his/her specific processing difficulties. The form of the perseveratory errors (and/or paraphasic errors) mirrors the basic processing difficulties of the subject; i.e., indicates the point at which processing breaks down (see Stark, 1984). In this context, following his discussion of perseveration as a symptom that reflects the primary deficits, Heilbronner (1906, p. 345) cites two relevant questions that refer to the primary deficits which trigger perseveration in the various disorders: (1) how the primary deficits themselves come about, and (2) which general conditions must be satisfied, in order for the incorrect response—which is solely to be considered the immediate and understandable consequence of the deficit—to take on the exact form of perseveration that it does.[38]

In neuropsychological textbooks, symptoms are analysed in terms of dichotomies such as: focal versus non-focal, localising versus non-localising, selective versus generalised or diffuse, specific versus nonspecific symptoms. In these dichotomies perseveration has often been listed under the second type as a non-specific or a generalised symptom. However, such bipartite divisions do not characterise the perseveratory phenomena adequately. Perseveration should be analysed in a more differentiated fashion, in line with Teuber and Weinstein's (1955) category type-2 effects of brain damage, or as Yates (1966) type-b changes (see also Teuber, 1955). Yates' tripartite division of the types of changes caused by brain damage postulates the following three types (1966, p. 112):

[38] Heilbronner's original German text: "Einmal wäre zu untersuchen, auf welche Weise in den verschiedenen Krankheitszuständen, die Haftenbleiben erzeugen, der primäre Ausfall (im weitesten Sinne) zustande kommt; ... Zum zweiten wäre genauer zu präzisieren, welche allgemeine Bedingungen erfüllt sein müssen, damit die Fehlreaktion, die ja allein als unmittelbare und verständliche Folge des Ausfalles aufgefasst werden darf, gerade in der Form des Haftenbleibens erfolgt" (Heilbronner, 1906, p. 345).

(a) a general deterioration in all aspects of functioning; but will also produce
(b) differential (group) effects, depending on the location, extent, etc. of the damage, and will produce
(c) highly specific effects if it occurs in certain highly specified areas of the brain.

This division accounts for the aforementioned discussion of perseveration as a focal versus general symptom observed in different clinical populations with brain damage. The focal, specific circumscribed perseveratory errors reflect the b-type of changes. On the other hand, the pervasive general deterioration observed in dementia—which can initially present itself as a focal sign—is best captured by a-type changes. As an example, agrammatic sentence production or paragrammatic language production can be cited for c-type changes, in contrast to perseverative responses, which are best characterised as b-type effects of brain damage.

The papers in this special issue of *Aphasiology* (and other papers by these authors on this topic), and in particular the collection of papers in the recently published special issue of *Seminars in Speech and Language* on perseveration edited by Buckingham and Christman (2004), provide a survey of the state of the art on modern studies.[39] Thus, it would go beyond the scope of this historical paper to discuss the recent publications on perseveration individually and in depth. However, reference will be made to particular ones when addressing the following aspects:

1. Specificity of perseveratory responses.
2. Patient selection and other methodological variables.
3. Degree of sophistication of the studies.
4. Modelling of hypothetical and actual data from control subjects and brain-damaged patients presenting with a specific (language) processing deficit.

A majority of the classical authors refer to the specificity of the perseveratory errors. For example, Kleist (1934) stresses that "... perseveration is present in only one area or is strongest, in that area in which the most severe focal symptoms are present" (p. 1334).[40] Von Soelder and Pick stress the specificity of the perseveratory responses with respect to the various stages in the process of producing language. Regarding the specificity of the perseveratory errors, most recent single-case studies highlight the specific deficits and their relationship to the observed perseveratory errors (Cohen & Dehaene, 1998; Crutch & Warrington, 2001; Martin & Dell, 2004; Martin, Roach, Brecher, & Lowery, 1998; Moses et al., 2004; Warrington & Leff, 2000). The assumed source of the errors is also postulated in the various publications. Regardless of the theoretical background of the various authors, the descriptions regarding the origin of perseveration can be related to one of the three classical accounts discussed in previous sections of this paper: (1) the deficit account,

[39] In addition, relevant papers that address various aspects of perseveration include (in alphabetical order): Albert and Sandson (1986); Allison (19966a, 1966b); Allison and Hurwitz (1967); Buckingham (1985); Cohen and Dehaene (1998); Crutch and Warrington (2001); Gotts and Plaut (2005); Gotts, della Rocchetta, and Cipolotti (2002); Hudson (1968); Moen (1993); Moses, Nickels, and Sheard (2004); Plaut and Shallice (1993); Sandson (1986); Sandson and Albert (1984); Warrington and Leff (2000).

[40] Kleist's original German text: "Für einen Zusammenhang zwischen Perseveration und kortikalen Funktionsausfällen sprechen ferner die Beobachtungen, in denen die Perseveration sich nur auf dem Gebiete zeigt oder dort am stärksten ist, wo auch die stärksten Herdsymptome liegen ..." (Kleist, 1934, p. 1334).

(2) the overactivation account, and (3) the underactivation or weak activation account, or as a combination of components of them.

In a review of the neuromechanisms proposed to account for perseveration, Hotz and Helm-Estabrooks (1995) enumerate three mechanisms that have most often been cited. They are impaired attention, memory dysfunction, or disordered motor patterns (p. 156). These mechanisms are in accord with the ideas put forward in publications by Sandson and Albert (1984, etc.). In recent publications, detailed descriptions of single cases are presented and the assumed processing deficits are specified with reference to the authors' preferred models of language processing.

Of the recent publications on verbal perseveration, Cohen and Dehaene's (1998) interpretation of verbal perseverations is singled out to elucidate similarities between classical and recent accounts, because these authors provide an overall theoretical account of the mechanisms involved and they discuss three cases showing perseveration on different specific stages of processing (see also Dell, Burger, & Svec, 1997). Moreover, they provide objective evidence for their innovative statistical account of perseveratory responses.[41]

Cohen and Dehaene's (1998) account of the tentative theoretical mechanism for the generation of perseverations reveals great overlap with the ideas put forward in the classical accounts: "… whenever a given processing level is deprived of its normal input, persistent activity inherited from previous trials is no longer overcome by current input, and is revealed in the form of perseverations" (p. 1641). The phrasing "deprived of its normal input" can be taken as indicative of a deficit as put forward by Heilbronner and Lissauer. The deficient input is characterised as being caused by a primary deficit, which also relates to Heilbronner's and Lissauer's account. The more complete summary of their mechanism (Cohen & Dehaene, 1998, p. 1655) bears resemblance to other ideas characteristic of the classical accounts:

> (i) persistence of activity from previous trials is a normal feature at many levels of the processing system;
>
> (ii) in normal subjects this persistent activity is overruled by the current input and is therefore not readily observable;
>
> (iii) whenever a processing level is deafferented from its normal input source, persistent activity is no longer systematically overcome by the current input and can exert a major influence on behaviour; hence, perseverations occur;
>
> (iv) the format of the perseverations (e.g. phonemes, words, etc.) corresponds to the specific format of the deafferented level, explaining the various types of verbal

[41] Several publications cited in Cohen and Dehaene also provide elaborate investigation of perseveration in healthy control subjects and aphasic clients. These include the publications of the group Dell, Martin, Schwartz, et al. and also the publications by Sandson and Albert. The former group has made formidable contributions to understanding the processing aspects in terms of connectionist modelling (see Martin & Dell, 2007 this issue). Sandson and Albert have published several publications that bear resemblance to ideas discussed in classical accounts. Albert and Sandson (1984) propose a taxonomy for perseveration consisting of three categories: stuck-in set, recurrent, and continuous perseveration. Relevant to this discussion is the recurrent perseveration, for which the authors hypothesise a process deficit that "involves a failure of the usual inhibition of memory traces" (p. 717). A variation of this proposal has also been put forward by Gloning (1974) as one of two basic mechanisms causing verbal perseveration, namely a defective erasing procedure (see also Hudson, 1968).

perseverations. In a nutshell, we suggest that perseverations result from persistent activity unmasked by deficient input.

Depending on the strength of the persistence of activity addressed in point (i), von Soelder's or Pick's account comes to mind. In this context, the authors note that "it is quite conceivable that previous responses remain activated at an abnormally high level due in particular to impairment of some inhibitory or check-off mechanism" (p. 1657), which is more consistent with von Soelder's account. However, Cohen and Dehaene (1998, p. 1658) also refer to their own theory and Pick's as passive accounts of perseveration:

> Interestingly, the debate between "passive" accounts of perseverations (Pick, 1903), such as ours, and more "active" theories dates back to the origins of this field of research (Hudson, 1968). Pick (1903), commenting on the perseveration of the word *locksmith,* claimed that "due to the weakness of the [present] associations, the representation of *locksmith*, which remained since the previous test below the threshold of consciousness, but available to it, crosses the threshold ... This representation is therefore *relatively* strengthened and can remain so for a certain amount of time." In our explanatory proposal, i.e. normal persistence plus deafferentation, we put emphasis on a minimal mechanism for perseverations. While this may not be the only mechanism, we believe that it is sufficient to account for a wide variety of pathological situations.

Point (ii) refers to the situation depicted in Figure 1. Point (iii) is reminiscent of the deficit account of perseveration. Their point (iv) addresses the specificity issue, which is alluded to in numerous classical publications, in particular Pick, von Soelder, Kleist, Heilbronner, Liepmann, etc. The deafferented level corresponds with the affected level in the classical accounts. Cohen and Dehaene (1998, p. 1642) state: "We suggest that a single mechanism, occurring at different stages of speech production, may explain not only lexical but also other types of verbal perseverations."

With regard to the duration of perseveration, Cohen and Dehaene (1998, p. 1655) refer to "exponential decay": "At any processing level, the probability that an error is a perseveration from a previous trial is a decreasing function of the lag between the two trials considered. This suggests that an exponentially decaying internal variable, such as an internal level of activation, is responsible for the recurrence of perseverations." Similar ideas are discussed in the classical literature by Heilbronner (1906, p. 306) among others.

With regard to the possibility that perseveration as observed in clinical populations is an exaggeration of normal phenomenon, von Soelder's ideas can be compared with those put forward by Cohen and Dehaene (1998). In their discussion of the literature, Cohen and Dehaene maintain that "... The very existence, in normal subjects, of exponentially decaying priming effects that last over several trials ... is of great consequence for interpreting the verbal perseverations produced by brain-damaged patients. It suggests that the persistent activation of words in the lexicon that underlies perseveration is indeed a normal phenomenon" (p. 1656). Von Soelder points out that "... also with healthy subjects there is an aftereffect of representations or concepts" (Ger.: "Vorstellungen"), which occasionally leads to perseveration. In this context, Von Soelder quotes examples from Meringer and Mayer's (1895) monograph (*Versprechen und Verlesen*) at length and comes to the conclusion that a comparison of their errors observed in healthy controls and the perseveratory responses of patients reveals that the differences are almost only quantitative (1899, p. 514). Von Soelder (1899, p. 514) summarises his discussion as follows:[42]

> From all this emerges, that a once activated language concept or representation does not disappear immediately, rather it persists for a while under the threshold of conscious awareness, it "lingers" and under circumstances can still become active. In the healthy subject und under normal circumstances this aftereffect disappears completely almost entirely due to the stronger effect of logical formation of associations. In the case of brain conditions, the most important of which were mentioned above, this aftereffect can assert itself so strongly, that it emerges as perseveration.

In recent years several other models have been introduced to account for errors produced by healthy controls and aphasic clients. One example is a recent model developed by Dell et al. (1997) to account for serial order errors. This model bears resemblance to the weak activation account put forward by Pick. In Dell et al.'s paper, perseveration occurs because the current target item is weakly activated. In this situation the previous utterances that are residually activated lead to intrusion.

Although great importance is to be attached to the classical studies on various aphasiological topics, when considering the merits and shortcomings of classical studies on perseveration it is not the case that they are without flaws. For example, in a survey of the rich history of classical publications on agrammatism, Stark and Dressler (1990) drew attention to the shortcomings of the much-cited studies on agrammatism. These shortcomings related to deficiencies in patient selection and other methodological aspects. For example, in the agrammatism literature, language data from a retarded child is cited as an example of telegraphic speech (Steinthal, 1871). This publication was thereafter cited as an example for agrammatism. Similar shortcomings hold for the classical perseveration literature. In terms of modern descriptions and taxonomies, it is sometimes difficult to know exactly what the overall deficits of the brain-damaged persons discussed in the studies actually were. Psychiatric and neurological clients are mixed, or the cases presented reveal several disorders, i.e., a mixture of psychiatric and neurological symptoms and disorders. Thus, although the theoretical insights of the classical studies are up to standard and are modern, the data presentation is at times difficult to follow.

In contrast, recent case studies reveal a more meticulous step-by-step demonstration and manipulation of variables to arrive at the underlying processing deficit(s) and the role specific variables play—see Gotts et al. (2002), Warrington and Leff (2000), Crutch and Warrington (2001), Cohen and Dehaene (1998), Martin, Roach, Brecher, and Lowery (1998). This hypothesis-driven test design structure is rarely present in the classical studies. The classical authors were actively interested in describing their patients' abilities and deficits to confirm or reject the theoretical ideas on perseveration current at the time, albeit in different terminology and with a

[42] Von Soelder's original German text: "Aus alledem geht hervor, dass eine geweckte Sprachvorstellung nicht sofort verschwindet, sondern unter der Bewusstseinsschwelle noch eine Zeit fortdauert,) 'nachklingt' und unter Umständen noch wirksam werden kann. Beim gesunden und unter normalen Verhältnissen verschwindet diese Nachwirkung fast ganz unter der kräftigeren Wirkung logischer Associationsbildung. Bei gewissen krankhaften Gehirnzuständen, deren wichtigste oben erwähnt worden, kann diese Nachwirkung sich so stark geltend machen, dass sie als Perseveration in Erscheinung tritt" (von Soelder, 1899, p. 514).

lesser degree of systematicity. However, when the differences between the current technological standards for lesion localisation (e.g., fMRI, CT scan; PET scan) are compared with those available to the classical aphasiologists, the classical aphasiologists accomplished a great deal in applying their clinical expertise. They did not limit descriptions to neuroanatomical characterisations, rather they expounded on the possible reasons for the observed responses. However, the next step of actually simulating perseveratory responses or modelling the observed pattern of performance was not (could not be) taken.

Modelling of hypothetical and actual data from control subjects and brain-damaged clients presenting with a specific (language) processing deficits is more prevalent in recent studies—see publications by Martin and Dell (2007 this issue); Gotts et al., 2002; Gotts and Plaut, 2004; Plaut and Shallice, 1993. Cohen and Dehaene's statistical analysis in terms of *lag distribution analysis* and *perseveration probability analysis* surpasses the degree of sophistication indicative of the classical studies, although their analyses apply to tasks requiring a single-word response. In this context, Heilbronner's reservations pertaining to the feasibility of being able to realise the perseveratory responses in tabular or statistical format due to the overall complexity of the data (task items and produced responses) and the interacting variables must be heeded. This is particularly relevant when the language tasks exceed, for example, word-level naming tasks, and include picture descriptions and/or spontaneous speech composed of extended samples of language production—see the case study of MH in this special issue of *Aphasiology* (Stark, 2007).

SUMMARY

The predictions of the three classical accounts and other older ideas on perseveration are indeed modern and relevant for an understanding of recent accounts of these phenomena. Therefore they should be considered when interpreting aphasic deficits—in particular perseveratory and/or paraphasic errors—and when providing language therapy to people with aphasia, who demonstrate a severe tendency to perseverate (e.g., using the method *Treatment for Aphasic Perseveration* or "TAP", by Helm-Estabrooks, Emery, & Albert, 1987). In summary, concepts put forward in the classical studies on the origin of perseveration are valid today, and are in several ways comparable to modern accounts of the phenomena.

POSTSCRIPT

Just before this paper went into print I received several stimulating comments from Hugh Buckingham. I could not do justice to some of them in this paper, but I would like to thank him and acknowledge his positive feedback. In a future paper on the topic I will respond to all of his remarks and suggestions, especially with regard to the continuity hypothesis.

REFERENCES

Albert, M. L., & Sandson, J. (1986). Perseveration in aphasia. *Cortex*, *22*, 103–115.

Allison, R. S. (1966a). Perseveration as a sign of diffuse and focal brain damage I. *British Medical Journal*, *2*, 1027–1032.

Allison, R. S. (1966b). Perseveration as a sign of diffuse and focal brain damage II. *British Medical Journal, 2*, 1095–1101.

Allison, R. S., & Hurwitz, L. J. (1967). On perseveration in aphasics. *Brain, 90*, 429–448.

Azcoaga, J. E. (1963). La fisiopatologia de los trastornos del lenguaje. *Acta Neurológica Latinoamericana, 9*, 125–139.

Brown, J. W. (1973). *Aphasia by Arnold Pick*. Springfield, IL: Charles C. Thomas.

Buckingham, H. W. (1985). Perseveration in aphasia. In S. Newman & R. Epstein (Eds.), *Current perspectives in dysphasia* (pp. 113–154). Edinburgh, UK: Churchill Livingstone.

Buckingham, H. W., & Christman, S. S. (Eds.). (2004). Perseveration in neurogenic communication disorders [special issue]. *Seminars in Speech and Language, 25*(4).

Cohen, L., & Dehaene, S. (1998). Competition between past and present assessment and interpretation of verbal perseverations. *Brain, 121*, 1641–1650.

Crutch, S., & Warrington, E. (2001). Refractory dyslexia: Evidence of multiple task-specific output stores. *Brain, 124*, 1533–1543.

DeBleser, R. (1987). From agrammatism to paragrammatism: German aphasiological traditions and grammatical disturbances. *Cognitive Neuropsychology, 4*, 187–256.

Dell, G. S., Burger, L. K., & Svec, W. R. (1997). Language production and serial order: A functional analysis and a model. *Psychological Review, 104*, 123–147.

Gairdner, W. T. (1866). *De la function de langage articulé avec une observation d'aphasie. Extrait des Archives générales de Médecine.* [translation and preamble by Jules Falret]. Paris: P. Asselin.

Gloning, K. (1974). Perseveration bei Aphasie. *Wiener Linguistische Gazette, 6*, 29–39.

Gloning, K. (1975). Zur Frage der "Semantischen" Paraphasie. In G. Drachman (Ed.), *Salzburger Beiträge zur Linguistik 1* (pp. 183–189). Tübingen: Gunter Narr.

Goldstein, K. (1948). *Language and language disturbances, Aphasic symptom complexes and their significance for medicine and theory of language.* New York: Grune & Stratton.

Goodglass, H., Gleason, J. B., Bernholtz, N. A., & Hyde, M. R. (1972). Some linguistic structures in the speech of a Broca's aphasic. *Cortex, 8*(2), 191–212.

Goodglass, H., & Kaplan, E. (1972). *The assessment of aphasia and related disorders.* Philadelphia: Lea & Febiger. (Second ed., 1983.).

Gotts, S. J., della Rocchetta, A. I., & Cipolotti, L. (2002). Mechanisms underlying perseveration in aphasia: Evidence from a single case study. *Neuropsychologia, 40*, 1641–1659.

Gotts, S. J., & Plaut, D. C. (2004). Connectionist approaches to understanding aphasic perseveration. *Seminars in Speech and Language, Perseveration in Neurogenic Communication Disorders, 25*(4), 323–334.

Gross, O. (1902). *Die Cerebrale Sekundärfunktion.* Leipzig: Vogel.

Heilbronner, K. (1895). Krankenvorstellung (Fall von "Asymbolie") *Allgemeine Zeitschrift für Psychiatrie, 51*, 1014–1015.

Heilbronner, K. (1897). Über Asymbolie. *Psychiatrische Abhandlungen, 3/4*, 1–60.

Heilbronner, K. (1906). Über Haftenbleiben und Stereotypie. *Ergänzungsheft der Monatsschrift für Psychiatrie, 18*, 293–371.

Helm Estabrooks, N., Emery, P., & Albert, M. L. (1987). Treatment of aphasic perseveration (TAP) program: A new approach to aphasia therapy. *Archives of Neurology, 44*, 1253–1255.

Hotz, G., & Helm-Estabrooks, N. (1995). Perseveration. Part 1: A review. *Brain Injury, 9*(2), 151–159.

Howard, D. (1985). Introduction to "On Agrammatism" (Ueber Agrammatismus) by Max Isserlin, 1922 (translated by H. Droller, D. Howard, & R. Campbell). *Cognitive Neuropsychology, 2*(4), 303–345.

Hudson, A. J. (1968). Perseveration. *Brain, 91*, 571–582.

Hughlings-Jackson, J. (1880). On affections of speech from disease of the brain. *Brain, 2*, 323–356.

Jasper, H. (1931). Is perseveration a functional unit participating in all behaviour processes? *Journal of Social Psychology, 2*, 28–51.

Jung, R. (1953). Allgemeine Neurophysiologie. Die Tätigkeit des Nervensystems . In G. v. Bergmann, G. W. Frey, & H. Schwiegk (Eds.), *Handbuch der Inneren Medizin, 5, Band, 1., Teil*, 1–159.

Kleist, K. (1934). *Gehirnpathologie vornehmlich auf Grund der Kriegserfahrungen.* Leipzig: J. A. Barth.

Liepmann, H. (1905). *Ueber Störungen des Handelns bei Gehirnkranken.* Berlin: Karger.

Lissauer, H. (1890). Ein Fall von Seelenblindheit nebst einem Beitrage zur Theorie derselben. *Archiv für Psychiatrie und Nervenkrankheiten, 21*, 222–270.

Luria, A. R. (1974). Language and brain: Towards the basic problems of neurolinguistics. *Brain and Language, 1*, 1–14.

Martin, N., & Dell, G. S. (2004). Perseverations and anticipations in aphasia: Primed intrusions from the past and future. *Seminars in Speech and Language, Perseveration in Neurogenic Communication Disorders*, *25*(4), 349–362.

Martin, N., & Dell, G. S. (2007). Common mechanisms underlying perseverative and non-perseverative sound and word substitutions. *Aphasiology*, *21*, 1002–1017.

Martin, N., Roach, A., Brecher, A., & Lowery, J. (1998). Lexical retrieval mechanisms underlying whole-word perseveration errors in anomic aphasia. *Aphasiology*, *12*(4/5), 319–333.

McNalty, A. (Ed.). (1961). *The British Medical Dictionary*. London: Caxton Publishing.

Meringer, R., & Mayer, K. (1895). *Versprechen und Verlesen. Eine psychologisch-linguistische Studie*. Stuttgart: Göschen.

Moen, I. (1993). Persveration in the speech of a patient with fluent anomic aphasia. *Clinical Linguistics and Phonetics*, *7*(1), 1–17.

Moses, M., Nickels, L., & Sheard, C. (2004). Disentangling the web: Neologistic perseverative errors in jargon aphasia. *Neurocase*, *10*(6), 452–461.

Müller, G. E., & Pilzecker, A. (1900). Experimentelle Beiträge zur Lehre vom Gedächtnis. *Zeitschrift für Psychologie und Physiologie der Sinnesorgane, Ergänzungsband 1*.

Neisser, C. (1895). Discussion zur Demonstration Heilbronner's in der Sitzung des Vereines ostdeutscher Irrenärzte zu Breslau den 1. Juli 1894. *Allgemeine Zeitschrift für Psychiatrie*, *51*, 1016.

Pick, A. (1892). Beiträge zur Lehre von den Störungen der Sprache. *Archiv für Psychiatrie*, *23*, 896–918.

Pick, A. (1900). Über die Bedeutung des akustischen Sprachzentrums als Hemmungsorgan des Sprachmechanismus. *Wiener Klinische Wochenschrift*, *37*, 823–827.

Pick, A. (1902). Beiträge zur Lehre von der Echolalie. *Jahrbuch für Psychiatrie und Neurologie*, *21*, 282–293.

Pick, A. (1903). Etude clinique sur les troubles de la conscience dans L'état postépileptique. *Annales médico-psychologiques*, *17*, 18–54. [Extrait: Janvier-Février, 1903: reprint of journal article used for quotation, pp. 1–37.]

Pick, A. (1906). Rückwirkung sprachlicher Perseveration auf den Assoziationsvorgang. *Zeitschrift für Psychologie und Physiologie der Sinnesorgane*, *42*, 241–257.

Pick, A. (1914). Perseveration und andere Mechanismen als Ursache agrammatischer Erscheinungen nebst Bemerkungen über die Beziehungen des "Verschreibens" zum "Versprechen". *Monatsschrift für Psychiatrie und Neurologie*, *35*, 407–420.

Pick, A. (1921). "Motorische" und "statische" Perseveration; zugleich ein Beitrag zur Lehre von den katatonem Erscheinungen. In A.Pick, Die Neurologische Forschungsrichtung in der Psychopathologie. *Abh. an dem Neurologie, Psychiatrie, und Psychologie und ihren Grenzbgebieten, Heft*, *13*, 94–141.

Pick, A. (1931). *Aphasia*. [See Rudolf Thiele: posthumous publication of Pick's article: This paper is the basis for Jason Brown's 1973 publication.]

Plaut, D. C., & Shallice, T. (1993). Perseverative and semantic influences on visual object naming errors in optic aphasia: A connectionist account. *Journal of Cognitive Neuroscience*, *5*(1), 89–117.

Poeck, K. (1978). Neurologie. *Ein Lehrbuch für Studierende und Ärzte, fünfte neu bearbeitete Auflage*. Berlin: Springer-Verlag.

Rieger, C. (1882). Über normale und kataleptische Bewegungen. *Archiv für Psychiatrie*, *13*, 427–481.

Rogers, K. (1935). Perseveration. *The Journal of Mental Science*, *81*, 138–144.

Rosenberg, M. (1912). Über gewisse Regelmäßigkeiten der Perseveration. *Zeitschrift für die gesamte Neurologie und Psychiatrie*, *8*, 123–132.

Sandson, J. (1986). *Varieties of perseveration*. Unpublished PhD Thesis, Cornell University.

Sandson, J., & Albert, M. L. (1984). Varieties of perseveration. *Neuropsychologia*, *22*(6), 715–732.

Sommer, R. (1893). Die Dyslexie als functionelle Störung. *Archiv für Psychiatrie*, *25*(3), 663–694.

Stark, J. (1984). *Verbale Perseveration bei Aphasie. Ein neurolinguistischer Ansatz*. Unpublished PhD Thesis, University of Vienna.

Stark, J. (2007). Syntax detached from semantics: Qualitative analysis of examples of verbal perseveration from a transcortical sensory aphasic patient. *Aphasiology*, *21*, 1114–1142.

Stark, J., & Dressler, W. U. (1990). Agrammatism in German: Two case studies. In L. Menn & L. K. Obler (Eds.), *Agrammatic aphasia: A cross-language narrative sourcebook* (pp. 261–441). Amsterdam: John Benjamins.

Steinthal, H. (1871). *Einleitung in die Psychologie und Sprachwissenschaft*. Berlin: Dümmler.

Teuber, H. L. (1955). Physiological psychology. *Annual Review of Psychology*, *6*, 267–296.

Teuber, H. L., & Weinstein, S. (1955). General and specific effects of cerebral lesions. *The American Psychologist*, *10*, 408–409.

Thiele, R. (1931). Aphasie von Arnold Pick. In A. Bethe, G. v. Bergmann, G. Embden, & A. Ellinger (Eds.), *Handbuch der normalen und pathologischen Physiologie, 15/2* (pp. 1416–1524). Berlin: Springer.

von Mayendorf, E. N. (1911). *Die aphasischen Symptome und ihre corticale Lokalisation*. Leipzig: Wilhelm Engelmann.

von Soelder, F. (1895). Über Perseveration. Vortrag in der Prager Wanderversammlung des Vereines für Psychiatrie und Nervenheilkunde in Wien am 5. Oktober 1895, ref. *Neurologisches Centralblatt, 14*, 958.

von Soelder, F. (1899). Über Perseveration, eine formale Störung im Vorstellungsablaufe. *Jahrbücher für Psychiatrie und Neurologie, 18*, 479–525.

Warrington, E. K., & Leff, A. P. (2000). Jargon dyslexia: A single case study of intact reading comprehension in a jargon dysphasic. *Neurocase, 6*, 499–507.

Yates, A. L. (1966). Psychological deficit. *Annual Review of Psychology, 17*, 111–144.

APHASIOLOGY, 2007, 21 (10/11), 960–974

Psychology Press
Taylor & Francis Group

Review Article

Chips, cheeks and carols: A review of recurrent perseveration in speech production

Melanie S. Moses
The University of Sydney, and Macquarie University, Sydney, Australia
Lyndsey A. Nickels
Macquarie University, Sydney, Australia
Christine Sheard
The University of Sydney, Australia

Background: Recurrent perseverative errors involve either the complete or partial repetition of a prior response to a new stimulus. They are commonly produced by speakers with aphasia and are difficult to remediate.
Aims: This paper reviews research on recurrent perseverative errors with a focus on different theoretical accounts.
Main Contribution: Comparisons are drawn between the literature on perseveration in the non-language-impaired population and in aphasia. In addition, theories that relate perseverative errors to underlying levels of language processing breakdown are described and contrasted with those that propose that they are primarily caused by impaired inhibition of recent memory traces.
Conclusions: Most recent studies have demonstrated systematic links between patterns of recurrent perseverative errors and underlying levels of language-processing breakdown in individual speakers with aphasia. For the comprehensive investigation of recurrent perseverative errors the examination of both whole word (i.e., *total*) and phonological (i.e., *blended*) perseverations is important, as is the use of case series rather than group designs.

Perseveration is the inappropriate repetition or continuation of an earlier response after a change in task requirements (Neisser, 1895), and has been observed in a wide variety of both physical and cognitive behaviours (Albert & Sandson, 1986; Helm-Estabrooks, Ramage, Bayles, & Cruz, 1998; Luria, 1965; Sandson & Albert, 1984). However, here we focus on recurrent perseveration in speech production, most commonly seen in speakers with aphasia, and illustrated in the example below. In

Address correspondence to: Dr Melanie Moses, c/o Dr Lyndsey Nickels, Macquarie Centre for Cognitive Science (MACCS), Macquarie University, Sydney, NSW 2109, Australia.
E-mail: mmoses@maccs.mq.edu.au

During the preparation of this paper, Dr Lyndsey Nickels was funded by an Australian Research Council QE2 Fellowship.

http://www.psypress.com/aphasiology DOI: 10.1080/02687030701198254

this example, Mavis, a woman with aphasia, was attempting to describe the Cookie Theft Picture from the Boston Diagnostic Aphasia Examination (Goodglass & Kaplan, 1983).

> This is a chi .. a chip, with a collar with a chee collar and this is a rack and a rack, a car and a car and a carol. What do you call that? And a carol .... and he's got a cheek and a chi chi cheek.

It is clear that this description includes unnecessary (and unwanted) repetition of sounds (e.g., ch), syllables (e.g., chi), and words (e.g., cheek, carol, rack, car): recurrent perseverative errors. What is not clear is why they occur. Furthermore, these recurrent perseverative errors are notoriously difficult to treat in aphasia language therapy (Morganstein & Certner-Smith, 2001). Hence, understanding their nature and source will potentially assist in both diagnosis and intervention approaches for people with aphasia.

Recurrent perseveration is defined as the inappropriate reproduction of a previous response following a subsequent stimulus (Sandson & Albert, 1984). A previous response may be either partially reproduced (blended perseveration) or completely reproduced (total perseveration) (Santo-Pietro & Rigrodsky, 1982), as demonstrated in Examples 1 and 2 in a picture-naming task.

Example 1

Picture 1. ball → *ball*

Picture 2. apple→ *ball (total perseveration)*

Example 2

Picture 1. book → *book*

Picture 2. car → *bar (blended perseveration)*

While perseverative errors, like non-perseverative errors, vary according to their relationship with previous responses, they also vary in their relationship to their respective targets. In Example 1, the perseverative error *ball* is identical to the preceding response, however, it is unrelated to its target, *apple* (i.e., an unrelated total perseveration). In contrast, in Example 1 *bar* is a partial perseveration of the previous response *book* and is also phonologically related to the target *car* (i.e., a phonologically related blended perseveration).

In this paper we review the literature on recurrent perseveration. First, in order to provide an understanding of how recurrent perseverative errors may be understood in terms of theories of normal language processing, we discuss studies with speakers without language impairment. This is followed by a discussion of the literature on recurrent perseverative errors produced by speakers with aphasia. A final section focuses specifically on people with jargon aphasia in whose speech output the perseveration of phonemes (blended perseveration) is particularly prominent.

RECURRENT PERSEVERATIVE ERRORS PRODUCED BY UNIMPAIRED SPEAKERS

While the production of recurrent perseverative errors has mainly been associated with people with aphasia, unimpaired speakers have also been found to produce these errors when performing language tasks, although less frequently (Buckingham, 1980; Ramage, Bayles, Helm-Estabrooks & Cruz, 1999). This suggests that studying the perseverative errors made by both populations may lead to converging evidence concerning their theoretical interpretation (Buckingham, 1980; Buckingham & Rekart, 1979). Even under favourable conditions, unimpaired speakers have been observed to produce small numbers of recurrent perseverative errors in certain language tasks. For example, Ramage et al. (1999) studied the frequency of different types of perseverative errors produced by individuals without brain impairment across different tasks (e.g., verbal definition, generative naming). The majority of recurrent perseverative errors occurred in a verbal definition task. Of the 60 participants studied, 46 produced at least one recurrent perseverative error, even though these errors accounted for only 1% of all responses across all tasks. Unimpaired speakers have been found to produce larger numbers of perseverative errors when conditions are less favourable such as when asked to name pictures prior to a deadline, or after earlier exposure to semantically related stimuli. There have been a number of different accounts of how these perseverative errors arise in the unimpaired language-processing system: one focuses on competing activation and the other on reduced language-processing efficiency. We will discuss each in turn.

Perseveration as a result of competing semantic activation

Some researchers have proposed that perseverative errors occur as a result of prior naming of semantically related items impairing subsequent naming, by competing with the target for selection. A number of studies by Vitkovitch and her colleagues found that when response deadlines were imposed, unimpaired participants sometimes perseverated on the names of semantically related pictures produced on a previous trial (Vitkovitch & Humphreys, 1991; Vitkovitch, Humphreys, & Lloyd-Jones, 1993; Vitkovitch & Rutter, 2000). For example, a picture of a donkey is named *zebra* after the participant has already named the picture of a zebra in the primed condition. Vitkovitch and Humphreys (1991) found that participants only produced perseverative errors in a picture-naming task when semantically related pictures were *named* in the prime condition. In contrast, participants did not perseverate on primes when the priming task was categorisation of semantically related pictures or reading aloud semantically related words. Vitkovitch and Humphreys (1991) hypothesised that perseverative errors are caused by increased levels of activation from primes in the links between semantics and phonology, this process being obligatory only to picture naming. They argued that this activation interferes with activation of the current target, resulting in the erroneous and perseverative selection of the prime. In studies by Vitkovitch and her colleagues (Vitkovitch & Humphreys, 1991; Vitkovitch, Kirby, & Tyrrell, 1996; Vitkovitch & Rutter, 2000) participants did not perseverate on items from the immediately preceding trial. In fact, Vitkovitch et al. (1996) found that perseverative errors only occurred after at least three intervening items. They concluded that this was due to the initial inhibition of persistent activation, which serves to prevent the immediate reselection of a prior target.

Wheeldon and Monsell (1994) demonstrated that naming semantically related primes slowed naming of a target picture presented after two intervening (unrelated) items (i.e., at a lag of 2). However, responses were slowed to a lesser degree when participants named pictures immediately preceded by the semantically related prime (i.e., at lag 0). Wheeldon and Monsell proposed that prior naming of a semantically related prime has both a facilitatory and inhibitory effect on subsequent picture naming but the time course of each effect differs. They suggested that due to overlap of conceptual features between prime and target, the semantically related prime initially facilitates production of the immediately following item. However, this facilitatory effect is very brief and rapidly decays, after which the semantically related prime actively competes and impairs the subsequent naming of a picture. While Vitkovitch and Humphreys (1991) proposed that the locus of competition from the prime is in the links between semantics and phonology, Wheeldon and Monsell (1994) proposed that the locus of the competition is more specifically at the level of lemma selection.[1] Hence, while the studies by Wheeldon and Monsell (1994) and Vitkovitch and Humphreys (1991) both found less interference from a semantically related prime at lag 0 (few perseverative errors and reduced slowing of reaction time), their accounts differed. Wheeldon and Monsell (1994) inferred an additional short-lasting facilitatory effect which "cancels out" some of the competition from the semantically related prime, while Vitkovitch and Humphreys (1991) argued for post-selection inhibition (see Dell, 1986, for a similar account).

Although the studies discussed so far have observed effects of priming by semantically related items on subsequent picture naming, a few studies have also examined these effects when participants perform other tasks (Arbuthnott, 1996; Campbell & Clark, 1989). Campbell and Clark (1989) examined a group of unimpaired participants answering multiplication problems under response deadlines. They found that participants made errors involving the reproduction of answers to preceding trials up to a lag of 10. After this, the effect (referred to as *error priming*, Campbell & Clark, 1989, p. 920) was less consistent. Campbell and Clark found that error priming from the immediately preceding trial was significantly below chance rate. Like Vitkovitch and Humphreys (1991), Campbell and Clark suggested that this was due to a short-lasting self-inhibitory effect, which counteracted the competition from previous trials to current trials, to avoid immediate reselection (see also Arbuthnott, 1996). They concluded that both competitive (referred to as *excitatory*) and self-inhibitory factors differentially influence the overall amount of activation that is received from prior trials. Like Wheeldon and Monsell (1994), Campbell and Clark (1989) proposed that the competitive influences of the prime have a differential effect on retrieval of the target over a longer lag period. They hypothesised that this process probably underlies error priming in other tasks that require retrieval from associative or semantic memory.

An automatic self-inhibitory process was also proposed by Arbuthnott (1996) to explain why unimpaired participants did not perseverate on the immediately preceding solutions to mathematical problems. Answers were facilitated (in speed

[1] Wheeldon and Monsell (1994) used the term "lemma" to refer to a level of lexical-semantic and syntactic information intervening between concepts and phonological forms (Levelt, 1989). The brief facilitatory effect was argued to be localised at a semantic level.

and accuracy) by what Arbuthnott (1996) termed a "repetition detection process" (p. 263), when problems were immediately preceded by the identical problem. However, this repetition detection process also caused participants to perseverate on immediately preceding trials that were most easily confused with repetition trials. The incidence of perseverative errors was independent of whether or not participants were aware that a repetition trial would or would not follow. This led Arbuthnott to conclude that the inhibition of perseveration was not under voluntary control. Rather, as with Campbell and Clark (1989), it was proposed that unimpaired speakers normally prevent perseverative errors by an automatic self-inhibitory process, which follows the heightened activation of a preceding target.

In summary, unimpaired speakers in general have been found to produce perseverative errors in picture naming following semantically related primes (Vitkovitch & Humphreys, 1991; Vitkovitch et al., 1993; Vitkovitch & Rutter 2000). These researchers have proposed that perseverative errors are caused by persistent activation of primed semantically related stimuli interfering with the mapping of semantic representations to the phonological form of a new target word. These studies have also suggested that the perseveration of an immediately preceding item is prevented either through transient facilitation of the target by the prime (Wheeldon & Monsell, 1994) or by automatic self-inhibition of the prime (Arbuthnott, 1996; Campbell & Clark, 1989).

Perseveration as a result of reduced language-processing efficiency

While semantically related perseverative errors have been commonly observed in priming studies, groups of unimpaired speakers have been found to produce unrelated items in speeded but un-primed conditions (e.g., 5.5% of errors, Group 2, Dell, Schwartz, Martin, Saffran, & Gagnon, 1997). Schwartz, Saffran, Bloch, and Dell (1994) elicited large numbers of perseverative and non-word errors in unimpaired participants attempting tongue twisters. However, with repeated practice, participants produced fewer perseverative and non-word errors and more non-perseverative and real-word errors, many of which were semantically related to their targets. Schwartz et al. (1994) simulated the same error pattern using Dell's (1986) computational model of word production. This was achieved by either increasing speech rate or decreasing connection strength between target nodes. Both of these manipulations were argued to simulate impaired activation of the target that is subsequently overcome by persistent activation from competing nodes. This resulted in large numbers of perseverative and non-word errors (i.e., a "bad" error pattern). Schwartz et al. (1994) simulated the practice effects observed in the tongue twister task; when the speech rate was decreased or connection strength increased, predominantly non-perseverative and real-word errors were produced (i.e., a "good" error pattern).

Priming will introduce a further source of error predisposing the system to produce perseverative errors, as the resting level of activation for previously produced items will be increased within theories of this type (Dell, 1986; Schwartz et al., 1994). However, after being selected for production, a node's level of activation is reset to zero, preventing its immediate reselection, explaining the absence of lag 0 perseverative errors in studies of unimpaired speakers. Nevertheless, due to the activation of neighbouring nodes, the node's level of activation quickly rebounds from zero as related nodes remain active (and hence re-activate the previously selected node) before gradually decaying over time. Schwartz et al. (1994) proposed that a previously selected unit is a source for perseveration in the interval after the rebound has occurred but before the excitation has died away. Although competition is said to be particularly strong in the case of semantically related words, activation from competing nodes is proposed to overcome that of target representations at any stage in word production when language-processing efficiency is compromised (Dell et al., 1997). Cohen and Dehaene (1998) also discussed how perseverative errors can occur in normal language production due to compromised language processing and normally existing amounts of persistent activation at any level of language processing. This results in perseveration of either words or phonological fragments of previous words. That activation can persist at a phonological encoding level, as at any other processing level, was also acknowledged by Levelt (1989). In contrast to proposals from priming studies, perseverative errors are argued to occur at any stage in word production where language processing is compromised, enabling normally existing amounts of persisting activation to overcome that of a weakened target representation (Cohen & Dehaene, 1998; Dell, 1986, Dell et al., 1997).

Consistent with these accounts, Moses, Nickels, and Sheard (2004a) elicited perseverative errors in 44 unimpaired participants in reading aloud and picture naming under speeded response deadlines. Different patterns of perseverative errors were produced across these tasks, reflecting each task's language-processing demands and the overall patterns of non-perseverative errors produced in each task. Moses et al. found that the majority of non-perseverative and perseverative errors produced in picture naming were semantically related to their targets, reflecting lexical processing difficulties. In contrast, in reading aloud most non-perseverative and perseverative errors were phonologically related to their targets, reflecting phonological encoding difficulties. It was also found that participants produced greater proportions of perseverative relative to non-perseverative errors in picture naming, the task eliciting most errors overall compared to reading aloud. Moses et al. (2004a) argued that the perseverative errors reflected both the level and degree to which language-processing efficiency was compromised by the response deadline in each task. They argued that the role of semantics in the production of perseverative errors has previously been overestimated, proposing that future studies should attempt to induce various levels of language-processing impairment to more accurately reflect the variety of impairment seen in speakers with aphasia.

Summary of two theoretical accounts

There are two different theoretical accounts of the cause of perseverative errors in unimpaired speakers. The *competing activation account* proposes that perseverative errors occur when naming of a picture is disrupted by activation of semantically related primes at lags greater than 0 (e.g., Vitkovitch & Humphreys, 1991; Vitkovitch et al., 1993; Wheeldon & Monsell, 1994). Studies from this perspective have maintained that the source of perseverative errors is in the mapping of the semantic representation to the phonological form of the word. In contrast, proponents of the *reduced language-processing efficiency account* maintain that perseverative errors can occur when language-processing efficiency is compromised at any processing level. This results in previously activated competitors reaching threshold before that of the target. In these studies, perseverative errors have been elicited by compromising language-processing efficiency through the use of fast response deadlines, rather than by manipulating priming conditions.

RECURRENT PERSEVERATIVE ERRORS PRODUCED BY PEOPLE WITH APHASIA

As with research on unimpaired speakers, there is debate in the literature as to the underlying cause of perseverative errors in speakers with aphasia. A number of studies have proposed that perseverative errors in aphasia result directly from failure to subconsciously inhibit prior activation of short-term memory (Allison, 1967; Hudson, 1969; Papagno & Basso, 1996; Sandson & Albert, 1984; Santo-Pietro & Rigrodsky, 1986; Yamadori, 1981). Yamadori (1981) suggested that perseverative errors could be explained in terms of "a slip of irrelevant (short-term) memory trace" (p. 594). Similarly, Santo-Pietro and Rigrodsky (1986) argued that perseveration occurs when previously retrieved items remain in working memory as stimulus traces that subsequently interfere with the ability to retrieve a new response from long-term memory.

Also consistent with an inhibitory cause of perseverative errors, Wepman (1972) proposed that perseverative errors occur when attentional capacities are compromised. In what he termed his "shutter principle" Wepman (1972) proposed that perseveration occurs as a result of the mind "shutting off" while the individual selects and formulates a response to a particular stimulus. Wepman (1972) claimed when a subsequent stimulus is presented, the person erroneously reproduces a response to the earlier stimulus that was activated while the shutter was open. However, there may be a number of problems with Wepman's "shutter principle". First, it does not appear to account for perseverative errors over a longer duration. Second, this theory cannot explain the perseveration of previous responses (as opposed to stimuli), as after responding to a previous item, the shutter should in theory have reopened.

In summary, these studies have proposed that perseverative errors occur primarily due to a failure to inhibit activation. From this perspective, although they frequently coexist, perseverative errors can be considered to occur relatively independently of language impairment associated with aphasia. In line with this account, Helm-Estabrooks, Emery, and Albert (1987) proposed a programme that, using principles of behaviour modification, aims specifically to reduce the production of perseverative errors in people with aphasia in the hope that language performance will subsequently improve.[2] By aiming to specifically treat the perseverative errors, this programme appears to support the inhibition account that perseverative errors are independent from other aspects of language processing.

More recently, research has demonstrated a probable link between the incidence of perseveration and the severity of aphasia; for example, Albert and Sandson (1986) and Sandson and Albert (1987) found that participants' scores on a confrontation naming task were negatively correlated with the number of perseverative errors. Hence they suggested that perhaps perseverative errors are triggered by disruption in the naming process. Similarly, Helm-Estabrooks et al. (1998) found that aphasia severity was positively correlated with incidence of perseverative errors in their group

[2] While claiming that the programme is designed to manipulate factors known to induce perseveration, the tasks used appear similar to those used to reduce other aphasic errors, e.g., a cueing hierarchy.

of participants with aphasia. Consequently, this has led to further investigation of the language conditions under which more or fewer perseverative errors occur. However, research findings remain inconsistent as to which language conditions precipitate perseveration. Some research has also shown that people with aphasia tend to produce more perseverative errors when performing complex and spontaneous tasks (e.g., naming an object), than on less complex and more automatic tasks, (e.g., repeating a spoken word or counting) (Helmick & Berg, 1976; Hudson, 1969; Santo-Pietro & Rigrodsky, 1982). Further research has shown that perseveration is more likely to occur when the response required is more predictable or constrained (e.g., picture naming) (Albert & Sandson, 1986). In contrast, other research has demonstrated that participants tend to produce more perseverative errors on tasks where a range of response options are possible (e.g., word list generation) (Papagno & Basso, 1996).

As discussed for unimpaired speakers, speakers with aphasia have also been found to produce more perseverative errors when response deadlines are imposed. Santo-Pietro and Rigrodsky (1982) showed that when time intervals between stimulus items were increased, the incidence of perseveration significantly decreased. In contrast, other types of errors were not influenced by the time between presentations of stimuli. Santo-Pietro and Rigrodksy (1982) discussed how in therapy settings, clinicians often increase the time between consecutive stimulus items to attempt to reduce their clients' tendency to perseverate.

Studies in aphasia have also suggested that semantic processing has a critical role in the production of perseverative errors. Both Albert and Sandson (1986) and Sandson and Albert (1987) found that the majority of recurrent perseverative errors that their participants with aphasia produced in picture naming were semantically related to the target. They proposed that prior responses that are semantically related to current targets are likely to be reactivated when access to a target is unsuccessful. This was believed to result from increased spreading activation from the previous targets to new semantically related targets. Santo-Pietro and Rigrodsky (1982) found that their 31 participants produced more perseverative errors when asked to name pictured items from their "semantically difficult" word list than from their "semantically easy" word list. However, the fact that semantic difficulty was determined according to frequency counts, suggests that other factors such as availability of the phonological form of the word may also have played a role.

Conditions under which most perseverative errors are produced therefore remain unclear. Despite having shown that different language tasks may elicit either more or fewer perseverative errors than others, many of these studies have reported group trends alone. Further, participants have mostly been grouped according to traditional aphasia syndrome classifications (e.g., Wernicke's and Broca's), providing limited insight into the systematic nature of perseverative error patterns specific to an individual's language-processing profile. (e.g., Helm-Estabrooks et al., 1998; Helmick & Berg, 1976; Hotz & Helm-Estabrooks, 1995; Sandson & Albert, 1987; Santo-Pietro & Rigrodsky, 1986; Yamadori, 1981). By examining group trends alone, only general links could be made regarding the presumed degree of language difficulty in a particular task and its subsequent impact on the production of perseverative errors. This inevitably limits the depth of analysis that can be performed, because within a traditional classification level, language profiles of people with aphasia are not homogeneous.

Current cognitive neuropsychological approaches to language processing emphasise the need to examine each individual's level of language processing breakdown rather than to group individuals on the basis of syndrome behaviours (Saffran, 1982). Important and detailed information may be derived from examining perseverative error patterns of a series of individuals with aphasia, which would more easily determine whether perseverative errors patterns are systematically linked to the level and degree of language processing breakdown.

Systematic links with underlying levels of language-processing breakdown

Recent research within a cognitive neuropsychological framework has begun to more specifically explore the linguistic influences on perseverative errors in individuals with differing levels of language-processing breakdown. There is a small but emerging body of evidence that, as with other types of aphasic errors, the perseverative errors made by people with aphasia reflect their underlying information-processing breakdown. Cohen and Dehaene (1998) demonstrated that different functional levels of language breakdown may be responsible for perseveration in aphasia. The incidence and types of perseverative errors produced by three participants with various levels of language impairment was examined across various language tasks. Perseverative errors were produced by each individual only on tasks that reflected their language-processing difficulties.

Participants produced either whole word (*total*) or phonological (*blended*) perseverations according to their individual levels of language-processing breakdown. For example, participant D.U.M. produced predominantly neologistic *blended* perseverative errors when reading aloud both real and non-words but not when naming pictures. On the basis of his error types, Cohen and Dehaene (1998) concluded that the locus of D.U.M.'s language processing breakdown was in the sublexical grapheme to phoneme route, common to both real and non-word reading aloud, but not used in picture naming. In contrast, another participant, R.A.V., produced whole word (*total*) perseverations in both picture naming and reading aloud, suggesting that the process of retrieving the lexical form was impaired. Cohen and Dehaene (1998) concluded that perseverative errors do not operate independently of language, but rather both their presence and type (i.e., whole word or phonological) are directly influenced by the processing demands of the task, as are non-perseverative errors. They proposed that two components are vital for the occurrence of perseverative errors: (1) weakened representation of a stimulus at any given processing level in addition to (2) normally existing persistent activation from previous responses. This clearly parallels the *reduced language-processing efficiency* account of perseverative errors proposed for unimpaired speakers, discussed earlier.

In line with this account, Moses, Nickels, and Sheard (2007 this issue) argued that the types of perseverative errors produced by their five aphasic participants reflected the level at which language processing was impaired for each participant in repetition, reading aloud, and picture-naming tasks. Evidence for this was first that similar distributions of lexical and non-lexical perseverative and non-perseverative errors were produced in each task, and second, the relative distribution of total and blended perseverative errors reflected the level at which language processing was most impaired. Moses et al. (2004a) reported similar trends in that their 44 unimpaired participants produced mainly total perseverations in a picture naming, reflecting compromised lexical-semantic processing, and produced mainly blended perseverations in a reading aloud task, reflecting compromised phonological encoding. While the patterns of *total* and *blended* perseverative errors were argued to reflect the level at which language processing is impaired, Moses, Nickels, and Sheard (2004b) argued that the binary coding of *total* versus *blended* perseveration may be overly simplistic (see below for further discussion of this study).

Martin, Roach, Brecher, and Lowery (1998) provided further evidence of a systematic link between perseverative errors and individual levels of language-processing breakdown. These researchers found that for their three participants with aphasia, subtypes of perseverative and non-perseverative lexical errors produced in a picture-naming task (i.e., mixed, semantic, formal, or unrelated errors) showed similar distributions. They concluded that perseverative errors are (at least partly) under similar influences to non-perseverative errors. Coming from a connectionist perspective, Martin et al. (1998) also concluded that perseverations are not solely due to activation from prior responses. Like Cohen and Dehaene (1998), they proposed that these errors appear to result from a combination of increased activation of words recently spoken (due to priming) and weak activation of the current intended utterance arising at any level of lexical representation.[3] Further evidence that perseverative errors can arise at various processing levels is the single case study by Hirsh (1998), who examined the perseverative error patterns produced by CJ, her participant with aphasia, in picture naming and reading aloud tasks. As targets eliciting the same perseverative errors were often semantically related, Hirsh (1998) suggested that CJ's perseverative errors were partly caused by difficulties arising in the mapping of semantics to the phonological form of the word, as proposed by Vitkovitch and Humphreys (1991). However, as many targets eliciting the same perseverative response by CJ were also phonologically related, Hirsh (1998) argued that phonological relatedness also plays a significant role in the production of perseverative errors. Both Hirsh (1998) and Moses et al. (2007 this issue) challenged Vitkovitch and Humphreys' (1991) theory on the grounds that it could not explain why their participants produced entire reproductions of prior neologisms, which are not represented at a lexical level. Although not specifically discussed, Hirsh (1998) also reported that the majority of CJ's perseverative errors were unrelated to the target, further suggesting that they arose at a processing level other than the mapping of semantics to phonology. By examining perseverative error patterns of individuals with aphasia, these studies (while of only a few individuals) have proposed that perseverative errors can arise at various processing levels as a result of underlying language impairment. This challenges theories that perseverative errors are solely caused by interference from primed competitors in the mapping between semantics and phonology (see earlier discussion of studies by Vitkovitch and colleagues and Wheeldon & Monsell, 1994).

Summary

Early accounts proposed that perseveration in aphasia was primarily caused by a problem inhibiting prior activation, irrespective of task or modalities. However, there is a growing body of literature providing evidence of more specific links to

[3] As Martin et al. (1998) only examined lexical errors, their conclusions are limited to levels of lexical representation.

language and underlying levels of language-processing breakdown. Recent studies have proposed that two vital components are required for perseverative errors to occur: (1) decreased activation of target lexical items resulting in (2) persistent activation from previously activated responses (e.g., Cohen & Dehaene, 1998; Martin et al., 1998). This theoretical account is most consistent with the *language-processing efficiency* account proposed to explain the production of perseverative errors in unimpaired speakers.

Cohen and Dehaene (1998) and Moses et al. (2007 this issue) proposed not only that the production of perseverations can be accounted for by the underlying language impairment, but also that conversely an examination of perseverative patterns of individual speakers with aphasia can assist clinicians in delineating underlying language deficits. In contrast to the treatment programme by Helm-Estabrooks et al. (1987), discussed earlier, Cohen and Dehaene (1998) suggested that by treating the specific language deficit itself there might be a corresponding reduction in perseveration, although they acknowledged the need for further studies to verify this proposal (see also Moses, Nickels, & Sheard, 2004c).

IMPORTANCE OF STUDYING *BLENDED* PERSEVERATIVE ERRORS

Cohen and Dehaene (1998) proposed that important information can be derived about an individual's language-processing breakdown from examining the full range of *blended* (including isolated phonemes) as well as *total* perseverative errors. However, *blended* perseverative errors have rarely been examined extensively, systematically, and across a variety of participants with different levels of language-processing impairment. Research has largely focused on *total* perseverations of whole words to the exclusion of *blended* perseverative errors (e.g., Helmick & Berg, 1976; Martin et al., 1998). Many studies do not even state how perseverative errors were coded, or discriminate between different types, making clear interpretation or replication of these studies difficult (e.g., Halpern, 1965; Hudson, 1969; Papagno & Basso, 1996). While some researchers have acknowledged the presence of *blended* perseverative errors (e.g., Allison & Hurwitz, 1967; Hudson, 1969; Martin et al., 1998), only a few have analysed these in any detail (e.g., Buckingham, 1985; Buckingham, Whitaker & Whitaker, 1978, 1979; Cohen & Dehaene, 1998; Hirsh, 1998; Santo-Pietro & Rigrodsky, 1982, 1986).[4]

The study of blended perseverative errors is particularly important in understanding the nature of neologistic errors, which typically characterise the language of people with jargon aphasia (Buckingham, 1987; Buckingham et al., 1978, 1979; Butterworth, 1992; Schwartz et al., 1994). In fact, most previous examination of blended perseverative errors has come from research on this population. Speakers with neologistic jargon aphasia have been frequently observed to perseverate on individual sounds or syllables from previous words or responses (e.g., Buckingham, 1985; Buckingham & Christman, 2004; Buckingham et al., 1978, 1979; Butterworth, 1979, 1992; Moses et al., 2004b; Schwartz et al., 1994). In previous sections of this

[4] The work of Buckingham and colleagues (e.g., Buckingham, 1985; Buckingham & Christman, 1996, 2004; Buckingham et al., 1978) has also examined the phonetic and stress properties of blended perseverative errors, providing valuable insight into the nature of the structure of the syllable and morphological processing. However, further discussion of these advances is beyond the scope of this paper.

review, these errors have been referred to as *blended* perseverative errors, consistent with research conducted by Santo-Pietro and Rigrodsky (1982, 1986). The exclusion of *blended* perseverations in previous studies has, no doubt, been partly due to the difficulty in defining and tracing the source of these errors, which is often less obvious than in the case of *total* perseverative errors (Martin et al., 1998). While advocating for their inclusion in analysis, Cohen and Dehaene (1998) recognised that the identification of *blended* perseverative errors may not always be evident on subjective inspection of the data. However, in an attempt to produce a detailed and rigorous analysis of the *blended* perseverative errors produced by their group of participants, Santo-Pietro and Rigrodsky (1982) used strict coding criteria shown below (Santo-Pietro & Rigrodsky, 1982, p. 187):

a) Initial consonant repetition occurring within 5 responses of the original utterance
b) Final consonant repetition occurring within 3 responses of the original
c) Vowel repetition occurring on the consecutive responses.

Santo-Pietro and Rigrodsky (1986) compared proportions of *total* and *blended* perseverative errors across three language tasks and found that, as a group, their participants produced similar proportions of *total* and *blended* perseverative errors in sentence completion and word reading, but significantly more *total* than *blended* perseverative errors in picture naming. Despite their attention to coding and reporting these differences, they did not provide possible explanations for this difference and no individual error patterns were analysed. In studies by Moses and colleagues (e.g., Moses et al., 2004a, 2004b, 2007 this issue), Santo-Pietro and Rigrodsky's (1982) stringent criteria for coding perseverative errors were adopted to minimise the false positive identification of perseverative errors. In each of these studies, Moses et al. have strongly advocated for the inclusion of both total and blended perseverative errors for comprehensive analysis of a speaker's underlying language-processing impairment. In their examination of neologisms produced by KVH, a man with neologistic jargon aphasia, Moses et al. (2004b) found that many of his neologisms contained phonemes perseverated from previous neologisms, and argued that there is an integral relationship between the production of neologisms and the perseveration of phonemes for speakers with jargon aphasia. Furthermore, while KVH's patterns of whole word (*total)* and phonological (*blended*) perseverations reflected his underlying language-processing impairment, the simple binary distinction of *total* and *blended* perseveration was found to be overly simplified for understanding the underlying nature of KVH's complex neologistic errors and further subdivisions of each error type were proposed.

Also recognising the need to adopt stringent coding criteria, Hirsh (1998) coded responses as blended perseverative errors (referred to as perseverations of subword segments) only if they shared 50% of phonemes (in approximately the same order) in common with a previous response. Martin et al. (1998) only analysed whole word (*total*) lexical perseverative errors, as their study examined the lexical influences on recurrent perseverative errors. However, they reported that one of their participants, W.R. with Wernicke's aphasia, produced "numerous neologistic blended perseverations" (N. Martin, personal communication, 7 February 2006). Martin et al. (1998) excluded W.R.'s blended perseverative errors on the basis that their source was too difficult to trace. Nevertheless, they acknowledged the value of investigating these errors further in future studies.

In summary, a few studies have attempted to quantitatively analyse the blended perseverative errors produced by speakers with aphasia, enabling more comprehensive investigation of the relationship between perseveration and underlying language-processing breakdown (e.g., Cohen & Dehane, 1998; Hirsh, 1998; Moses et al., 2004a, 2004b, 2007 this issue; Santo-Pietro & Rigrodsky, 1982, 1986). While it is recognised that coding of blended perseverations may potentially be arbitrary, exclusion of these errors from analysis is problematic, as valuable data may clearly be lost. Further attempts to include *blended* perseverative errors, particularly in the analysis of speakers with jargon aphasia, should clearly be pursued.

CONCLUSION AND FUTURE DIRECTIONS

There is growing evidence that perseverative errors are linked with the degree and type of language impairment in aphasia. However, this relationship may not be as straightforward as initially proposed and is dependent on the examination of both *total* and *blended* perseverative errors. Only by including both perseverative error types can we have a truly comprehensive investigation of the relationship between perseverative and non-perseverative errors. The integral relationship between the production of neologisms and the perseveration of phonemes must also be recognised in attempting to understand the underlying nature of neologistic jargon aphasia. Clearly, we need more studies that systematically analyse the nature of perseverative errors. These analyses require use of a wide range of tasks that tap into different levels of language processing and comparison across a series of individuals with aphasia. Such analyses will continue to pave the way for a more detailed understanding of the nature of perseverative errors and the factors that influence their occurrence in speakers with aphasia.

As perseveration is a significantly disabling communication deficit in people with aphasia and is not readily changed by therapy (Morganstein & Certner-Smith, 2001), increased knowledge of the underlying nature of this deficit is essential to developing efficacious therapy techniques. Recent studies suggest that the identification and coding of perseverative errors may help clinicians profile an individual's language-processing breakdown, which may provide directions for treatment (Cohen & Dehaene, 1998). In this vein, rather than treating perseverative errors in isolation, perhaps treatment programmes should aim to remediate the underlying language impairment of which perseveration is symptomatic (see Moses et al., 2004c for further discussion). More intricate and systematic analysis of these problematic and somewhat resilient perseverative errors will clearly assist researchers and clinicians in both their assessment and ultimately their treatment of the disabling communication disorder that is aphasia.

REFERENCES

Albert, M. L., & Sandson, J. (1986). Perseveration in aphasia. *Cortex*, *22*, 103–115.

Allison, R. S., & Hurwitz, L. J. (1967). On perseveration in aphasics. *Brain*, *90*, 429–448.

Arbuthnott, K. D. (1996). To repeat or not to repeat: Repetition facilitation and inhibition in sequential retrieval. *Journal of Experimental Psychology: General*, *125*, 261–283.

Buckingham, H. W. Jr. (1980). On correlating aphasic errors with slips of the tongue. *Applied Linguistics*, *1*, 199–220.

Buckingham, H. W. (1985). Perseveration in aphasia. In S. Newman & R. Epstein (Eds.), *Current perspectives in dysphasia* (pp. 113–154). Edinburgh, UK: Churchill Livingston.

Buckingham, H. W. (1987). Phonemic paraphasias and psycholinguistic production models for neologistic jargon. *Aphasiology*, *1*, 381–400.

Buckingham, H. W., & Christman, S. S. (1996). Perseverative blends and splicing: Evidence for theories of syllable constituency. *Brain and Cognition*, *32*, 323–325.

Buckingham, H. W., & Christman, S. S. (2004). Phonemic carryover perseveration: Word blends. *Seminars in Speech and Language*, *25*(4), 363–373.

Buckingham, H. W. Jr., & Rekart, D. (1979). Semantic paraphasia. *Journal of Communication Disorders*, *12*, 197–209.

Buckingham, H. W. Jr., Whitaker, H. A., & Whitaker, H. A. (1978). Alliteration and assonance in neologistic jargon aphasia. *Cortex*, *14*, 365–380.

Buckingham, H. W. Jr., Whitaker, H. A., & Whitaker, H. A. (1979). On linguistic perseveration. In H. Whitaker & H. A. Whitaker (Eds.), *Studies in neurolinguistics* (Vol. 4, pp.329–352). New York: Academic Press.

Butterworth, B. (1979). Hesitation and the production of verbal paraphasias and neologisms in jargon aphasia. *Brain and Language*, *8*, 133–161.

Butterworth, B. (1992). Disorders of phonological encoding. *Cognition*, *42*, 261–286.

Campbell, J. I., & Clark, J. M. (1989). Time course of error priming in number-fact retrieval: Evidence for excitatory and inhibitory mechanisms. *Journal of Experimental Psychology: Learning, Memory and Cognition*, *15*, 920–929.

Cohen, L., & Dehaene, S. (1998). Competition between past and present: Assessment and interpretation of verbal perseverations. *Brain*, *121*, 1641–1659.

Dell, G. S. (1986). A spreading activation theory of retrieval in sentence production. *Psychological Review*, *93*, 283–321.

Dell, G. S., Schwartz, M. F., Martin, N., Saffran, E. M., & Gagnon, D. (1997). Lexical access in aphasic and nonaphasic speakers, *Psychological Review*, *104*, 801–838.

Goodglass, H., & Kaplan, E. (1983). *The assessment of aphasia and related disorders* (2nd ed.). Philadelphia: Lea & Febiger.

Halpern, H. (1965). Effect of stimulus variables on verbal perseverations of dysphasic subjects. *Perceptual and Motor Skills*, *20*, 421–429.

Helm-Esterbrooks, N., Emery, P., & Albert, M. L. (1987). Treatment of Aphasic Perseveration (TAP) program. A new approach to aphasia therapy. *Archives of Neurology*, *44*, 1253–1255.

Helm-Estabrooks, N., Ramage, A., Bayles, K. A., & Cruz, R. (1998). Perseverative behaviour in fluent and non-fluent aphasia. *Aphasiology*, *12*, 7–8.

Helmick, J. W., & Berg, C. B. (1976). Perseveration in brain-injured adults. *Journal of Communication Disorders*, *9*, 143–156.

Hirsh, K. W. (1998). Perseveration and activation in aphasic speech production. *Cognitive Neuropsychology*, *15*, 377–388.

Hotz, G., & Helm-Estabrooks, N. (1995). Perseveration. Part I: A review. *Brain Injury*, *9*, 151–159.

Hudson, A. J. (1969). Perseveration. *Brain*, *91*, 571–582.

Levelt, W. J. (1989). *Speaking: From intention to articulation*. Cambridge, MA: MIT Press.

Luria, A. R. (1965). Two kinds of motor perseveration in massive injury of the frontal lobes. *Brain*, *88*, 1–12.

Martin, N., Roach, A., Brecher, A., & Lowery, J. (1998). Lexical retrieval mechanisms underlying whole-word perseveration errors in anomic aphasia. *Aphasiology*, *12*, 319–333.

Morganstein, S., & Certner-Smith, M. (2001). Thematic language stimulation therapy. In R. Chapey (Ed.), *Language intervention strategies in aphasia and related language disorders* (4th ed., pp. 383–396). Philadelphia: Lippincott, Williams & Wilkins.

Moses, M. S., Nickels, L. A., & Sheard, C. (2004a). "I'm sitting here feeling aphasic!" A study of recurrent perseverative errors elicited in unimpaired speakers". *Brain and Language*, *89*, 157–173.

Moses, M. S., Nickels, L. A., & Sheard, C. (2004b). Disentangling the web: Neologistic perseverative errors in jargon aphasia. *Neurocase*, *10*(6), 1–10.

Moses, M. S., Nickels, L. A., & Sheard, C. (2004c). That dreaded word *perseveration*. Understanding might be the key. *Australian Communication Quarterly*, *6*(2), 70–74.

Moses, M. S., Sheard, C., & Nickels, L. A. (2007). Insights into recurrent perseverative errors in aphasia. A case series approach. *Aphasiology*, *21*, 975–1001.

Neisser, A. (1895). Krankenvorstellung (Fall von 'Asymbolie'). *Allgemeine Zeitschrift Für Psychiatrie*, *51*, 1016–1021.

Papagno, C., & Basso, A. (1996). Perseveration in two aphasic patients. *Cortex*, *32*, 67–82.

Ramage, A., Bayles, R., Helm-Estabrooks, N., & Cruz, R. (1999). Frequency of perseveration in normal subjects. *Brain and Language*, *66*, 329–340.

Saffran, E. M. (1982). Neuropsychological approaches to the study of language. *British Journal of Psychology*, *73*, 317–337.

Sandson, J., & Albert, M. L. (1984). Varieties of perseveration. *Neuropsychologia*, *22*, 715–732.

Sandson, J., & Albert, M. L. (1987). Perseveration in behavioural neurology, *Neurology*, *37*, 1736–1741.

Santo-Pietro, M. J., & Rigrodsky, S. (1982). The effects of temporal and semantic conditions on the occurrence of the error response of perseveration in adult aphasics. *Journal of Speech and Hearing Research*, *25*, 184–192.

Santo-Pietro, M. J., & Rigrodsky, S. (1986). Patterns of oral-verbal perseveration in adult aphasia. *Brain and Language*, *29*, 1–17.

Schwartz, M. F., Saffran, E. M., Bloch, D. E., & Dell, G. (1994). Disordered speech production in aphasic and normal speakers. *Brain and Language*, *47*, 52–88.

Vitkovitch, M., & Humphreys, G. W. (1991). Perseverant responding in speeded naming of pictures: It's in the links. *Journal of Experimental Psychology: Learning, Memory and Cognition*, *17*, 664–680.

Vitkovitch, M., Humphreys, G. W., & Lloyd-Jones, T. (1993). On naming a giraffe a zebra: Picture naming errors across different object categories. *Journal of Experimental Psychology: Learning, Memory and Cognition*, *19*, 243–259.

Vitkovitch, M., Kirby, A., & Tyrrell, L. (1996). Patterns of excitation and inhibition in picture naming. *Visual Cognition*, *3*, 61–80.

Vitkovitch, M., & Rutter, C. (2000). The effects of response stimuli interval on error priming in sequential object naming. *Visual Cognition*, *7*, 645–670.

Wepman, J. M. (1972). Aphasia therapy: A new look. *Journal of Speech and Hearing Disorders*, *37*, 203–214.

Wheeldon, L. R., & Monsell, S. (1994). Inhibition of spoken word production by priming a semantic competitor. *Journal of Memory and Language*, *33*, 332–356.

Yamadori, A. (1981). Verbal Perseveration in aphasia, *Neuropsychologia*, *19*, 591–594.

APHASIOLOGY, 2007, 21 (10/11), 975–1001

Psychology Press
Taylor & Francis Group

Insights into recurrent perseverative errors in aphasia: A case series approach

Melanie S. Moses

The University of Sydney and Macquarie University, Sydney, Australia

Christine Sheard

The University of Sydney, Australia

Lyndsey A. Nickels

Macquarie University, Sydney, Australia

Background: Recurrent perseverative errors are most commonly produced by speakers with aphasia (Albert & Sandson, 1986). While some research has proposed that recurrent perseverative errors are primarily caused by an impaired ability to inhibit a prior response, most recent research proposes that these errors occur as a direct result of underlying language impairment at any specified processing level (e.g., Cohen & Dehaene, 1998).

Aims: This investigation was designed to further explore the hypothesis that the type of recurrent perseverative errors produced reflects the level of language-processing breakdown. Two specific questions were addressed: (1) Is the distribution of types of perseverative error similar to that of non-perseverative errors within different language tasks? (2) Do the relative proportions of *total* and *blended* perseverative errors reflect an individual's language-processing profile?

Methods & Procedures: The recurrent perseverative error patterns of five individuals with aphasia with varying levels of language-processing breakdown were examined across three language tasks (repetition, reading aloud, and picture naming).

Outcomes & Results: The incidence of different types of recurrent perseverative errors was found to be influenced by the processing demands of individual tasks, relative to each participant's language-processing breakdown. However, certain findings challenged current theories, such as the large proportion of perseverative errors that were unrelated to their targets and some participants' entire reproduction of prior neologisms across different responses. Different theoretical accounts are explored to attempt to understand these error patterns.

Conclusions: This study supports theories proposing that recurrent perseverative errors are a direct result of underlying language-processing breakdown in aphasia (Cohen & Dehaene, 1998; Martin, Roach, Brecher, & Lowery, 1998). It is argued that examination

Address correspondence to: Dr Melanie Moses, c/o Dr Lyndsey Nickels, Macquarie Centre for Cognitive Science (MACCS), Macquarie University, Sydney, NSW 2109, Australia.
E-mail: mmoses@maccs.mq.edu.au

We would like to thank KCC, KVH, DRS, SMM, and TOW, the participants with aphasia, for their enthusiasm and hours of hard work. Thank you to the War Memorial Hospital and the Royal Rehabilitation Centre Sydney for allowing us to use clients from their centres. Finally, we would also like to thank Professor David Howard for his statistical support. During the preparation of this paper, Dr Lyndsey Nickels was funded by an Australian Research Council QE2 Fellowship.

http://www.psypress.com/aphasiology DOI: 10.1080/02687030701198312

of both whole word (*total*) and phoneme (*blended*) perseverative errors is necessary for a comprehensive analysis of the proposed relationship between perseveration and language-processing impairment.

One of the persistent problems associated with aphasia is the phenomenon of recurrent perseveration, which involves the inappropriate involuntary partial or complete repetition of an earlier response following a subsequent stimulus (Helm-Estabrooks, Ramage, Bayles, & Cruz, 1998; Sandson & Albert, 1984).[1] Recurrent perseveration presents as a significant barrier to the remediation of aphasia and contributes greatly to the overall resulting communicative disability. Therefore increased knowledge of the underlying nature of perseverative errors will assist clinicians in their treatment of this problematic symptom.

Perseverative errors may involve the reproduction of either an entire response or of a single or multiple phonemes from an earlier response. Santo-Pietro and Rigrodsky (1982) labelled these different perseverative errors as *total* and *blended* perseverative errors respectively and will be referred to as such throughout this paper. Some research asserts a primary inhibitory cause for recurrent perseveration (e.g., Allison, 1966; Hudson, 1968; Papagno & Basso, 1996; Santo-Pietro & Rigrodsky, 1986; Yamadori, 1981), where earlier responses are thought to actively inhibit later attempts. However, there is growing evidence that perseverative errors are specifically linked to underlying levels of language-processing breakdown (e.g., Cohen & Dehaene, 1998; Hirsh, 1998; Martin et al., 1998). For example, in a study of three aphasic individuals Cohen and Dehaene (1998) found that perseverative errors were produced only on tasks that reflected each individual's language-processing difficulties. Moreover, the type of perseveration produced also reflected the level of language impairment: whole-word (total) perseverations occurred with impaired lexical retrieval and phonological (blended) perseverations with phonological impairment. Cohen and Dehaene (1998) proposed that two components are vital for the occurrence of perseverative errors: (1) weakened representation of a stimulus at any given processing level, and (2) normally existing persistent activation from previous responses.

Similarly, Martin et al. (1998) argued that perseverative errors reflected level of impairment. However, rather than examining the relationship of the error to its source (i.e., total vs blended), they examined the nature of the relationship between the error and the target. For example, are error and target semantically related, phonologically related, or unrelated? When they compared target–error relationships across perseverative and non-perseverative errors produced on a picture-naming task, they found that their three participants produced similar distributions of errors. However, Martin et al. restricted their analysis to lexical errors and total perseverations, excluding blended perseverative errors. We would argue that in order to fully evaluate the hypothesis that perseverative errors reflect language-processing impairment, both total and blended perseverations must be included. Nevertheless, there is a bias in the literature towards examining total perseverations alone and excluding blended perseverations (e.g., Helmick & Berg, 1976, Martin et al., 1998). Although the coding of blended perseverations can be arbitrary, a

[1] From this point forward, we use the term *perseverative errors* to refer to recurrent perseverative errors.

limited number of studies have adopted stringent coding criteria (e.g., Cohen & Dehaene, 1998; Hirsh, 1998; Moses, Nickels, & Sheard, 2004b; Santo-Pietro & Rigrodsky, 1982, 1986). Moses, Nickels, and Sheard (2004a, 2004b) argued that the examination of blended perseverative errors is particularly important when studying speech production in people with jargon aphasia, for whom these errors are particularly prominent (see also Buckingham, 1985; Buckingham, Whitaker, & Whitaker, 1978, 1979; Butterworth, 1979). Unless both types of perseverative errors are investigated, our understanding of how perseverative errors reflect different levels of language-processing breakdown is necessarily limited.

As the underlying linguistic nature and cause of recurrent perseverative errors remain largely unexplored, this study conducts a systematic analysis of both whole-word (*total*) and phoneme (*blended*) perseverative errors across a range of speech production tasks. Specifically, we test the hypothesis that the patterns of perseverative errors produced will reflect the language-processing profiles rather than being the consequence of a separate cognitive mechanism operating independently of language. Testing this hypothesis requires the examination of the relationship between language-processing impairment, task requirements, and type of perseverative error. In order to do this, it is not sufficient that this is examined in a single case, or by averaging across a group: only a case series will provide the necessary evidence. This detailed and systematic analysis of these problematic and resilient errors should assist in both the assessment and ultimately the treatment of recurrent perseverative errors in the clinical setting.

We address two specific questions in different analyses with a case series of individuals with aphasia.

1. *Is the distribution of types of perseverative error similar to that of non-perseverative errors within different language tasks?*

In other words, is the relationship of the error to the target similar across perseverative and non-perseverative errors? If similar distributions of error types are found, this supports the hypothesis that perseverative errors reflect underlying language-processing breakdown.

2. *Do the relative proportions of total and blended perseverative errors reflect an individual's language-processing profile?*

Cohen and Dehaene's (1998) account predicts that more *blended* perseverative errors will occur with phonological-level impairment and more *total* perseverative errors with semantic- and/or lexical-level breakdown. This analysis examines how far these predictions hold.

METHOD

Participants

The perseverative patterns of five individuals with aphasia are presented. All had aphasia resulting from acquired neurological damage. All were monolingual English speakers with no prior language impairment, were medically stable, and at least 4 months post-onset. They were selected on the basis that they displayed perseverative errors as identified by their treating speech pathologist. The participants were not selected on the basis of any traditional aphasia classification. However, the Western Aphasia Battery (Kertesz, 1982) was administered to all, in order to establish a replicable classification of their aphasia for descriptive purposes.

Participant 1: KCC

This 63-year-old man suffered a left cerebral vascular accident (CVA) in April 1998, 21 months before testing, resulting in severe dysfluent aphasia. He was classified as having Broca's aphasia (AQ = 38.2) (WAB; Kertesz, 1982), characterised by severely dysfluent and agrammatic verbal output, with marked word-finding difficulties. In conversation, KCC utilised a limited repertoire of single words, social greetings, and the stereotyped phrase "The way we go". His speech was highly perseverative and often echolalic in conversation. Audiological examination revealed a bilateral mild sensori-neural hearing loss for frequencies higher than 2000 Hz. This hearing loss did not impact on his ability to comprehend speech in the one-to-one clinical setting.

Participant 2: KVH

This 71-year-old man suffered a left basal ganglia CVA in January 2000. At the time of testing, he presented with very severe fluent jargon aphasia. KVH was classified on the WAB as having Conduction aphasia (AQ = 59.6), which had resolved from an initial WAB classification of Wernicke's aphasia. KVH's spontaneous speech was fluent and contained much neologistic and semantic jargon, which he rarely attempted to self-correct. KVH demonstrated some difficulties comprehending more complex speech, however he managed well at a basic conversational level. Audiological examination revealed that although KVH's hearing was adequate for frequencies within the speech range, he demonstrated some mild sensori-neural high-frequency loss, consistent with expectations for normal ageing. His vision was unimpaired.

Participant 3: DRS

This 53-year-old woman suffered a left middle cerebral artery aneurysm in April 1999, 2 years prior to testing. At the time of testing, DRS presented with a moderate to severe fluent jargon aphasia. DRS was classified on the WAB as having conduction aphasia (AQ = 62.7), which had resolved from an earlier WAB classification of Wernicke's aphasia. She had fluent, grammatical speech and communicated quite effectively in conversation despite producing many semantic, phonological, and neologistic errors when labelling items. DRS often compensated for her expressive difficulties by writing down the word she was trying to say or by drawing it. DRS demonstrated some difficulties in adequately comprehending conversational speech, although she functioned well within context. Her hearing and vision were within normal limits.

Participant 4: SMM

This 63-year-old woman suffered from a sudden onset of aphasia approximately 18 months prior to testing, from a condition of unknown origin. MRI showed primary changes to the left posterior parietal region. The exact date of this episode is not known but she first presented for medical assessment in 1999. The most recent MRI (conducted in February 2002) resulted in a diagnosis of primary progressive aphasia.

SMM presented with a very severe expressive and receptive aphasia. She was classified on the WAB as having Wernicke's aphasia with grammatical verbal output full of neologistic and semantic jargon. She compensated by using circumlocution and gesture. SMM demonstrated significant auditory comprehension difficulties at both single-word and conversational levels, and written language was used to aid her comprehension of spoken language. Her hearing and vision were within normal limits. Her communication status remained stable during the period of testing and there were no differences in her successive performances across trials of each research task.

Participant 5: TOW

This 76-year-old man suffered a left lacunar infarct in the basal ganglia in February 1996, approximately 4 years prior to testing, resulting in severe dysfluent aphasia. TOW was classified as having a conduction aphasia (WAB, AQ = 57.42), characterised by grammatical yet very hesitant conversational speech. He demonstrated considerable frustration with his speaking difficulties and often made multiple attempts to self-correct his erroneous responses (i.e., characteristic of conduite d'approache). TOW's comprehension was adequate at a conversational level. TOW presented with a mild pure tone sensori-neural hearing loss in the right ear, consistent with normal ageing, however he did not appear to have difficulties comprehending simple sentences. TOW used glasses for reading.

Background language assessments

An initial series of assessments were administered in order to establish each individual's level of impairment(s) according to an information-processing framework from Nickels (2000) and similar to Kay, Lesser, and Coltheart (1992) (see Figure 1). Assessment tasks included selected subtests from the Psycholinguistic Assessment of Language-processing in Aphasia (PALPA; Kay et al., 1992), The Pyramids and Palm Trees Test (PPT; Howard & Patterson, 1992), and the Castles Word and Nonword Reading Test (Coltheart & Leahy, 1996).

Research tasks and procedure

Participants performed repetition, reading aloud, and picture naming of pictureable nouns, each comprising the same 126 items presented in different pseudo-random orders (see Appendix A). The items were taken from the Snodgrass and Vanderwart (1980) set of 260 object pictures and were selected from range of semantic categories. Target words varied from 1 to 5 syllables (mean = 1.76, $SD = 0.91$). Items in the repetition task were presented by the examiner, whose mouth was obscured to prevent lip reading. In reading aloud, written stimuli were presented individually on a laptop screen in Times New Roman font size 72. Pictures for naming were enlarged and presented individually on half-A4-sized laminated cards. Although no strict time constraint was imposed in which to respond, participants were encouraged to attempt one response per item. If no response had been provided after 20 seconds, the next item was presented. Participants performed each task twice, with at least 1 week between each administration. Responses were combined across both trials and are reported as proportions of the combined total number of items. Participants were given only one task per session, to minimise priming effects and the chance of perseverating from items in different tasks.

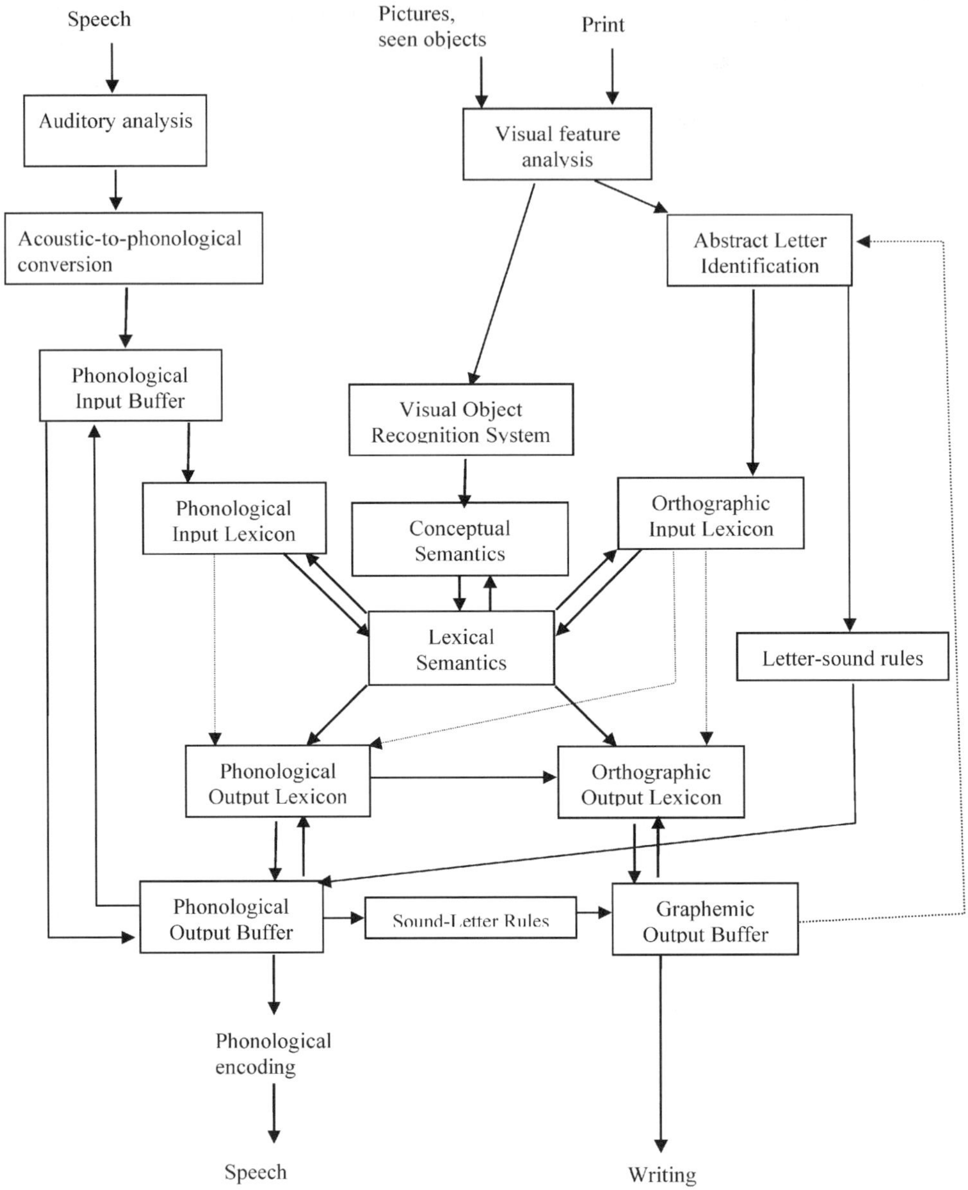

Figure 1. A sketch of the cognitive processes involved in the comprehension and production of single words Nickels (2000). Note: Dotted lines represent those links that are more controversial and/or less well established in the literature. Nickels (2000) is explicit that this is a sketch and should not be interpreted as a complete or final model, but simply as one that represents sufficient detail to interpret the performance of many individuals with aphasia.

Coding of errors

Responses were transcribed on-line and checked retrospectively from the recordings by a speech pathologist. A second speech pathologist independently coded responses from one trial of each research task for each research participant. Coding agreement was reviewed according to the coding criteria (below) and independently recoded until a minimum of 90% point-by-point inter-rater agreement was reached. Only the first full (stressed) response to each target was analysed, consistent with the procedures of Dell, Schwartz, Martin, Saffran and Gagnon (1997), Hirsh (1998), and Santo-Pietro and Rigrodsky (1986).

Errors were coded on three levels:

1. Their relationship to the target (see Table 1).
2. Whether they were *perseverative* or *non-perseverative*.
3. If they were perseverative, as either a *total* or *blended* perseverative error (see Table 2).

Responses were coded as perseverative if they involved either a partial or complete repetition of a prior response (Sandson & Albert, 1984). This was based on

TABLE 1
Target error coding criteria

Error	*Description*	*Example*
Lexical (real word) errors		
Semantic	Real word that was semantically related to target	dog → cat
Formal	Real word that shared either the initial phoneme or at least 50% or more phonemes with target (following a combination of Dell et al., 1997 and Hirsh, 1998).	dog → desk pan → pen
Mixed	Real word that was both semantically and phonologically related to target	motorcycle → bicycle
Visual	Real word of an item similar in visual form to the target	orange → ball
Unrelated	Real word that was not related to the target in any obvious way	dog → apple
Non-lexical (nonword) errors		
Phonological	Non-word that shared either the initial phoneme or at least 50% of phonemes with target	dog → deg
Neologistic	Non-word sharing less than 50% of phonemes with the target and with a different initial phoneme	dog → kib
	Nonsensical combination of real words or non-word + real word	ostrich → four west pliers → special lig
Other errors		
Don't know	Indication that response was unknown or if item was not responded to at all	"I don't know" or silence
Description	Attempts to describe as opposed to name item	finger → when you point

TABLE 2
Perseverative error coding criteria

Perseverative error	*Criteria*
Total	Exact repetition of prior response Could be a total repetition of a previous response but may only form a part of a new compound word response (e.g., *pen* → writing *pen*)
Blended	50% phonemes in common with a prior response in approximately the same order (Hirsh, 1998) OR 1. Same initial phoneme with five responses 2. Same final phoneme within three responses 3. Same main vowel on consecutive responses (Santo-Pietro & Rigrodsky, 1982)

the most recent match to a prior response in a perseverative set or chain. The criteria for classification are presented in Table 2 and are consistent with those used by Hirsh (1998) and Santo-Pietro and Rigrodsky (1982).[2] Both "don't know" and "description" responses were coded as non-perseverative.

RESULTS

Delineation of levels of language-processing breakdown

Preliminary and research language task scores are reported in Tables 3 and 4 respectively, followed by a more detailed discussion of each participant's hypothesised level of language-processing breakdown from analysis of the *non-perseverative errors* (in order to allow for later comparison with perseverative errors in Analysis 1) (see Table 5 for non-perseverative errors). Table 6 (later) summarises each participant's primary level of output language-processing breakdown.

There were no significant differences between the accuracy of Trials 1 and 2 of each task for any participant, with the exception of DRS and KVH whose reading aloud performance improved across Trials 1 and 2 (see Appendix B). This either reflects a task practice effect or a degree of day-to-day variability.

Participant KCC

Preliminary language test interpretation

Phonological processing. Overall, KCC had mild auditory processing deficits affecting his discrimination of word and nonword minimal pairs similarly (Fisher Exact Test, $p < .451$). This may have been exacerbated by his mild pure tone hearing loss. Despite only mild auditory analysis difficulties, KCC had considerable difficulty repeating nonwords, suggesting possible additional phonological encoding

[2] The coding of blended perseverative errors is acknowledged to be arbitrary and hence there is the possibility that false identification of these errors may sometimes occur. To minimise potential false positive miscoding, items sharing initial phonemes were not placed within five intervening items, nor within three intervening items for those with the same final phoneme, nor consecutively for those with the same main vowel.

TABLE 3
Preliminary language test scores (reported as proportions)

Test	*N*	*KCC*	*KVH*	*DRS*	*SMM*	*TOW*
Phonological processing						
PALPA 1						
(nonword minimal pair discrimination)	72	.85	–	.83	–	.67
PALPA 2						
(real word minimal pair discrimination)	72	.90	.76	.86	.72	.75
PALPA 5						
(auditory lexical decision)						
TOTAL	160	.92	.85	.92	.67	.81
Real words	80	.91	.96	.85	.91	.79
Nonwords	80	.93	.74	.99	.43	0.84
High frequency	40	.95	.95	.93	.93	.90
Low frequency	40	.88	.98	.78	.90	.68
High imageability	40	1.00	1.00	.98	.98	.85
Low imageability	40	.83	.93	.73	.85	.73
PALPA 8						
(nonword repetition)	30	.53	.33	.20	.00	.40
Semantic processing						
Pyramids & Palm Trees	52	.85	.71	.98	.85	.87
PALPA 47						
(Spoken word–picture matching)	40	.90	.93	.85	.90	.95
PALPA 48						
(Written word–picture matching)	40	.90	.88	.98	.90	1.00
PALPA 49						
(auditory synonym judgements)						
TOTAL	60	.68	.75	.73	–	.65
High imageability	30	.73	.87	.90	–	.77
Low imageability	30	.63	.63	.57	–	.53
Orthographic processing						
Castles Irregular & Regular Word and Nonword Reading Test						
TOTAL	90	.47	.06	.73	.53	.43
Regular words	30	.63	.07	.50	.77	.67
Irregular words	30	.67	.07	.43	.50	.50
Nonwords	30	.10	.03	.03	.33	.13
PALPA 25						
(visual lexical decision)						
TOTAL	120	.89	.83	.95	.79	.78
Real words	60	.92	.95	.92	.85	.72
Nonwords	60	.87	.70	.98	.73	.83
High frequency	30	.90	.97	1.00	1.00	.70
Low frequency	30	.93	.93	.83	.70	.73
High imageability	30	.93	1.00	.93	.97	.83
Low imageability	30	.90	.90	.90	.73	.60

TABLE 4
Overall scores on research tasks

Participant	*Repetition*	N [a]	*Reading aloud*	*N*	*Picture naming*	*N*
KCC	.75	248	.58	248	.21	248
KVH	.60	252	.04	252	.08	252
DRS	.71	252	.60	252	.35	252
SMM	.09	252	.61	252	.25	252
TOW	.59	250	.75	250	.45	250

[a] The difference in *N* for KCC and TOW was due to items unintentionally being omitted from the task.

TABLE 5
Distribution of non-perseverative errors across tasks

		Repetition	*Reading aloud*	*Picture naming*
Participant	*Error*	*NP*	*NP*	*NP*
KCC	semantic	0	0	12
	formal	5	10	8
	unrelated	0	5	10
	mixed	0	3	2
	visual	0	0	2
	phonological	36	23	6
	neologistic	2	3	8
KVH	semantic	0	0	6
	formal	10	6	5
	unrelated	1	4	16
	mixed	0	3	1
	visual	0	0	1
	phonological	15	18	3
	neologistic	3	22	40
DRS	semantic	0	2	15
	formal	6	13	11
	unrelated	4	1	6
	mixed	0	10	13
	visual	0	0	1
	phonological	22	37	17
	neologistic	4	6	20
SMM	semantic	0	0	16
	formal	8	10	11
	unrelated	0	0	4
	mixed	0	0	3
	visual	0	0	0
	phonological	19	64	11
	neologistic	7	0	6
TOW	semantic	0	0	8
	formal	14	13	15
	unrelated	2	0	8
	mixed	1	1	5
	visual	0	0	28
	phonological	30	6	7
	neologistic	6	3	1

TABLE 6
Main locus of output impairment for all participants

	KCC	*KVH*	*DRS*	*SMM*	*TOW*
Primary location of output impairment	Semantic (SS)	Lexical access (SS → POL)	Phonological encoding (POB)	Phonological encoding (POB) & semantics (SS)	Phonological encoding (POB)

difficulties (investigated later in more detail). Auditory lexical decision was relatively preserved, but with significant imageability and frequency effects, suggesting a reliance on accessing meaning of whole word forms.

Semantics. KCC's performance suggests a semantic system deficit. Evidence includes equally impaired performance on auditory and written word to picture matching, and poor performance on Pyramids and Palm Trees and auditory synonym judgements.

Orthographic processing. Significantly poorer reading of nonwords than words indicates severely impaired sublexical orthographic processing (Castles Regular and Irregular Word and Nonword Reading Test: Fisher Exact Test, $p < .0001$). Given this pattern, as would be expected, there was no regularity effect in word reading (Fisher Exact Test, $p = 1.000$). KCC's visual lexical decision was relatively preserved and his score was similar to that on auditory lexical decision (McNemar's Test, $p = 1.00$), with no effects of imageability on performance.

Research task interpretation

Repetition. KCC produced relatively few errors in this task. Most non-perseverative errors were phonological, reflecting some mild difficulties at the phonological output buffer and subsequent phonological encoding. Real word repetition was significantly better than non-word repetition (Fisher Exact Test, $p = .017$), suggesting an advantage when he was able to use a lexical route.

Reading aloud. As with repetition, most non-perseverative errors in reading aloud were phonological, again suggesting phonological encoding difficulties. However, compared with repetition, there were more formal errors, reflecting a greater reliance on using the lexical route in reading. There was a significant effect of imageability on overall accuracy (Wald = 6.362, $p = .012$), suggesting an influence of semantics on reading accuracy.

Picture naming. KCC made most errors in spoken naming. This task required access to his impaired semantic system via pictures, which unlike repetition and reading tasks provide no additional lexical or sublexical phonological information. There was a significant effect of frequency on overall accuracy (Wald = 9.690, $p = .002$). Picture naming resulted in a considerable number of semantic errors, reflecting this task's obligatory access to the semantic system. As in the other tasks, KCC also made some phonological errors reflecting his mild phonological encoding impairment.

Summary

Based on the preliminary tests and analysis of his non-perseverative error patterns, KCC's primary processing difficulties in word production appeared to stem from a semantic impairment resulting in impaired activation of the phonological form. KCC had some additional mild problems at the level of the phonological output buffer and the subsequent phonological encoding processes affecting both real and non-word production.

Participant KVH

Preliminary language test interpretation

Phonological processing. Both auditory analysis and auditory lexical decision were impaired. Although KVH's hearing was adequate for speech, audiological testing found some mild high-frequency loss, possibly affecting his discrimination of individual sounds. KVH was able to process some phonological information in non-word repetition, evident in the fact that 90% of all errors were phonologically related to their targets.

Semantics. Difficulties were evident accessing semantics via both spoken and written modalities and from pictures alone, suggesting a conceptual semantic deficit. This is further supported by his impaired performance on auditory synonym judgements.

Orthographic processing. Impaired performance was demonstrated on both visual lexical decision and written word to picture matching, suggesting breakdown at the orthographic input lexicon and access to the already impaired semantic system. Word and nonword reading aloud were profoundly impaired. While there were no effects of regularity or lexicality on accuracy (as KVH performed so close to floor) there were more phonologically related responses to regular words (14/30) and nonwords (13/30) than there were to irregular words (8/30). This suggests that KVH was more successful in accessing at least partial phonological information for regular and non-words for which he could use sub-lexical processing not available to the same extent as for irregular words. This pattern points to an impairment accessing the phonological form of the word via a lexical reading route (see below for further discussion).

Research task interpretation

Repetition. This elicited the least number of errors of the three tasks. Most of the non-perseverative errors were either phonological or formal, reflecting mild phonological encoding difficulties.

Picture naming. This task elicited a larger number of errors than repetition. KVH made a small number of semantically related non-perseverative errors reflecting the obligatory access of the semantic system in this task, however, most of his non-perseverative errors were neologistic and a large number were unrelated (real word) errors. In contrast to repetition, there were very few phonological errors in naming, suggesting that his larger number of neologistic errors reflected more than just phonological difficulties. There was a significant effect of imageability on overall accuracy (Wald = 4.818, $p = .028$), further suggesting a lexical-semantic impairment

Reading aloud. KVH produced a similar number of errors in this task as he did in picture naming (Fisher Exact Test, $p = .083$). Most non-perseverative errors in this task were neologistic or phonological. Although there was no effect of imageability on overall accuracy, when examining non-perseverative errors compared to correct responses, there was an effect of imageability on overall accuracy (Wald = 3.905, $p = .048$), suggesting the influence of semantic processing in this task.

Summary

KVH demonstrated most difficulty at a lexical processing level. In picture naming, this breakdown reflected impaired activation of semantics and subsequent insufficient activation of the phonological form. In reading aloud, KVH's impairment at the orthographic input lexicon similarly resulted in reduced activation of the phonological form for output. KVH's phonological encoding deficits further impact on performance in all output modalities. Where possible, KVH benefited from using sublexical processing to read aloud and repeat regular and non-words. However, he could not do this for picture naming or reading aloud irregular words. In both reading aloud and picture naming, KVH produced large numbers of neologisms. In contrast, relatively few neologisms were produced in repetition. If his phonological encoding difficulties were the primary cause of KVH's abundant neologisms, we would have expected similar numbers of neologisms in repetition, as all three tasks rely on phonological encoding. Although KVH clearly has phonological encoding difficulties, these do not appear to be his primary source of breakdown. An alternative explanation for KVH's neologisms is that they reflect compensation for an underlying lexical processing impairment, as proposed by Butterworth (1979, 1992) to explain the pervasive abstruse neologistic errors commonly observed in people with jargon aphasia. (See Moses et al., 2004a, for a more detailed discussion of the source of KVH's neologistic errors.) We therefore propose that KVH's language was breaking down at both a phonological encoding but more particularly at a lexical processing level, having a profound effect on his ability to accurately respond.

Participant DRS

Preliminary language test interpretation

Phonological processing. DRS's auditory processing skills were significantly impaired. Minimal pair discrimination was poor, as was repetition of non-words where there was a significant effect of syllable length on accuracy. These results indicate a severe breakdown at the levels of auditory analysis and phonological encoding. There was a significant effect of imageability on accuracy in auditory lexical decision, which was mildly impaired, suggesting that DRS accessed her semantic system to help her distinguish words from non-words in the auditory modality.

Semantics. DRS's conceptual semantics was within normal limits. While she had moderate difficulties in accessing meaning from the auditory modality, access via orthography was relatively intact, suggesting that the semantic system itself was preserved for at least concrete stimuli.

Orthographic processing. DRS was virtually unable to read aloud non-words, with a significant effect of lexicality on accuracy (Fisher Exact Test, $p < .0001$) suggesting that her sublexical grapheme–phoneme orthographic route was more impaired than her ability to recognise whole words at the lexical level. As might be expected, DRS showed no regularity effect (Fisher Exact Test, $p = .796$). Visual lexical decision was mildly impaired yet not significantly differently from auditory lexical decision (McNemar's Test, $p = .754$). However, unlike auditory lexical decision, there was no imageability effect, suggesting that DRS was not as reliant on her semantic system to identify written words as she was to identify spoken words.

Research task interpretation

Repetition. DRS produced significantly fewer errors in real word repetition than she did in non-word repetition (Fisher Exact Test, $p < .0001$), suggesting that she benefited from accessing the lexical route. This was further supported by the significant effect of frequency on overall accuracy in real word repetition (Wald = 5.576, $p = .018$). However, as in non-word repetition, most non-perseverative errors in this task were phonological and there was a significant effect of syllable length on accuracy (Wald = 15.699, $p < .0001$), reflecting pervasive phonological encoding difficulties.

Reading. Again, most non-perseverative errors again were phonological or formal. Nonetheless, the presence of mixed and semantic errors indicated a reliance on semantic and lexical processing, supported also by an effect of imageability on overall accuracy (Wald = 4.691, $p = .03$). There was also a significant effect of syllable length on overall accuracy (Wald = 10.221, $p < .0001$), reflecting DRS's phonological encoding difficulties.

Picture naming. In contrast to repetition and reading aloud, there was a higher proportion of semantic non-perseverative errors in picture naming, which, together with the significant effects of frequency (Wald = 8.854, $p = .003$) and imageability (Wald = 15.513, $p < .0001$) on accuracy, reflected the obligatory semantic processing in this task. In addition there were large numbers of both phonologically related and neologistic errors.

Summary

DRS's primary breakdown was in phonological processing for both speech perception and production. She had difficulties in auditory phonological analysis and lexical decision tasks as well as in phonological encoding for speech production tasks. The large number of phonological errors in all tasks (and large numbers of neologisms in picture naming) and significant effects of syllable length on accuracy in repetition and reading aloud further suggest impaired phonological encoding. In picture naming, given her intact semantic processing, the large numbers of semantically related errors and significant effects of frequency and imageability on accuracy, suggest impaired access to the phonological form. This is consistent with greater accuracy in reading aloud and repetition where additional phonological information can facilitate output.

Participant SMM

Preliminary language test interpretation

Phonological processing. SMM's auditory discrimination was profoundly impaired, suggesting a severely impaired auditory phonological analysis. She was also unable to repeat any nonwords.

Semantics. Regardless of modality, SMM performed poorly on the range of semantic tasks, suggesting that both conceptual and lexical semantics were severely impaired.

Orthographic processing. Although impaired, SMM's lexical decision was significantly better in the written than auditory modality (McNemar's Test, $p = .025$). She read regular words aloud significantly better than both nonwords (Fisher Exact Test, $p = .002$) and irregular words (Fisher Exact Test, $p = .03$, one-tailed). These results suggest that SMM could read better when able to use a combination of both the lexical and sublexical sources of phonological information.

Research task interpretation

Repetition. This was the least accurate task. Most non-perseverative errors were phonological. There was no significant difference between her performance on real and non-word repetition (Fisher Exact Test, $p = .149$), suggesting common loci of impairment in auditory phonological analysis, subsequent phonological lexical encoding and its linkage to meaning, and also in the phonological output buffer as demonstrated by an effect of syllable length on overall accuracy (Wald = 4.548, $p = .033$).

Reading aloud. SMM produced fewest errors in this task. The majority of her non-perseverative errors were again phonological. Together with a significant effect of syllable length on accuracy (Wald = 17.131, $p < .0001$), these also reflected a phonological encoding impairment.

Picture naming. Unlike the other tasks, SMM produced semantically related non-perseverative errors in picture naming where there were significant effects of frequency (Wald = 11.044, $p = .001$) and imageability (Wald = 9.767, $p = .002$) on overall accuracy. These results indicate lexical retrieval difficulties, probably stemming from her impaired semantic processing. The fact that SMM produced formal and phonological errors, suggested that sometimes she was able to partially activate information about the phonological form of target lexical items, while her production of so many neologisms remained testimony to the severe general breakdown of her phonological encoding across all three research tasks.

Summary

SMM's language was profoundly impaired at the levels of the auditory analysis and all subsequent phonological encoding processes. She also had a severe central semantic system deficit. However her severe phonological encoding impairment was her major source of error in word production. This impairment had greatest impact on repetition where SMM was forced to rely on auditory processing alone, as she had poor access to semantics. In contrast when reading aloud, she could derive additional sublexical phonological information from the more concrete written stimuli and so performed relatively better in that most of her errors were merely phonological rather than neologistic.

Participant TOW

Preliminary language test interpretation

Phonological input. TOW demonstrated marked difficulties with minimal pair discrimination, suggesting impairment at the level of auditory phonological analysis. His mild hearing loss may also have impacted on these results. Auditory lexical decision was also impaired, with a trend towards an effect of frequency on accuracy (Fisher Exact Test, $p = .057$, 1 tailed), suggesting a lexical-level impairment. There was a trend towards better repetition of real words than non-words (Fisher Exact Test, $p = .052$, 1 tailed), suggesting that his sublexical route was more impaired than his lexical route.

Semantics. TOW performed well on spoken and written word to picture matching but was impaired on Pyramids and Palm trees, and auditory synonym judgements, where low-imageability items were not significantly above chance (Binomial $p = .428$). Overall, the results still implicate a mild semantic impairment.

Orthographic processing. Visual lexical decision was impaired to a similar degree as auditory lexical decision (McNemar's Test, $p = .626$). There was no significant regularity effect (Fisher Exact Test, $p = .295$), but there was a significant lexicality effect (regular and irregular combined vs non-words: Fisher Exact Test, $p < .0001$). These results further suggest that his lexical route was less impaired than his sub-lexical route.

Research task interpretation

Repetition. Most non-perseverative errors were phonological or formal and there was a trend towards a significant effect of syllable length on overall accuracy (Wald = 3.522, $p = .06$), indicating difficulties at the level of the phonological output buffer and subsequent phonological encoding processes.

Reading aloud. As with repetition, most non-perseverative errors were phonological or formal, with a significant effect of syllable length on accuracy (Wald = 7.030, $p = .008$), further suggesting phonological encoding difficulties.

Picture naming. Again, phonological and formal errors were the most common error types. However, unlike in the other tasks, there were some semantic errors, reflecting additional lexical-semantic processing difficulties. There was a significant effect of frequency (Wald = 9.133, $p = .003$) and a trend towards an effect of syllable length on overall accuracy (Wald = 3.077, $p = .079$), also indicating breakdown at both lexical and phonological encoding levels of processing.

Summary

TOW's results indicate breakdown primarily at the levels of the auditory phonological analysis, phonological output buffer, and subsequent phonological encoding processes. He had an additional mild semantic-level impairment. While TOW performed well on tasks requiring lexical semantic input, the integrity of his semantic system may have been insufficient to activate the phonological form of the word, as was evident in picture naming.

Experimental analyses

Having profiled each participants' language-processing impairment, we now examine the perseverative error patterns they produced in each task in order to test the hypothesis that perseverative errors reflect levels of language-processing breakdown (see Table 6).

Analysis 1. Comparison of lexical and non-lexical non-perseverative and perseverative errors

For each participant, the numbers of perseverative and non-perseverative errors were compared after grouping them according to whether they were lexical or non-lexical. Comparisons were made of lexical and non-lexical error groups rather than individual error types due to the small numbers of errors of some types. Lexicality of an error reflects the level of language processing impaired in the task and may be less sensitive to smaller differences between the individual perseverative and non-perseverative error types. For example, both semantic and formal errors arise at a lexical processing level whereas neologisms and phonological errors by definition are produced at a sublexical level. If the distributions of lexical and non-lexical errors were similar for perseverative and non-perseverative errors across the tasks, this would suggest that perseverative errors reflect the participants' level of language-processing breakdown. Table 7 presents the breakdown of perseverative and non-perseverative errors in all tasks for each participant. Proportions of all perseverative and non-perseverative errors are reported except for "don't know" and descriptions.

DRS and SMM showed no significant differences in the distribution of lexical and non-lexical perseverative and non-perseverative errors in any task. KVH showed only a marginally significant difference in repetition, due to the large numbers of unrelated perseverative errors. Both KCC and TOW showed significant differences in the distributions of lexical and non-lexical perseverative and non-perseverative errors in picture naming, their most error-prone task. As with KVH, this was due to large numbers of unrelated perseverative errors produced.

Analysis 2. Comparison of total and blended perseverative errors

In the second analysis the relative proportions of *total* and *blended* perseverative errors were compared across the tasks to further determine whether their

TABLE 7
Comparison of non-perseverative (NP) and perseverative (P) errors across tasks [a]

No. Errors		*Repetition*		*Reading aloud*		*Picture naming*	
Participant	*Error*	*NP*	*P*	*NP*	*P*	*NP*	*P*
KCC	Semantic	0	0	0	0	12	15
	Formal	5	1	10	6	8	4
	Unrelated	0	1	5	10	10	55
	Mixed	0	0	3	2	2	2
	Visual	0	0	0	0	2	1
	Phonological	36	14	23	11	6	4
	Neologistic	2	0	3	3	8	1
	Lexical	5	2	18	18	34	77
	Non-lexical	38	14	26	14	14	5
		$p = .271$		$p = .246$		$p = .001$**	
KVH	Semantic	0	2	0	5	6	6
	Formal	10	9	6	10	5	6
	Unrelated	1	14	4	32	16	48
	Mixed	0	0	3	0	1	0
	Visual	0	0	0	0	1	0
	Phonological	15	8	18	37	3	3
	Neologistic	3	6	22	105	40	70
	Lexical	11	25	13	47	29	60
	Non-lexical	18	14	40	142	43	73
		$p = .049$*		$p = 1.000$		$p = .556$	
DRS	Semantic	0	2	2	2	15	21
	Formal	6	3	13	9	11	12
	Unrelated	4	7	1	1	6	4
	Mixed	0	0	10	2	13	1
	Visual	0	0	0	0	1	2
	Phonological	22	9	37	12	17	13
	Neologistic	4	9	6	7	20	25
	Lexical	10	12	26	14	46	40
	Non-lexical	26	18	43	19	37	38
		$p = .310$		$p = .670$		$p = .637$	
SMM	Semantic	0	14	0	0	16	22
	Formal	8	19	10	3	11	23
	Unrelated	0	43	0	1	4	14
	Mixed	0	1	0	0	3	10
	Visual	0	1	0	0	0	2
	Phonological	19	53	64	19	11	3
	Neologistic	7	59	0	1	6	17
	Lexical	8	78	10	4	34	71
	Non-lexical	26	112	64	20	17	20
		$p = .058$		$p = .741$		$p = .165$	
TOW	Semantic	0	0	0	0	8	10
	Formal	14	5	13	6	15	10
	Unrelated	2	2	0	0	8	16
	Mixed	1	1	1	1	5	4
	Visual	0	0	0	6	28	12

(Continued)

TABLE 7
(Continued)

No. Errors		*Repetition*		*Reading aloud*		*Picture naming*	
Participant	*Error*	*NP*	*P*	*NP*	*P*	*NP*	*P*
	Phonological	30	19	6	3	7	5
	Neologistic	6	20	3	0	1	1
	Lexical	17	8	14	13	64	52
	Non-lexical	36	39	9	3	8	6
		$p = .107$		$p = .369$		$p = .03$*	

[a] Fisher Exact Test reported.
* Statistically significant at the $p < .05$ level.
** Statistically significant at the $p < .001$ level.

distributions reflected each participant's level of language-processing breakdown. For this analysis, perseverative errors were coded as either *total* or *blended*, according to their relationship with the source of the perseveration (i.e., whether the response involved a complete or partial reproduction of a prior response repectively; see also Table 2. This was in contrast to the previous analyses, which examined the relationship with the target stimulus). Table 8 presents the relative proportions of *total* and *blended* perseverative errors produced by each participant across the tasks.

In general, the relative proportions of *total* and *blended* perseverative errors reflected the level of processing that was particularly impaired in each task for the different participants. KCC and KVH produced predominantly *blended* perseverative errors in repetition, reflecting mild phonological encoding difficulties. In contrast, KCC produced mainly *total* perseverative errors in picture naming, reflecting his more severely impaired lexical retrieval difficulties. KCC produced similar proportions of *total* and *blended* perseverative errors in reading aloud, reflecting both his difficulties accessing the lexical word form in addition to his phonological encoding difficulties. DRS, SMM, and TOW all produced large proportions of blended perseverative errors in each task, reflecting their primary phonological encoding deficits. However, both SMM and TOW produced large proportions of total perseverative errors in picture naming, reflecting their additional semantic impairments.

While the distributions of total and blended perseverative errors largely reflected the individual's language-processing profiles, there were some unexpected findings that challenged current theories. Firstly, KVH produced unpredictably large

TABLE 8
Proportions of *total* and *blended* perseverative errors across tasks

	Repetition			*Reading aloud*			*Picture naming*		
Participant	*N*	*Total*	*Blended*	*N*	*Total*	*Blended*	*N*	*Total*	*Blended*
KCC	16	0.12	0.88	32	0.44	0.56	82	0.82	0.18
KVH	39	0.38	0.62	18	0.21	0.79	13	0.34	0.66
DRS	30	0.17	0.83	33	0.21	0.79	78	0.26	0.74
SMM	19	0.34	0.66	24	0.08	0.92	91	0.64	0.36
TOW	47	0.13	0.87	16	0.19	0.81	58	0.38	0.62

proportions of *blended* perseverative errors in picture naming and reading aloud where he demonstrated difficulties accessing the lexical form of the word. However, we propose that, as the majority of *blended* perseverative errors in these tasks were neologistic, they may have reflected the generation of a response when no word was available for output; in other words to fill a "lexical gap". These could, for example, be produced either as a result of persistent activation at a phoneme level or from a default mechanism that generates neologisms (Butterworth, 1979, 1992; see Moses et al., 2004a, for detailed discussion of KVH's pattern of errors). Therefore, KVH's production of large proportions of *blended* perseverative errors in picture naming and reading aloud may after all be consistent with the hypothesis that the type of perseverative error reflects the processing demands of the task, just as for non-perseverative errors.

The next unexpected finding was that KVH and SMM produced *total* perseverations of neologistic responses in their most error-prone tasks; reading aloud and picture naming for KVH and repetition for SMM. As non-words do not (by definition) have a lexical representation, this challenges the theory that total perseverative errors reflect impaired lexical processing.[3] These errors can again be accounted for according to Butterworth's (1979, 1992) neologism generating device, which specifies that neologisms can be reproduced when the device is engaged in rapid succession. An alternative account is that these total neologistic perseverative errors occurred as result of short-lived persistent activation at a phoneme level or a default generation of phonemes (Butterworth, 1979, 1992; Butterworth, Swallow, & Grimston, 1981; Dell et al., 1997; see also Hirsh, 1998, and Moses et al., 2004b, for further debate regarding these accounts). Either account appears plausible given that all but one of KVH's neologistic *total* perseverative errors was sourced to the immediately preceding response. Similarly for SMM, 63% (10/16) of her neologistic total perseverative errors were sourced to the immediately preceding response and 81% (13/16) occurred within six intervening responses. Further examination of SMM's neologistic *total* perseverative errors revealed that 56% were close phonological approximations of frequently occurring responses, "apple" and "spring", possibly reflecting a phonological distortion of a erroneously selected word.[4]

A further unexpected finding for SMM was that despite the predominance of *blended* perseverative errors in repetition, a considerable number of *total* perseverative errors were also produced in this task. Further investigation revealed that 49% of these *total* perseverative errors were the repeated response, "apple". A possible explanation is that, being unable to encode virtually any auditory phonological information needed to repeat a word, SMM may have produced the more easily activated word "apple" in an attempt to fill the response slot.

[3] We acknowledge that whilst we would have predicted most total perseverations to involve the "classic" reproduction of whole words (as decribed by Cohen & Dehaene, 1998), this was not necessarily the case as our coding criteria for total and blended perseveration did not specify the lexicality of the error. That is, total perseverations need not be lexical and blended perseverations need not be non-lexical. Hence, although most total perseverations were lexical, a number of neologisms were classified as "total perseverations" as they invoved a complete reproduction of a prior neologism. The main challenge was that these neologisms cannot simply result from retrieval of the same lexical item (see also Hirsh, 1998).

[4] Howard, Patterson, Franklin, Orchard-Lisle, and Morton (1985) proposed that neologisms can reflect distortions of lexical errors.

GENERAL DISCUSSION

We have examined the language processing of five aphasic individuals with output characterised by recurrent perseverative errors. The functional localisation of their impairments was followed by two analyses that investigated the hypothesis that the production of perseverative errors reflects underlying language-processing impairment (e.g., Cohen & Dehaene, 1998; Martin et al., 1998).

In Analysis 1, patterns of lexical and non-lexical perseverative errors were found to be similar to the patterns of non-perseverative errors within each language task. These findings support the theory that perseverative errors are directly influenced by the language-processing demands of a task, as are non-perseverative errors (e.g., Cohen & Dehaene, 1998; Martin et al., 1998, Moses, Nickels, & Sheard, 2004c). However, there were some differences between the distribution of perseverative and non-perseverative errors, most notably the larger numbers of unrelated perseverative errors produced by some participants in picture naming. These errors may have reflected a tendency for these participants to stereotypically reproduce a particular word for multiple stimuli (although their verbal output was not limited to these responses). There is debate in the literature as to whether or not to code these errors as perseverative on the basis that they may reflect other cognitive impairments (e.g., Cohen & Dehaene, 1998). However, we argue that these errors may in fact reflect a more severe manifestation of the underlying language-processing deficit, whereby certain previous responses are reproduced in place of an inaccessible target or any target-related information.

In Analysis 2, it was demonstrated that the distribution of *total* and *blended* perseverative errors produced in each task further reflected the level at which language processing was impaired for each participant. The unpredictably large proportion of neologistic blended perseverative errors produced by KVH in picture naming and reading aloud was argued to be consistent with Butterworth's (1979, 1992) neologism-generating theory, where neologisms are produced by a process of perseveration of phonemes from previous responses. It was further argued that this theory can also explain the *total* perseverations of prior neologisms produced by both KVH and SMM. Hirsh (1998) drew a similar conclusion in attempting to explain CJ's complete perseveration of non-lexical responses. However, we acknowledge the scepticism surrounding an account such as the neologism-generating device that has a sole function of error production (e.g., Ellis, 1985). An alternative explanation for these errors could be that they are reproduced due to short-term activation at a phonological encoding level (see Moses et al., 2004a, for detailed discussion).

Vitkovitch and Humphreys (1991) argued that perseverative errors are caused by persistent activation in the links between semantics and phonology. However, our data challenge this proposal, as it cannot account for the large numbers of non-lexical perseverative errors produced by the participants in the current study (where the source of perseveration was argued to be at a phonological encoding level; for further discussion see Hirsh, 1998; Moses et al., 2004c). Moses et al. (2004b) argued against Vitkovitch and Humphreys' (1991) theory on the grounds that unimpaired participants *non-perseverative* errors are also predominantly semantically related. Hence, the perseverative errors patterns were argued to reflect the nature of the language-processing demands of picture naming, where lexical-semantic processing is obligatory and clearly most susceptible to errors overall for the speakers without aphasia.

CONCLUSIONS

We have demonstrated that the perseverative errors produced by the five participants did not appear to be produced independently of their language-processing breakdown. Rather, we conclude that these errors were directly influenced by the level of each participant's language-processing breakdown, thereby corroborating and extending on findings from other recent studies (e.g., Cohen & Dehaene, 1998; Martin et al., 1998). More specifically, we have demonstrated that the incidence of different types of perseverative errors is influenced by the processing demands of language tasks, relative to an individual's language-processing breakdown. In addition, we argue that blended perseverative errors can and must be included in any comprehensive analysis of perseverative errors.

Our findings contradict proposals that perseverative errors are caused by impaired inhibition of previously activated responses (Allison, 1966; Hudson, 1969; Papagno & Basso, 1996; Santo-Pietro & Rigrodsky, 1986; Yamadori, 1981), as we would have expected patterns of perseverative errors to have been constant across the various language tasks. Rather our results are most in line with recent literature specifying that perseverative errors occur as a result of impaired language processing coupled with normally existing amounts of persistent activation at any given level of language processing (Cohen & Dehaene, 1998; Martin et al., 1998).

While impaired language processing is proposed to be the primary cause of perseverative errors, we recognise that other factors, not explored in this paper, may play a role in the production of perseverative errors. Finally, we suggest that a case series design is highly valuable in demonstrating the variable nature of perseverative errors specific to an individual's language-processing profile. In contrast, group designs based, for example, on traditional aphasia classification types assume homogeneity between participants, which might oversimplify the complexity of their symptoms. Consequently, they cannot explore the specific nature of perseverative errors in the context of specific levels of language-processing breakdown beyond a certain level for fear of violating this statistical assumption.

In sum, systematic examination of an individual's perseverative error patterns may make a valuable contribution to our understanding of their language-processing profile. While it may be tempting to think of perseveration as a separate "problem" in the clinical setting, the results of the current study suggest that perhaps these errors should be viewed more as symptomatic of the underlying language impairment (Moses et al., 2004c). Hence, rather than attempting to remediate perseverative errors per se, we would suggest that, as always, treatment should aim to remediate the underlying language impairment as the source of the perseverative errors. Future studies focusing on the remediation of language-processing impairments could verify this proposal further by examining changes in the degree of perseverative errors as participants' abilities to retrieve language targets improve.

REFERENCES

Albert, M. L., & Sandson, J. (1986). Perseveration in aphasia. *Cortex, 22*, 103–115.

Allison, R. S. (1966). Perseveration as a sign of diffuse and focal brain damage. *British Medical Journal, 2*, 1095–1101.

Buckingham, H. W. (1985). Perseveration in aphasia. In S. Newman & R. Epstein (Eds.), *Current persectives in dysphasia* (pp. 113–154). Edinburgh, UK: Churchill Livingston.

Buckingham, H. W., Whitaker, H. A., & Whitaker, H. A. (1978). Alliteration and assonance in neologistic jargon aphasia. *Cortex*, *14*, 365–380.

Buckingham, H. W., Whitaker, H. A., & Whitaker, H. A. (1979). On linguistic perseveration. *Studies on Neurolinguistics*, *4*, 329–335.

Butterworth, B. (1979). Hesitation and the production of verbal paraphasias and neologisms in jargon aphasia. *Brain and Language*, *8*, 133–161.

Butterworth, B. (1992). Disorders of phonological encoding. *Cognition*, *42*, 261–286.

Butterworth, B., Swallow, J., & Grimston, M. (1981). Gestures and lexical processes in jargonaphasia. In J. W. Brown (Ed.), *Jargonaphasia.* New York: Academic Press.

Cohen, L., & Dehaene, S. (1998). Competition between past and present: Assessment and interpretation of verbal perseverations. *Brain*, *121*, 1641–1659.

Coltheart, M., & Leahy, J. (1996). Assessment of lexical and non-lexical reading abilities in children: Some normative data. *Australian Journal of Psychology*, *48*, 136–140.

Dell, G. S., Schwartz, M. F., Martin, N., Saffran, E. M., & Gagnon, D. (1997). Lexical access in aphasic and nonaphasic speakers. *Psychological Review*, *104*, 801–838.

Ellis, A. W. (1985). The production of spoken words: A cognitive neuropsychological perspective. In A. W. Ellis (Ed.), *Progress in the psychology of language* (Vol. 2). Hove, UK: Lawrence Erlbaum Associates Ltd.

Helm-Estabrooks, N., Ramage, A., Bayles, K. A., & Cruz, R. (1998). Perseverative behaviour in fluent and non-fluent aphasia. *Aphasiology*, *12*, 7–8.

Helmick, J. W., & Berg, C. B. (1976). Perseveration in brain-injured adults. *Journal of Communication Disorders*, *9*, 143–156.

Hirsh, K. W. (1998). Perseveration and activation in aphasic speech production. *Cognitive Neuropsychology*, *15*, 377–388.

Howard, D., & Patterson, K. (1992). *Pyramids and Palm Trees Test.* Bury St. Edmunds, UK: Thames Valley Test.

Howard, D., Patterson, K., Franklin, S., Orchard -Lisle, V., & Morton, J. (1985). Treatment of word retrieval deficits in aphasia. A comparison of two therapy methods. *Brain*, *108*, 817–829.

Hudson, A. J. (1969). Perseveration. *Brain*, *91*, 571–582.

Kay, J., Lesser, R., & Coltheart, M. (1992). *Psycholinguistic Assessment of Language Processing in Aphasia.* Hove, UK: Lawrence Erlbaum Associates Ltd.

Kertesz, A. (1982). *Western Aphasia Battery.* New York: Grune & Stratton.

Martin, N., Roach, A., Brecher, A., & Lowery, J. (1998). Lexical retrieval mechanisms underlying whole-word perseveration errors in anomic aphasia. *Aphasiology*, *12*, 319–333.

Moses, M. S., Nickels, L. A., & Sheard, C. (2004a). Disentangling the web: Neologistic perseverative errors in a person with jargon aphasia. *Neurocase*, *10*(6), 452–461.

Moses, M. S., Nickels, L. A., & Sheard, C. (2004b). "I'm sitting here feeling aphasic!" A study of recurrent perseverative errors elicited in unimpaired speakers". *Brain and Language*, *89*, 157–173.

Moses, M. S., Nickels, L. A., & Sheard, C. (2004c). That dreaded word *perseveration.* Understanding might be the key. *Australian Communication Quarterly*, *6*(2), 70–74.

Nickels, L. A. (2000). *A sketch of the cognitive processes involved in the comprehension and production of single words.* Retrieved on 10th June 2004 from http://www.maccs.mq.edu.au/~lyndsey/model.doc

Papagno, C., & Basso, A. (1996). Perseveration in two aphasic patients. *Cortex*, *32*, 67–82.

Sandson, J., & Albert, M. L. (1984). Varieties of perseveration. *Neuropsychologia*, *22*, 715–732.

Santo-Pietro, M. J., & Rigrodsky, S. (1982). The effects of temporal and semantic conditions on the occurrence of the error response of perseveration in adult aphasics. *Journal of Speech and Hearing Research*, *25*, 184–192.

Santo-Pietro, M. J., & Rigrodsky, S. (1986). Patterns of oral-verbal perseveration in adult aphasia. *Brain and Language*, *29*, 1–17.

Snodgrass, J. G., & Vanderwart, M. (1980). A standardised set of 260 pictures: Norms for name agreement, image agreement, familiarity, and visual complexity. *Journal of Experimental Psychology: Human Learning and Memory*, *6*, 174–215.

Vitkovitch, M., & Humphreys, G. W. (1991). Perseverant responding in speeded naming of pictures: It's in the links. *Journal of Experimental Psychology: Learning, Memory and Cognition*, *17*, 664–680.

Yamadori, A. (1981). Verbal perseveration in aphasia. *Neuropsychologia*, *19*, 591–594.

APPENDIX A

Research task stimuli

Picture naming

Item	*Stimulus*	*Item*	*Stimulus*	*Item*	*Stimulus*
1	chisel	43	doll	85	hanger
2	necklace	44	screw	86	pencil
3	fork	45	envelope	87	cup
4	sail boat	46	chair	88	bowl
5	pig	47	donkey	89	glasses
6	spoon	48	sea horse	90	hammer
7	apple	49	rhinoceros	91	box
8	record player	50	asparagus	92	eye
9	clock	51	lamp	93	celery
10	nut	52	penguin	94	boot
11	light switch	53	suitcase	95	carrot
12	zebra	54	vase	96	rabbit
13	glove	55	ear	97	dog
14	fish	56	jacket	98	book
15	cigar	57	paintbrush	99	swing
16	comb	58	nose	100	butterfly
17	leg	59	trousers	101	desk
18	rolling pin	60	nail	102	cannon
19	tomato	61	frog	103	belt
20	skirt	62	leopard	104	onion
21	pliers	63	needle	105	peacock
22	house	64	foot	106	door
23	watermelon	65	iron	107	brush
24	crocodile	66	bowl	108	piano
25	lock	67	jumper	109	garbage bin
26	gorilla	68	chain	110	mountain
27	heart	69	motorcycle	111	candle
28	clown	70	strawberry	112	button
29	drum	71	barn	113	duck
30	finger	72	eagle	114	elephant
31	spinning wheel	73	baseball bat	115	plug
32	windmill	74	pram	116	star
33	corn	75	lemon	117	pot
34	harp	76	french horn	118	goat
35	flower	77	helicopter	119	bread
36	pipe	78	rocking chair	120	shoes
37	hand	79	pineapple	121	bottle
38	saw	80	scissors	122	cake
39	orange	81	sheep	123	deer
40	violin	82	flute	124	bird
41	camel	83	swan	125	refrigerator
42	ostrich	84	knife	126	toe

Reading aloud

Item	*Stimulus*	*Item*	*Stimulus*	*Item*	*Stimulus*
1	knife	43	record player	85	box
2	scissors	44	piano	86	nail
3	motorcycle	45	chisel	87	pliers
4	gorilla	46	iron	88	elephant
5	swan	47	lamp	89	refrigerator
6	corn	48	cigar	90	lock
7	rolling pin	49	boot	91	jacket
8	goat	50	donkey	92	book
9	frog	51	fish	93	garbage bin
10	clock	52	pig	94	camel
11	strawberry	53	comb	95	french horn
12	pencil	54	violin	96	bowl
13	needle	55	rocking chair	97	nut
14	drum	56	bottle	98	eagle
15	spinning wheel	57	jumper	99	pram
16	crocodile	58	penguin	100	cake
17	asparagus	59	fork	101	glove
18	envelope	60	light switch	102	house
19	peacock	61	cannon	103	celery
20	dog	62	barn	104	leopard
21	rhinoceros	63	necklace	105	helicopter
22	swing	64	vase	106	belt
23	pineapple	65	tomato	107	desk
24	windmill	66	pipe	108	heart
25	clown	67	chair	109	toe
26	duck	68	ear	110	ostrich
27	hammer	69	orange	111	baseball bat
28	watermelon	70	pot	112	sea horse
29	cup	71	hand	113	button
30	screw	72	flute	114	harp
31	trousers	73	nose	115	leg
32	bread	74	lemon	116	shoes
33	onion	75	hanger	117	bow
34	suitcase	76	rabbit	118	sailboat
35	zebra	77	foot	119	plug
36	chain	78	skirt	120	deer
37	apple	79	bird	121	star
38	glasses	80	flower	122	candle
39	spoon	81	saw	123	eye
40	carrot	82	paintbrush	124	doll
41	mountain	83	finger	125	brush
42	butterfly	84	door	126	sheep

Repetition

Item	*Stimulus*	*Item*	*Stimulus*	*Item*	*Stimulus*
1	violin	43	jumper	85	drum
2	bow	44	suitcase	86	french horn
3	pram	45	chair	87	pliers
4	elephant	46	refrigerator	88	flute
5	ostrich	47	piano	89	leopard
6	rabbit	48	asparagus	90	goat
7	spoon	49	pipe	91	shoes
8	zebra	50	desk	92	garbage bin
9	sheep	51	tomato	93	knife
10	rocking chair	52	carrot	94	comb
11	pencil	53	celery	95	fork
12	vase	54	swing	96	sailboat
13	boot	55	bread	97	jacket
14	deer	56	motorcycle	98	penguin
15	lemon	57	finger	99	orange
16	gorilla	58	belt	100	fish
17	iron	59	cup	101	peacock
18	helicopter	60	saw	102	cannon
19	watermelon	61	box	103	swan
20	scissors	62	lamp	104	bottle
21	trousers	63	foot	105	light switch
22	crocodile	64	doll	106	eye
23	glove	65	hand	107	plug
24	needle	66	bird	108	camel
25	baseball bat	67	onion	109	button
26	nut	68	windmill	110	lock
27	hanger	69	house	111	rolling pin
28	rhinoceros	70	corn	112	pig
29	strawberry	71	paintbrush	113	skirt
30	necklace	72	heart	114	barn
31	door	73	apple	115	donkey
32	nose	74	chain	116	eagle
33	record player	75	frog	117	harp
34	hammer	76	spinning wheel	118	brush
35	bowl	77	chisel	119	leg
36	flower	78	pineapple	120	sea horse
37	toe	79	glasses	121	candle
38	clown	80	ear	122	butterfly
39	screw	81	cigar	123	dog
40	mountain	82	clock	124	book
41	duck	83	nail	125	cake
42	envelope	84	star	126	pot

APPENDIX B

Trial 1 vs Trial 2 responses across tasks

	Repetition			*Reading aloud*			*Picture naming*		
Participant	*T1* N = *126*	*T2* N = *126*	*T1 vs T2*	*T1* N = *126*	*T 2* N = *126*	*T1 vs T2*	*T 1* N = *126*	*T 2* N = *126*	*T1 vs T2*
KCC	99	87	.074	65	78	.280	29	24	1.000
KVH	70	81	.178	1	9	.021	8	11	.581
DRS	93	85	.216	65	85	.002**	42	47	.441
SMM	10	13	.607	75	79	.566	32	32	1.000
TOW	70	78	.312	90	98	.280	56	57	1.000

**McNemar's Test (two-tailed) reported.

APHASIOLOGY, 2007, 21 (10/11), 1002–1017

Psychology Press
Taylor & Francis Group

Common mechanisms underlying perseverative and non-perseverative sound and word substitutions

Nadine Martin
Temple University, PA, USA

Gary S. Dell
University of Illinois, USA

Background: Perseverations of sounds and words are common errors in aphasia. Understanding their mechanisms is of considerable interest to theories of word retrieval and also to treatment of anomia. Here, we explore the hypothesis that perseveration errors are generated by the same mechanisms as non-perseverative errors: weak activation of the intended word in the context of a competition from other activated words.
Aims: In analyses of perseverative and non-perseverative naming errors of 94 individuals with aphasia, we aimed to show that the only difference between the two kinds of errors is that perseverated words and sounds have an increased probability of being retrieved instead of the target word because of their residual activation potential from their prior activation.
Methods and Procedures: Correlational analyses were conducted to test (1) an interactive activation model's (Schwartz, Dell, Martin, Sobel, & Gahl, 2006) account of the occurrence of sound and whole-word perseverations, (2) distributions of perseverative and non-perseverative across error categories, and (3) the relationship between weakened connection strength between semantic and lexical representations and the occurrence of "no response" errors.
Outcomes and Results: Our analyses indicate that whole-word perseverative and non-perseverative errors are associated with weak spreading of activation between semantics and the target word form, and that sound perseverations and non-perseverations are associated with weak spreading of activation between the target word form and its corresponding sounds. Additionally, distributions of perseverative and non-perseverative errors across error categories are strongly associated. Finally, the occurrence of "no response" type errors is associated with weak semantic activation and the occurrence of whole-word perseverations.
Conclusions: The data from this study support a model of word and sound perseverations in which their occurrence is attributed to the same mechanisms as non-perseverative errors: weakened activation of the intended word in the context of a

Address correspondence to: Nadine Martin PhD, Temple University, Department of Communication Sciences, 1701 North 13th Street, Philadelphia, PA 19122, USA. E-mail: nmartin@temple.edu

This research was supported by grants from the National Institutes of Health (National Institute of Deafness and Communication Disorders) R01 DC01924 to Temple University (PI: N. Martin) and R01 DC00191 to Moss Rehabilitation Research Institute (PI: M.F. Schwartz). We thank Paula Sobel and Adelyn Brecher who were responsible for patient testing, scoring, and data management. We are also grateful to Dana Bitetti, Lianne DiMarco, Stephanie Tempest, and Francine Kohen for their assistance in data organisation and analyses. Finally, we thank Myrna Schwartz for helpful discussions that contributed to the overall work.

http://www.psypress.com/aphasiology DOI: 10.1080/02687030701198346

competitive activation process in which other word forms that are related to the target word have potential to be retrieved instead of the target. Potential perseverated words and sounds participate in this process, but have an additional boost to their activation levels because of residual activation potential.

Speech errors have proven to be a rich source of data that reveals the nature of linguistic representations and the cognitive mechanisms underlying the production of words and sentences. For example, studies of the semantic and phonological relationships between a word intended to be spoken and a substituted word indicate that production of a word involves at least two stages: retrieval of the word as an abstract syntactic-semantic entity, and then retrieval of its sounds (Garrett, 1975; Levelt, Roelofs, & Meyer, 1999). Semantic word substitutions such as "clam" spoken instead of "snail" are assumed to occur during the first stage, and phonological substitutions such as "snore" for "snail" have been attributed to the second stage (Fromkin, 1971). Moreover, "mixed" word substitutions, which share both meaning and sounds of a target word (such as saying "snake" for "snail"), are relatively more probable than word substitutions that share either meaning or sounds with the target word (Dell & Reich, 1981; Harley, 1984; Martin, Weisberg, & Saffran, 1989; Martin, Gagnon, Schwartz, Dell, & Saffran, 1996), indicating some mechanism whereby semantic and phonological domains jointly influence word production. Studies of all of these error types suggest a competitive activation process in which the target word must compete with other semantically and/or phonologically related words that become active through the retrieval process.

The competition is not limited to a target word's semantic and phonological neighbours, however. It also involves words that have been spoken recently or are intended to be spoken in the very near future. The activation of these representations is elevated because of their recent or anticipated utterance. If the prior utterance is selected in error, this is a perseverative intrusion (e.g., "Today's class will be about the class … I mean the **test**"). If the upcoming utterance is retrieved too soon, this is an anticipatory intrusion (e.g., "Today's test … today's **class** will be about the test"). This study is concerned with the first of these, the perseverative intrusion or perseveration, of sounds or words spoken prior to the current target sounds or word, and how they relate to non-perseverative sound and word substitutions.

We have argued elsewhere (Martin & Dell, 2004; Martin, Roach, Brecher, & Lowery, 1998) that perseverative and non-perseverative sound and word intrusions arise in part from the same mechanism, a competitive activation process in which a non-target sound or word accumulates more activation than the target sound or word at the moment that the sound or word is selected for production. In both the perseverative and non-perseverative cases, the intruding sound or word has exceeded the activation level of the target word. This is not normally a likely event. However, there are factors that lessen the target word's activation, and when this happens, the stage is set for other words or sounds to intrude. The activation of potential non-perseverative intrusions would be elevated primarily because of their similarity with the target word (semantic and phonological similarity for words and phonological similarity for sounds). The activation levels of possible perseverative intrusions would be elevated because of residual activation potential stemming from their prior utterance, which gradually recedes over time (Cohen & Dehane, 1998).

When we use the term "residual activation potential", we are deliberately conflating two notions. One is residual activation itself. When a unit in a spreading activation system is being processed, that processing is represented by its representation possessing an activation level over its normal baseline. Most spreading activation systems assume that it takes some time for that activation to return to its baseline. The other is that recent use may render the item more accessible by, for example, changing (either temporarily or permanently) other properties of the system that lead to activation, such as connection weights or item thresholds. Either way, a recently retrieved item has greater potential to compete in subsequent utterances.

In the present study we provide speech error data that support the claim that perseverations are caused by (1) weak activation of the intended word or sound and (2) residual activation potential of a prior word or sound utterance. Consequently, any factor that weakens the intended linguistic unit, or contributes to that of a prior unit promotes the probability of a perseveration. For example, a low-frequency word target should be vulnerable to perseverations of high-frequency words that were recently spoken, and data indicate that this is the case (Gotts, della Rocchetta, & Cipolotti, 2002; Hirsh, 1998). Moreover, the probability of a perseveration should be further enhanced if the two share semantic or phonological features, and again the data are supportive (Martin et al., 1998). The data presented here extend the support for this two-factor approach to perseverations by examining errors from a large-scale study of naming error patterns of 94 aphasic individuals (Schwartz et al., 2006)

Our account of perseverative errors is derived in theory from two computational models, one of single-word retrieval (Foygel & Dell, 2000; Schwartz et al., 2006) and another that deals with the serial order of words (Dell, Burger, & Svec, 1997a). Below, we describe each of these models briefly and the mechanisms by which errors occur.

TWO-STEP INTERACTIVE ACTIVATION MODEL OF WORD RETRIEVAL

Figure 1 depicts the hypothesised network structures that underlie the retrieval of a word from meaning (based on model in Foygel & Dell, 2000; Schwartz et al., 2006). The model's network has three layers of representation, semantic, lexical, and phonological. Word retrieval in production occurs via a spreading activation process through the three layers. This spreading is bidirectional, forward from semantic to lexical to phonological layers and feeding back in the reverse direction. Word and phoneme retrieval are competitive. After a certain amount of time, the most active word unit is selected and then given an extra boost of activation. Somewhat later, the most active phonological nodes are selected.

Our account of speech errors assumes that production of correct and erroneous utterances depends on a probabilistic process inherent in spreading activation; although the most active units are always chosen, at each moment in time, activation levels are perturbed by random noise. Correct utterances are, of course, highly probable and in reality, most prevalent. However, the intent to produce a word leads to the activation of the intended word and its sounds as well as activation of words and sounds that share properties with the target word. This happens simply because words that are similar in meaning share semantic units and words that are similar in sound share phonological units, and the shared units are conduits for the

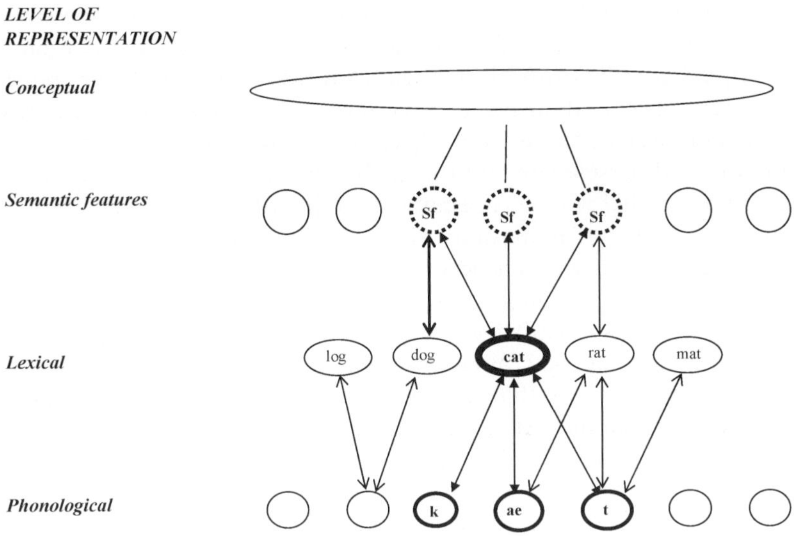

Figure 1. An interactive activation model of single word retrieval.

transmission of activation. The influence of semantic and phonological relatedness combines with other factors such as frequency, age of acquisition, and imageability that also contribute to the activation levels of the target word and its competitors. When a competitor is more active than the target, an error is chosen instead of the target. Perseverative sound and word substitutions work exactly the same way, except that residual activation potential also contributes to the probability of a word being retrieved in error.

A MODEL OF SERIAL ORDER

Dell et al.'s (1997a) model adds a mechanism for activating word sequences to the word retrieval model. It incorporates three components or functions that control serial order in speech production: turning off past utterances, activating current utterances, and priming upcoming utterances. The two components most related to perseverations are the turning off of previous utterances (to prevent them from being reselected) and the activation of the current target sounds and words, which must be sufficient to surpass other competing words. These three functions are widely accepted as necessary to control serial order (e.g., Houghton, 1990). More controversial, however, is the question of which component breaks down when there is a perseveration. Some models invoke a disinhibition account, which proposes that there is a failure of the function that is supposed to turn off past utterances (e.g., Arbuthnott, 1996; Yamadori, 1981).

Although this account can explain the existence of perseverations, it would have to include an additional disturbance affecting the activation of the current target utterance in order to account for high perseverative rates in some individuals with language impairment and the occurrence of non-perseverative errors. Additionally, the disinhibition account needs to explain whether some or all spoken words become disinhibited and, if the latter, why some disinhibited words intrude as perseverations and others do not. One possibility is that the disturbance in inhibition is partial and leaves varying amounts of residual activation that may or may not be sufficient to displace the current target word. However, several studies have demonstrated a systematic time-lag relationship between a target word and the most recent occurrence of a word that displaces that target (Cohen & Dehane, 1998; Gotts et al., 2002). This systematic relationship between the temporal window separating target and potential perseverate and the probability of that perseveration occurring is more easily reconciled with a systematic decaying function of activation potential than momentary failure of inhibition.

Dell et al. (1997a) provide an account of perseverations within their model of serial order by appealing to the two factors that we referred to earlier; weak target activation and residual activation potential. Perseverative sound and word substitutions are first enabled by some disturbance in activation of the current target word in the same way that non-perseverative sound and word substitutions are. Second, the probability of a perseverative intrusion is increased because its representations (semantic, lexical, and phonological) have been recently activated. Although the model does assume that some mechanism deactivates representations that are spoken, some degree of residual activation potential remains, and this residual increases the likelihood that previous representations are spoken later. Most importantly, though, unlike the disinhibition account, failure of the deactivation process is not assumed to be a major cause of perseverations in the serial order model. Finally, the increased probability associated with a previous item is further modulated by long-term factors such as the word's feature overlap with the intended utterance and its word frequency relative to the target word.

In this study, we report error data produced by 94 individuals with aphasia in response to a single-word picture-naming test (Schwartz et al., 2006). The corpus of responses includes both perseverative and non-perseverative word and sound errors. Although the task involves single-word utterances, one can still examine perseverative influences that arise from previous trials. Here we do so, and obtain support for the hypothesis that perseverative and non-perseverative word and sound errors share common underlying mechanisms. The error patterns are analysed in the context of the first model we presented, the interactive two-step model of word retrieval. Specifically, the aphasic naming deficits were modelled as lesions to two parameters of the model: the s parameter (semantic-lexical connection strength) and/or p (lexical-phonological connection strength) parameter. In the present study, we predicted that (1) lesions of the s parameter are associated with rates of both perseverative and non-perseverative whole-word substitutions, and (2) lesions of the p parameter are associated with perseverative and non-perseverative sound substitutions. That is, individuals whose overall naming error pattern is characterised best in the computational model with a semantic lesion, are more likely to produce whole-word errors whether they are perseverative or non-perseverative. The similarity of the perseverative and non-perseverative errors in both cases is the critical prediction. Additionally, we examined the distribution of perseverative and non-perseverative errors across error classes including semantic, formal, mixed, and unrelated word errors and nonword errors, predicting that the distributions would be similar. Finally, we anticipated that "no response" type errors would be associated with occurrences of whole-word perseverations, reflecting weak activation of the connections between semantics and the word form representation of the intended word. Such a relationship would support the hypothesis that weak activation of a target word is part of the mechanism by which whole-word perseverative intrusions occur (Dell et al., 1997a; Schwartz, Saffran, Dell & Bloch, 1994).

METHOD

Participants

The 94 individuals with aphasia who participated in Schwartz et al. (2006) and Dell, Martin, and Schwartz (2007) also participated in this study. Aetiology of aphasia for 93 of the participants was a cerebral vascular accident, and for 1 participant a gunshot wound. The average age of our participants was 59 and the age range was 22 to 86 years. Mean education level was 13.2 years with a range from 7 to 25 years. The average number of months post-onset was 38.2 and ranged from 1 to 195 months post-onset. A total of 40% of our participants were female and 39% were African-American. All participants were administered the *Western Aphasia Battery* (*WAB*; Kertesz, 1982). By the WAB classification, our sample included 33% with Broca's aphasia, 31% with anomic aphasia, 19% with conduction aphasia, 15% with Wernicke's aphasia, and 2% with transcortical sensory aphasia.

Participants were tested under a research protocol that was approved by the Institutional Review Boards of Temple University and Albert Einstein Healthcare Network (AEHN). They provided written informed consent before enrolling in the study, and they were paid for their participation.

Assessment of picture naming

The *Philadelphia Naming Test* (*PNT*; Roach, Schwartz, Martin, Grewal, & Brecher, 1996) was administered to each participant. This test consists of 175 pictures of objects. The object names are one to four syllables long and range in frequency from 1 to 2110 occurrences per million (Francis & Kucera, 1982).

The pictures are presented on a Macintosh computer using MacLaboratory software (Chute, 1990). A picture appears on the screen and the participant is given 30 seconds to name the picture. The examiner says the name after the participant has given a response or at the end of 30 seconds, after which the next trial is initiated. The participant's responses are tape-recorded and roughly transcribed during the session. The tapes are also transcribed later by a certified speech pathologist. Eight response categories are relevant to current predictions:

Correct response. This category includes responses with all phonemes correct. Additionally, for some participants with articulatory impairments (apraxia, dysarthria) we developed a lenient score which ignored minor articulatory distortions that were consistently produced by a participant, and deviations from the target word by the addition, deletion, or substitution of a single consonant.

Semantic error. This is a whole-word error that holds one of the following relationships with the target word: synonymous, associative, categorical (coordinate, subordinate, or superordinate).

Formal error. This is a whole-word error that is phonologically related to the target word. An error word is phonologically related when the target and error begin or end with the same phoneme, when they have a phoneme in common in corresponding syllable or word positions, or when they share more than one phoneme (excluding unstressed vowels) in any part of the word.

Mixed error. This is a whole-word error that is both semantically and phonologically related to the target word.

Nonword error. This category includes nonwords that are phonologically similar to the target (e.g., bucket → /bae-kIn/) and those that are not (e.g., bucket → /do-fIn/).

Unrelated error. This is a whole-word error that has no semantic or formal overlap with the target word.

No response. This error category includes instances when the participant offers no response to the picture.

Description. This category includes phrase and sentence responses that describe the picture or the concept it represents, but do not include an attempt to name it.

Perseverative sound and word errors

In Schwartz et al. (2006) each of the word and sound response categories could also include a second classification if they were perseverations. In such instances the response was coded as one of the categories above and then as a whole-word perseveration or a sound perseveration. Whole-word errors were classified as perseverations if the error was produced in any previous response within the testing session. Sound errors were coded as perseverations if the sound occurred in the previous response.

Fitting the models to the data

Schwartz et al. (2006) used two versions of the interactive activation model to fit to the naming data: the weight-decay (WD) model and the semantic-phonological (SP) model. The WD model fits naming data by altering parameters of connection weight and decay rate globally throughout the semantic-lexical-phonological network. This model has been tested as an account of naming impairment in aphasia in several studies (Martin, Dell, Saffran, & Schwartz, 1994; Dell, Schwartz, Martin, Saffran, & Gagnon, 1997b). In the present paper we focus on the account of aphasic naming in the SP version of the model, which lesions only the parameter of connection weight, but does so separately for semantic-lexical connections (s weight) and lexical-phonological connections (p weight). To fit the data, free parameters s and p were assigned to the model to generate error proportions that approximated as closely as possible those of the patient. Only the proportions of correct responses, and semantic, formal, mixed, unrelated, and nonword errors are used in the model-fitting process. "No response" errors and descriptions are removed from the data before the fitting begins. It is also important to note that whether or not a given error was perseveratory was not considered. For example, the proportion of semantic errors included both perseverations and non-perseverations. The closeness of the fits was evaluated with a chi square goodness of fit value. The parameters were identified by using a pre-stored variable-resolution map of the parameter space. Details of this fitting procedure can be found in Dell, Lawler, Harris, and Gordon (2004), and the fitting routine itself can be used by following the procedures noted in http://langprod.cogsci.uiuc.edu/cgi-bin/webfit.cgi)

The distribution of each participant's naming responses across response categories as well as the fits of those data to the weight-decay and semantic-phonological models can be found in Table 2 of Schwartz et al., (2006).

In the analyses below, we looked first at accuracy of naming in relation to two sets of variables: (1) the s weight and p weight parameters used to fit naming response patterns of the 94 participants to the interactive activation model, and (2) the rates of word and sound perseverations produced by each participant. We then examined the model's predictions concerning the relationship between lesioned s and p weight parameters and occurrences of perseverative and non-perseverative word and sound errors and "no response" errors. These predictions are outlined with each analysis.

In other analyses we investigated relationships among perseverative and non-perseverative errors to determine whether their distributions across error classes (e.g., semantic, formal, nonword) were similar within participants, suggesting a common mechanism underlying the occurrence of perseverative and non-perseverative errors. Finally, we investigated whether word or sound perseverations were associated with "No response" type errors. Such an association would be consistent with the idea that weak activation of targets, indexed by no responses, also sets the stage for perseverations.

RESULTS

Model's predictions of naming responses

The five analyses below examine the model's predictions of naming accuracy and occurrences of various error types.

Analysis 1. Integrity of s and p parameters and accuracy of naming response. As might be expected, the size of both the s weight and the p weight predict accuracy of naming (s weight and correctness: $r = .653$, $p < .0000001$; p weight and correctness: $r = .368$, $p < .0001$, indicating that the stronger connection weights are associated with greater accuracy.

Analysis 2. Rates of word and sound perseverations and overall accuracy in naming. Significant negative correlations were obtained between rates of whole-word perseverations and accuracy ($r = -.676$, $p < .0000001$) and between rates of sound perseverations and accuracy ($r = -.589$, $p < .00000001$) indicating that patients who made more perseverations were less accurate in overall naming.

Analysis 3. Model's predictions of word and sound perseverations. The model characterises word retrieval impairments as some degree of reduction in semantic weight (the s parameter) and/or reduction in phonological weight (the p parameter). In this analysis, we correlated the s and p weights used to characterise each patient's naming response distribution with their overall rates of word and sound perseverations. We predicted that the s parameter would correlate negatively with rates of word-level perseverations, reflecting an association between weak links from semantic to lexical representations and occurrences of word-level perseverations. We further predicted that the p parameter would correlate negatively with rates of sound perseverations reflecting an association of weakened links between lexical and sound representations and occurrences of sound perseverations. In line with our predictions, whole-word perseverations were negatively associated with the value of the s parameter. Sound perseverations correlated negatively and significantly with both s and p values, although as expected, the association was more apparent in the p parameter (see Table 1).

Analysis 4. Model's predictions of rates of perseverative and non-perseverative whole-word errors in picture naming. Here we correlated the s and p values with rates of four categories of whole-word errors (semantic, mixed, formal, and unrelated paraphasias). The lexical errors were divided into perseverative and non-perseverative types within each error category to test the hypothesis that a reduction in s, but not p, would be associated with whole-word errors regardless of whether they were perseverative or non-perseverative. The results, noted in Table 2, support this hypothesis. With one exception, perseverative and non-perseverative whole-word substitutions are negatively correlated with semantic weights, indicating that weaker semantic connection weight is associated with a greater number of whole-word errors. The one exception is the rate of non-perseverative formal paraphasias. These were negatively associated with reductions of both s and p weights. This outcome is consistent with the general consensus that a subset of the formal

TABLE 1
Analysis 3: Perseveration type

Parameter	*Word*	*Sound*
s weight	−.499**	−.122
p weight	−.333**	−.444**

Analysis 3. Pearson correlations between rates of whole-word and sound perseverations with the s- and p-weight parameters of the interactive activation model used to fit naming response distributions of 94 subjects on the *Philadelphia Naming Test* (Roach et al., 1996). $^{**}p < .001$, $^{*}p < .05$

TABLE 2
Analysis 4: Response category

Parameter	*Semantic*	*Formal*	*Mixed*	*Unrelated*
Perseverative				
s weight	−.320**	−.367**	−.269**	−.447**
p weight	.064	−.178	.065	−.144
Non-perseverative				
s weight	−.375**	−.383**	$-.184^{+}$	−.544**
p weight	.028	−.423**	.099	−.227*

Analysis 4. Pearson correlations between rates of four categories of perseverative and non-perseverative whole-word substitutions and the s- and p-weight parameters of the interactive activation model used to fit naming response distributions of 94 subjects on the *Philadelphia Naming Test* (Roach et al., 1996). $^{**}p < .001$, $^{*}p < .05$, $+p = .08$

paraphasias are errors at the stage of phonological retrieval, not word retrieval (Dell et al., 1997b; Schwartz et al., 2006).

Analysis 5. Model's predictions of rates of perseverative and non-perseverative nonword errors in picture naming. Here we correlated s and p with rates of pure nonword errors and with nonword errors that involved a sound perseveration. This pattern of correlations contrasts with that involving word errors, in that it is the p, not the s, parameter that is most important. As Table 3 indicates, occurrences of both pure and perseverative nonword errors correlate negatively with the p parameter. The correlations of the nonword errors with s are also negative, but considerably smaller.

Analysis 6. Model's predictions of "no response" errors. Sometimes when an individual has difficulty retrieving a name, they give no response at all. Accompanying this "no response" might be a statement such as "I know it but I can't say it". These responses could be due to weak activation of the word from semantics (reduced s weight) or weak activation spreading from the word to its corresponding phonemes (reduced p weight). Dell et al. (2004) hypothesised that these kinds of responses reflect events in which the word level is insufficiently active to be selected. Because the semantic-lexical connections are more influential in this activation than the lexical-phonological connections, we predicted that "no responses" would be more strongly associated with s, than with p. We correlated s and p weights used to model each participant's naming response pattern with rates of no responses and descriptive responses. The latter response type is very similar to the "no response" error except that the participant provides some descriptive information about the pictured object that he/she cannot name. Table 4 shows the

TABLE 3
Analysis 5: Nonword error type

Parameter	*Perseverative*	*Non-perseverative*
s weight	−.265**	−.149
p weight	−.440**	−.552**

Analysis 5. Pearson correlations of rates of perseverative and non-perseverative nonword errors with the s- and p-weight parameters of the interactive activation model used to fit naming response distributions of 94 subjects on the *Philadelphia Naming Test* (Roach et al., 1996). $^{**}p < .001$, $^{*}p < .05$

TABLE 4
Analysis 6: Response type

Parameter	*Descriptions*	*No Response*
s weight	−.364**	−.372**
p weight	−.048	−.023

Analysis 6. Pearson correlations of rates "No response" and Descriptive (circumlocutions) responses with the s- and p-weight parameters of the interactive activation model used to fit naming response distributions of 94 subjects on the *Philadelphia Naming Test* (Roach et al., 1996). $^{**}p < .001$, $^{*}p < .05$

relevant data. As predicted, the rates of descriptive and no response errors are significantly negatively correlated with s, but not p. Thus, the weaker the semantic-lexical connection weights, the more likely there is to be a no response type error.

Analysis 7. Distributions of perseverative and non-perseverative word and sound errors across error categories. If perseverative and non-perseverative whole-word substitutions share some common underlying mechanism, they should tend to be observed together in the same patients. The same is true for nonword errors. Nonword errors with no perseverated sounds from an immediately preceding response should be positively correlated with nonword errors that do include a sound perseveration from the prior response. We included in the analyses of formal paraphasias both word-level and sound-level perseverations because, as noted earlier, evidence suggests that formal paraphasias can result from mis-selection of the lexical representation or mis-selection of a phoneme with an outcome that by chance is a real word. For the other categories of word error, we only looked at occurrences of whole-word perseverations. Finally, the nonword perseverations by their very nature included only sound-level perseverations.

Table 5 shows a matrix of correlations between non-perseverative and perseverative word errors of four types (mixed, semantic, formal, and unrelated) and non-perseverative and perseverative nonword errors. For all categories of error, the rates of perseverative and non-perseverative occurrences are positively and significantly correlated. This pattern indicates that a participant's distribution of word and nonword errors is similar for perseverative and non-perseverative errors even if the absolute rates of each are different.

Figure 2 shows the plots of regression line fits associated with the correlations of perseverative and non-perseverative errors in six categories of error. Although there is some variability across error types, the plots show that occurrences of perseverative and non-perseverative errors are generally associated. This variability will be discussed further in the General Discussion.

The correlation matrix in Table 5 also shows some associations between perseverative and non-perseverative errors of different classes. These all fall generally into an expected pattern. Mixed errors, which include a semantic relationship with the target, are associated with semantic perseverations. Formal paraphasias, which are sound-based word errors, are associated with perseverative

TABLE 5
Analysis 7: Response types

Non-perseverations:	*Perseverations: Response type*					
Response type	*Mixed*	*Semantic*	*Formal (Word)*	*Formal (Sound)*	*Unrelated*	*Nonword*
Mixed	.257*	.285*	.130	−.174	.064	−.216
Semantic	.420**	.334**	.104	−.170	.050	−.218
Formal	.065	.025	.349**	.619**	.198	.679**
Unrelated	.224*	.050	.681**	.578**	.727**	.412**
Nonword	−.080	−.194	.045	.526**	−.031	.657**

Analysis 7. Matrix of Pearson correlations between among of perseverative and non-perseverative word errors in four response categories and perseverative and non-perseverative nonword errors produced by 94 participants on the *Philadelphia Naming Test* (Roach et al., 1996). $^{**}p < .001$, $^{*}p < .05$

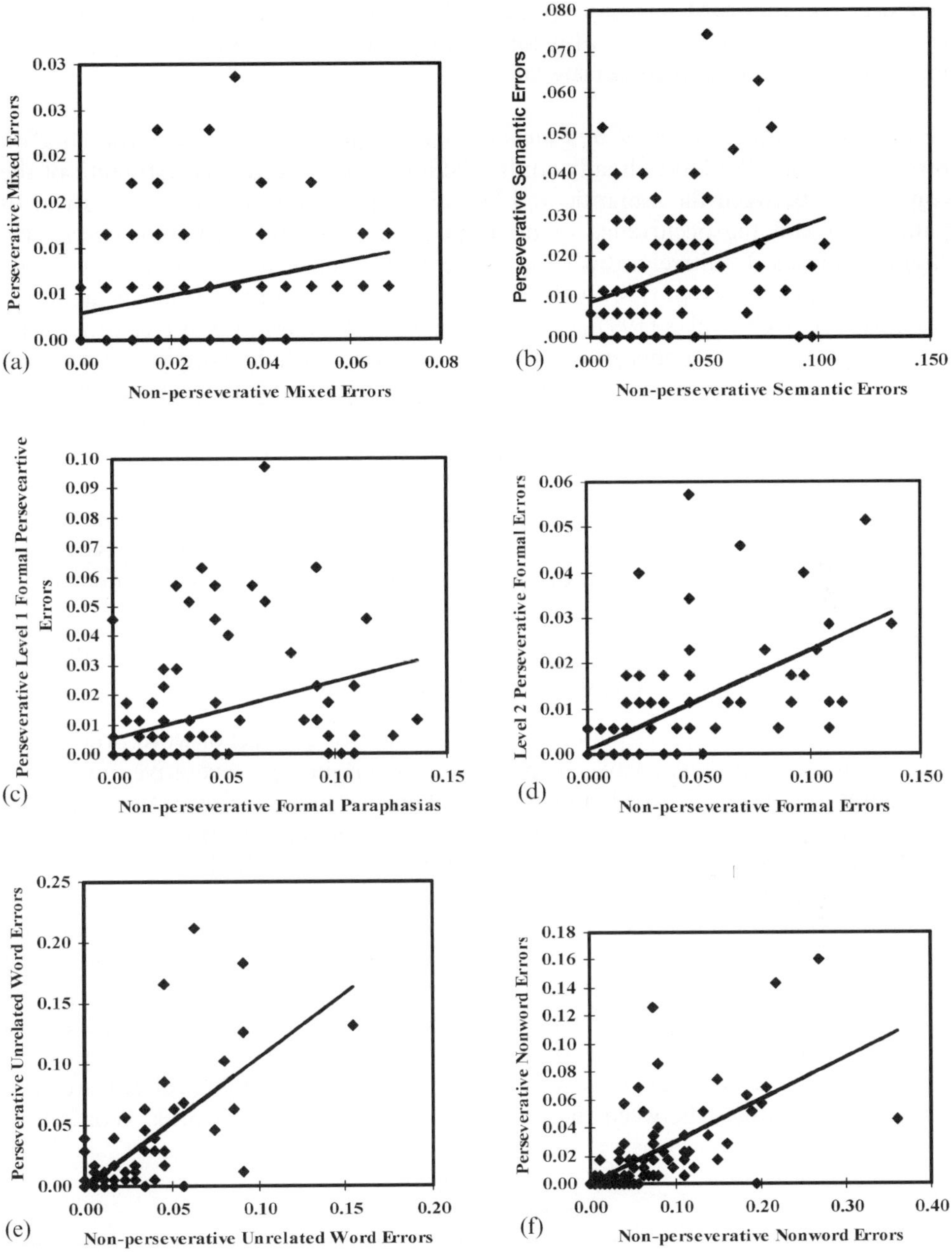

Figure 2. (a) Rates of perseverative and non-perseverative mixed errors: Plot of regression line fit. (b) Rates of perseverative and non-perseverative semantic errors: Plot of regression line fit. (c) Rates of perseverative (whole-word overlap) and non-perseverative formal paraphasias: Plot of regression line fit. (d) Rates of perseverative (sound overlap) and non-perseverative formal paraphasias: Plot of regression line fit. (e) Rates of perseverative and non-perseverative unrelated whole-word errors: Plot of regression line fit. (f) Rates of perseverative (sound overlap) and non-perseverative nonword errors: Plot of regression line fit.

sound-based nonword errors. Overall, these results are consistent with the hypothesis that the occurrence of whole-word substitutions is governed by the same mechanisms as whole-word perseverations.

Analysis 8. Rates of word and sound perseverations and the occurrence of "no response" errors. We have already confirmed a link between reduced strength of the connections between the semantic and lexical levels of representation (the s weight parameter) and the occurrence of no response type errors, including descriptive circumlocutions. Intuitively, this relationship makes sense; if one cannot access the word form from semantics, it is difficult to initiate production of a word. Additionally, Dell et al.'s (1997a) model of serial order implicates a role of reduced strength to these same connections in the occurrence of whole-word perseverations. The rationale is that weak connection strength supporting the current intended utterance provides a context in which a prior utterance with some residual activation potential could surpass the activation level of the current target and intrude as a perseveration. On the basis of this hypothesised mechanism, we predicted that whole-word perseverations would correlate positively with rates of no responses and descriptive circumlocutions. As Table 6 indicates, these two error types are significantly correlated with occurrences of word perseverations but not sound perseverations.

GENERAL DISCUSSION

The analyses reported in this paper provide evidence for a model of word production that assumes continuity between processes underlying perseverative and non-perseverative sound and word substitutions. That is to say, perseverative and non-perseverative intrusions are generated by the same malfunction of the word production system; weak activation of the target word and sounds in the context of competition from other sounds and words activated via spreading activation. Competition between a target word and other words in the lexicon is initiated by several factors. Chief among these is the spreading of activation from the target word to other words in the lexicon that share semantic and phonological features with that target word. In the interactive activation model, words that share semantic features of the target are activated in the initial feedforward spreading of activation throughout the lexical network, and words that share phonological features are activated by feedback between the phonological and lexical networks. Words that

TABLE 6
Analysis 8: Perseveration

Type	*Descriptions*	*No Response*
Word (whole-word perseverations)	.222*	.408**
Sound (sound perseverations)	.138	.034

Analysis 8. Pearson correlations between rates of "No Response" and Descriptive (circumlocutions) responses and rates of Word and Sound perseverative errors produced by 94 participants on the *Philadelphia Naming Test* (Roach et al., 1996). $^{*}p < .05$, $^{**}p < .001$

have been activated recently because they have been spoken are also subject to the same influences that contribute to competition between the target word and other words in the lexicon. However, these same words have an additional boost to their activation levels because they have been activated recently. This factor is what distinguishes perseverative from non-perseverative substitutions.

This conclusion is supported by the data from this study. In all of our analyses, perseverative and non-perseverative errors behaved similarly. The interactive model's predictions about lesions leading to particular classes of errors were consistent for both perseverative and non-perseverative errors within each class of error. Moreover, the relationships between lesioned parameters and error types make sense. Reduced semantic weights should be associated with higher rates of word errors as this kind of lesion affects competition at the word level. In the same vein, reduced phonological weights should be associated with sound-level errors because reduced strength of the links between words and sounds affects competition at the sound level.

Additionally, the correlational analyses of the perseverative and non-perseverative errors indicate that they show similar distributions across error categories within participants. Of course, it is important to note that the correlations are not perfect and, for error categories that are infrequent such as semantic and mixed errors, they are somewhat small (see Figure 2 for scatter plots of perseverative and non-perseverative errors for the error categories). Some of this variability is just noise in the data. However, we acknowledge that we cannot rule out the possibility that some variation is due to individuals having greater or less perseverative tendencies—tendencies that are independent of the size of their semantic and phonological lesions. Our point is only that such an independent tendency is not an overwhelming factor for our sample. If it were, it would work against the correlations that we found between perseverative and non-perseverative error rates for the categories.

Two findings from this study are important with respect to the model of perseveration that we are advocating (Dell et al., 1997a). The first is the relationship between reduced s weights (between semantics and the word form) and the occurrence of "no response" errors and description errors. Second is the relationship between perseverations and these same classes of error. The weak connections between semantic and lexical levels of representation make it difficult to activate the target representation. In this case, the speaker would produce an erroneous response, refrain from offering a response at all, or describe whatever he/she knows about the pictured object without producing the name. The finding that whole-word perseverations are associated (1) with reduced semantic weights, and (2) with "no response" and descriptive errors, provides further corroborating evidence that they are a normal outcome of a system with an impairment affecting strength of activation of the word that is intended to be spoken. In unimpaired speakers, that strength can be reduced because of speed stress or unfamiliarity with the word or sound sequence, and in aphasic speakers, the strength of activation is reduced because of the brain damage (Schwartz et al., 1994).

Although these findings have theoretical implications as we have discussed, they are also of clinical interest. Perseveration is not an uncommon occurrence in aphasia. Diagnostic information concerning the locus of breakdown in the language system can be inferred from the patterns of association between word and nonword perseverative and non-perseverative errors as well as the association between "no response" type errors and whole-word perseverations. For example, if it is observed that "no response" errors and whole-word perseverations are both present, we could infer that the breakdown in word retrieval is occurring in the connections between semantic and lexical representations, and that the impairment is affecting the ability to successfully activate the targeted word representation. If there are fewer of these word-level errors and sound errors are more predominant, we would likely see few word-level perseverations, but might observe sound-level perseverations. This clustering of error patterns can be informative about the locus of the deficit in word retrieval and consequently guide the treatment approaches that a clinician might take in working with a client.

CONCLUSION

The analysis of perseverative and non-perseverative word and sound substitutions presented here supports a model of perseveration that involves, at minimum, two components: one that is shared with the mechanism that generates non-perseverative word and sound errors, and one that is responsible for the perseverative influence itself. In other words, perseverative and non-perseverative errors are at least as much alike as they are different. Patterns of both perseverative and non-perseverative errors clearly reflect the locus of impairment in the word retrieval system. Whole-word errors (perseverative and non-perseverative), no responses, and descriptions reflect unsuccessful activation of the word form from semantics. Sound errors (both perseverative and non-perseverative) reflect weak spreading of activation from a word representation to its constituent sounds.

REFERENCES

Arbuthnott, K. D. (1996). To repeat or not to repeat: Repetition facilitation and inhibition in sequential retrieval. *Journal of Experimental Psychology: General, 125*, 261–283.

Chute, D. L. (1990). *MacLaboratory for Psychology* (computer program). Devon, PA.: MacLaboratory.

Cohen, L., & Dehaene, S. (1998). Competition between past and present. Assessment and interpretation of verbal perseverations. *Brain, 121*, 1641–1659.

Dell, G. S., Burger, L. K., & Svec, W. R. (1997a). Language production and serial order: A functional analysis and a model. *Psychological Review, 104*, 123–147.

Dell, G. S., Lawler, E. N., Harris, H. D., & Gordon, J. K. (2004). Models of errors of omission in aphasic naming. *Cognitive Neuropsychology, 21*, 125–146.

Dell, G. S., Martin, N., & Schwartz, M. F. (2007). A case-series test of the interactive two-step model of lexical access: Predicting word repetition from picture naming. *Journal of Memory and Language, 56*, 490–520.

Dell, G. S., & Reich, P. A. (1981). Stages in sentence production: An analysis of speech error data. *Journal of Verbal Learning and Verbal Behavior, 20*, 611–629.

Dell, G. S., Schwartz, M. F., Martin, N., Saffran, E. M., & Gagnon, D. A. (1997b). Lexical access in aphasic and non-aphasic speakers. *Psychological Review, 104*(4), 801–838.

Foygel, D., & Dell, G. S. (2000). Models of impaired lexical access in speech production. *Journal of Memory and Language, 43*, 182–216.

Francis, W. N., & Kucera, H. (1982). *Frequency analysis of English usage: Lexicon and grammar*. Boston, MA: Houghton-Mifflin.

Fromkin, V. A. (1971). The non-anomalous nature of anomalous utterances. *Language, 47*, 27–52.

Garrett, M. F. (1975). The analysis of sentence production. In G. H. Bower (Ed.), *The psychology of learning and motivation* (pp. 133–175). San Diego, CA: Academic Press.

Gotts, S. J., della Rocchetta, A., & Cipolotti, I. L. (2002). Mechanisms underlying perseveration in aphasia: Evidence from a single case study. *Neuropsychologia, 40*, 1930–1947.

Harley, T. A. (1984). A critique of top-down independent levels models of speech production: Evidence from non-plan internal speech errors. *Cognitive Science*, *8*, 191–219.

Hirsh, K. W. (1998). Perseveration and activation in aphasic speech production. *Cognitive Neuropsychology*, *15*(4), 377–388.

Houghton, G. (1990). The problem of serial order: A neural network memory of sequence learning and recall. In R. Dale, C. Mellish, & M. Zock (Eds.), *Current research in natural language generation*. London: Academic Press.

Kertesz, A. (1982). *Western Aphasia Battery*. New York: Grune & Stratton.

Levelt, W. J. M., Roelofs, A., & Meyer, A. S. (1999). A theory of lexical access in speech production. *Behavioral and Brain Science*, *22*, 1–75.

Martin, N., & Dell, G. S. (2004). Perseverations and anticipations in aphasia: Primed intrusions from the past and future. *Seminars in Speech and Language Pathology*, *25*, 349–362.

Martin, N., Dell, G. S., Saffran, E. M., & Schwartz, M. F. (1994). Origins of paraphasias in deep dysphasia: Testing the consequences of a decay inpairment in an interactive spreading activation model of language. *Brain & Language*, *47*, 609–660.

Martin, N., Gagnon, D., Schwartz, M. F., Dell, G. S., & Saffran, E. M. (1996). Phonological facilitation of semantic errors in normal and aphasic speakers on a picture naming task. *Language and Cognitive Processes*, *11*, 257–282.

Martin, N., Roach, A., Brecher, A., & Lowery, J. (1998). Lexical retrieval mechanisms underlying whole-word perseveration errors in anomic aphasia. *Aphasiology*, *12*, 319–333.

Martin, N., Weisberg, R. W., & Saffran, E. M. (1989). Variables influencing the occurrence of naming errors: Implications for models of lexical retrieval. *Journal of Memory and Language*, *28*, 462–485.

Roach, A., Schwartz, M. F., Martin, N., Grewal, R. S., & Brecher, A. (1996). The Philadelphia Naming Test: Scoring and rationale. *Clinical Aphasiology*, *24*, 121–133.

Schwartz, M. F., Dell, G. S., Martin, N., Gahl, S., & Sobel, P. (2006). A case series test of the two-step interactive model of lexical access: Evidence from picture naming. *Journal of Memory and Language*, *54*, 228–264.

Schwartz, M. F., Saffran, E. M., Bloch, D., & Dell, G. S. (1994). Disordered speech production in aphasic and normal speakers. *Brain and Language*, *47*, 52–88.

Yamadori, A. (1981). Verbal perseveration in aphasia. *Neuropsychologia*, *19*, 591–594.

APHASIOLOGY, 2007, 21 (10/11), 1018–1038

Psychology Press
Taylor & Francis Group

Case study: Where do aphasic perseverations come from?

Tess Ackerman

Leeds East Primary Care Trust, and University of York, UK

Andrew W. Ellis

University of York, UK

Background: Perseverations are common in the speech of people with aphasia but the phenomenon has been the subject of relatively little investigation. We had the opportunity to study an aphasic patient who produced a large number of perseverations in naming, reading, and repetition tasks.
Aims: To gain a better understanding of the origins and causes of perseverative errors in a man with aphasia (MM) through a detailed analysis of his errors across naming, reading, and repetition, combined with a thorough assessment of his language disorder.
Methods & Procedures: MM was given a cognitive neuropsychological assessment of his language-processing system. He was then asked to name 140 black and white drawings of objects and to repeat and read aloud the same 140 object names. Each of these tasks was done on two occasions.
Outcomes & Results: MM showed major semantic impairment combined with some phonological and orthographic deficits. He was better at reading object names than repeating them, and worst at object naming. Analysis of his errors showed differences between naming, repeating, and reading. Whole-word perseverations were most common in object naming, where they were predominantly unrelated to the target items.
Conclusions: MM's aphasia and perseverations are discussed in terms of the theory put forward by Martin and Dell (2007, this issue). We endorse the proposition that perseverations should be understood within the wider context of aphasic breakdown, and that no special mechanisms may be required to explain perseverative errors. But the lack of any influence of lexical responses like word frequency on MM's performance, and the fact that perseverations mostly resulted in unrelated errors, are problematic for the Martin and Dell framework. They suggest that MM's perseverations mostly occurred when his semantic and phonological system were deprived of any useable input, with the target being unable to influence the response. Under such circumstances, either no response was available, or MM made an unconstrained and therefore unrelated response, in which case the endogenously driven reactivation of recent responses (whole words or fragments) was likely to fill the void with a perseverative error.

Perseverative errors are common in aphasia but have received relatively little attention within aphasiology, at least until recently. An early study by Sandson and

Address correspondence to: Andrew Ellis, Department of Psychology, University of York, York YO10 5DD, UK. E-mail: awe1@york.ac.uk

We are grateful to MM for agreeing to participate in this study, which formed part of the first author's postgraduate study at the University of York, supported by a major scholarship from the Hospital Saving Association Charitable Trust, and by the Leeds Community and Mental Health Trust and the Leeds East Primary Care Trust.

http://www.psypress.com/aphasiology DOI: 10.1080/02687030701198361

Albert (1984) noted that perseverations can occur in non-linguistic tasks as well as in language use, and drew a distinction between three different forms of perseveration. "Continuous perseveration" was illustrated by a patient who, when asked to draw a daisy, put an inappropriately large number of petals on his drawing. "Stuck-in-set perseveration" occurred when a patient was unable to switch from one approach or task to another. Recurrent perseverations were defined as the unintentional repetition of a response in the absence of the stimulus that initially elicited it. They were illustrated with reference to an aphasic patient who defined the word bed as "lay on", then, when asked to define ship, replied "lay on, no ship, bed", with perseverations on the previous error (lay on) and the previous target (bed). The next-but-one target word was "breakfast", which the patient defined as "breakfast, bed, bacon", perseverating again on "bed".

Allison and Hurwitz (1967) tested 24 aphasic patients for perseveration in verbal and non-verbal tasks. Of these patients, 16 showed signs of perseveration, although none of them perseverated in all of the tasks, indicating that perseveration is not a general tendency but may affect some tasks and not others. The 31 aphasic individuals tested by Santo Pietro and Rigrodsky (1982) all showed some degree of perseveration in picture naming, word reading, or sentence completion, although the percentage of perseverative responses varied from 7% to 70%. Yamadori (1981) and Albert and Sandson (1986) also noted widespread perseverative errors in their aphasic patients.

The present paper is concerned with the phenomenon of recurrent perseveration in aphasia. Hirsh (1998) noted four characteristics of this form of perseveration that are pertinent to any attempt to explain how and why it comes about. First, whole words are the commonest unit for perseveration, but parts of words and whole nonwords may also perseverate (Buckingham, Whitaker, & Whitaker, 1979; Santo Pietro & Rigrodsky, 1986). Second, a response need not have been correct in the first instance for it to be perseverated: both errors and correct responses can be perseverated, as can items presented as targets that were not responded to correctly in the first instance (Buckingham et al., 1979; Santo Pietro & Rigrodsky, 1986; Yamadori, 1981). Third, a word can appear as a perseveration to the item that immediately follows it, but it is common for one or more other items to intervene before the perseveration occurs (Buckingham, 1985; Sandson & Albert, 1984; Yamadori, 1981). Fourth, perseverating words may be semantically or phonologically related to the target word that evokes them, but are often unrelated (see Papagno & Basso, 1996; Sandson & Albert, 1984; Santo Pietro & Rigrodsky, 1986).

Hirsh (1998) reported the case of an aphasic patient, CJ, who was tested a year or more after a left-hemisphere CVA and who made perseverative errors in both naming pictures of objects and reading the written names of those objects aloud. CJ's accuracy in the two tasks was very similar (naming 22% correct; reading aloud 23% correct). Approximately 35% of his errors in both tasks involved perseveration, including perseverations of whole words (e.g., lion → "hour" followed later by owl → "hour") and perseverations of part-words or part-nonwords (e.g., giraffe → "villion" followed later by lemon → "willion"). Most perseverated responses were made only once or twice, but some responses were repeated up to 10 times. An average of 7 to 10 items intervened between productions of the same response, with a range from 0 to 58 intervening items in naming and 0 to 61 items in reading aloud. Although some perseverated responses in naming and reading were semantically related to the target word that elicited them (about 12%), and a further 18% in naming and 23% in reading were phonologically related to the target word, the majority of perseverated responses (64% in both tasks) bore no apparent relation to the item that CJ was trying to name or read when the error occurred. Some authors have reported patients in whom the majority of perseverative errors were related to the target items that induced them (e.g., Martin, Roach, Brecher, & Lowery, 1998) while other authors have reported lesser effects of target–error relatedness (e.g., Moses, Nickels, & Sheard, 2004; Papagno & Basso, 1996). Finally, Hirsh (1998) reported an effect of word frequency on CJ's naming and reading accuracy: items that resulted in correct responses were more frequent than items that resulted in either perseverative or non-perseverative errors. Santo Pietro and Rigrodsky (1982) reported a similar effect of frequency, although Halpern (1965) found only influence of word length, with items that resulted in correct responses tending to be shorter than items that resulted in perseverations. Martin et al. (1998) were unable to detect an influence of word frequency in their three aphasic patients.

Hirsh (1998) argued that an account based on a semantic interaction between the target and persisting activation from a previous, related word would not explain most of CJ's whole-word perseverations satisfactorily, just as it would not explain his nonword perseverations (such as carrot → "myralin" followed later by pumpkin → "myralin"). Nonword perseveration, Hirsh suggested, implied persisting activation at the level of phonemes (see also Moses et al., 2004). Important recent developments in our understanding of the processes underlying perseverative errors include the publication of accounts that explain such errors in terms of damage to component processes within implemented computational models (Gotts & Plaut, 2004; Martin & Dell, 2007 this issue). We will return to such models in the Discussion section of this paper.

The present paper reports a case study of an aphasic man, MM, who made frequent perseverations in naming, and also made perseverative errors in repetition and reading aloud. He perseverated both whole words and fragments of words and nonwords. At this point we refer the reader to Table 1 for an impression of the extent to which MM's attempts to name a sequence of object pictures were compromised by frequent perseverations. In Sample 1, MM produced a semantic error in response to the second item in a series of pictures (a picture of a lion, which MM called a "tiger"). He went on to produce the word "tiger" as a whole-word perseveration on items 13, 25, 29, and 30. With the possible exception of spider → "tiger", these were all unrelated word errors. But fragments of "tiger" also occurred in his responses on trials 7, 10, 11, 12, 14, and 27. Sample 2 highlights perseverations involving the word "umbrella", which was produced first as a correct naming response, but then occurred a further 20 times as a whole-word perseveration in addition to contributing to nonwords with perseverative fragments (e.g., "sumbrella", "humbrehat"). Both whole- and part-word perseverations could span one or more intervening items: in the lower sample, "umbrella" occurred as a perseverative error to item 42 (sock) then not again until item 82, where it was produced as an unrelated perseverative response to the target kangaroo.

The aim of our investigation was to understand more about the causes of MM's perseverations, and to do that in the context of an assessment of the status of his language-processing system more generally. That assessment provides the context in which to consider the pattern of whole-word and fragmentary perseverative errors in naming, repetition, and reading. We will begin by characterising MM's language processing, and in particular his processing of single words, through a consideration of his performance on a wide-ranging cognitive neuropsychological assessment. That

TABLE 1
Perseverations in MM's naming of a series of object pictures

Item no.	*Target*	*Response*	*Item no.*	*Target*	*Response*
Sample 1					
2	Lion	*tiger*	17	Box	(no response)
3	Whistle	wiskle	18	Whale	seng
4	Clock	wis	19	Vase	sig
5	Violin	three	20	Crab	sai
6	Bath	bath	21	Bell	sung
7	Telescope	*tiggen*	22	Rabbit	shabbit
8	Giraffe	five	23	Soldier	(no response)
9	Torch	talk	24	Yo-yo	(no response)
10	Umbrella	*tig*	25	Spider	*tiger*
11	Sheep	*tigger*	26	Candle	sigle … wax
12	Bellows	*tie*	27	Van	*tie*
13	Mermaid	*tiger*	28	Chain	cheen
14	Window	*tig*	29	Flag	*tiger*
15	Swan	saik	30	Stool	*tiger*
16	Moon	noon			
Sample 2					
10	Umbrella	*umbrella*	42	Sock	*umbrella*
11	Sheep	lamb	43	Cheese	tebatow
12	Bellows	*umbrella*	…		
13	Mermain	*umbrella*	…		
14	Window	*umbrella*	81	Balloon	ballow
15	Swan	*umbrella*	82	Kangaroo	*umbrella*
16	Moon	moose	83	Boy	footballer
17	Box	*umbrella*	…		
18	Whale	*umbrella*	92	Bowl	bowl
19	Vase	can't remember	93	Caravan	*umbrella*
20	Crab	*umbrella*	94	Squirrel	girl
21	Bell	*umbrella*	95	Microscope	telephone
…			96	Carrot	(no response)
25	Spider	(no response)	97	Pram	*umbrella*
26	Candle	*umbrella*	…		
27	Van	*umbrella*	104	Sandwich	sandwich
…			105	Hat	*humbrehat*
32	Cat	cat	106	Queen	rest
33	Slide	*umbrella*	107	Comb	*umbrella*
34	Owl	*umbrella*	…		
35	Ruler	Rule	110	Foot	f … l … left foot
36	Cigarette	*sumbrella*	111	Camera	*cambrella*
37	Piano	am	112	House	*humbrehat*
38	Cloud	*umbrella*	113	Pen	*umbrella*
39	Door	window	114	Tractor	*umbrella*
40	Snail	snow	115	Leg	foot
41	King	king			

will be followed by an analysis of his attempts to name, repeat, and read the same set of 140 items, comparing accuracy on the different tasks, consistency across administrations, the issue of whether the properties of the different items affected his ability to process them correctly, and his error patterns (both perseverative and non-perseverative). The underlying motivation is the belief shared with Martin and Dell (2007 this issue) that perseverations are not best studied in isolation, but need to be understood in the context of a patient's wider profile of preserved and impaired functions, and the pattern of errors in general.

CASE REPORT

MM was an 80-year-old, right-handed, retired aeronautical engineer who had suffered a stroke in 1997. A CT scan carried out soon after the stroke showed a left intracerebral haematoma, with extension into the lateral and third ventricles. A second CT scan confirmed the presence of a left basal ganglia haematoma. MM's spontaneous speech was fluent but lacked content, and had limited functional use. He mainly produced stereotypical social phrases such as "I can't remember" or "How are you?". Attempts to produce content words resulted in the production of phonologically related words and nonwords, neologisms, or no response at all. He often perseverated on phrases, single words, or nonwords, or on parts of words. He frequently indicated that he was aware of his perseverations when they occurred, sometimes following a perseveration with "No!". At the same time, he was usually unable to inhibit the perseveration. The part-word perseverations he produced resulted in the production of phonologically related nonwords (neologisms) in his speech. He gave the impression of being more aware of his whole-word perseverations than his part-word perseverations. His lack of recognition of some of his part-word perseverations, and the confusion they caused to his listeners, made them particularly damaging to his communication.

The tests reported here were carried out between 2000 and 2002, when MM's language abilities had stabilised. In February 2001, MM was asked to describe the Cookie Theft picture from the Boston Diagnostic Aphasia Examination (Goodglass, Kaplan, & Weintraub, 1983). The picture shows a rather distracted mother washing dishes at a sink that is overflowing. Behind her a boy is standing on a stool in order to get at biscuits (cookies) in a cupboard. The stool he is standing on is about to topple over. A young girl, presumably his sister, is watching him. In describing the picture, MM said:

> Well, so what do I look? The unyer the disappointing the wotting that the er wotting wotting is wotting foal on the flow flower...tuz are falling on the...tuz the telly the telephen ... I can't remember...verses no I can't remember what is the time...can laiving at the ...time...no I can't remember...is bolling spoiling is boiling all together...no I can't remember...children.. spilling of ...two kookez cookies but there's a spawling on the way falling falling ...of the light. I can't...it's not good fellips.

There is perseveration of words (e.g., falling; time) and of the nonword "wotting". The neologism "spawling" appears to be a blend of "falling" and "spoiling". The familiar, well-used phrase "I can't remember" is articulated correctly and used four times.

Cognitive neuropsychological assessment

Table 2 shows the results of the cognitive neuropsychological assessment given to MM. The results indicated a number of impairments within his language-processing system.

A low-level auditory-phonetic impairment is suggested by MM's difficulties with the nonword minimal pairs task (indicating whether pairs of spoken nonwords are

TABLE 2
MM's performance on tests administered as part of the cognitive neuropsychological assessment

SPEECH PERCEPTION
Nonword minimal pairs (PALPA Battery: Kay et al., 1992)
Score: 58/72 (Control mean 70/72)
Auditory lexical decision (PALPA Battery: Kay et al., 1992)
Words: 76/80 (Control mean 77.6/80); Nonwords: 70/80 (Control mean 76/80)
Repetition of mixed words and nonwords (PALPA Battery: Kay et al., 1992)
Words: 40/80
High frequency, high imageability 12/20
High frequency, low imageability 11/20
Low frequency, high imageability 8/20
Low frequency, low imageability 9/20
Nonwords: 14/80
Repetition of nonwords (PALPA Battery: Kay et al., 1992)
Score: 5/24

OBJECT RECOGNITION AND NAMING
Object decision (BORB: Riddoch & Humphreys, 1993)
Real objects: 47/64; Non-objects 62/64
Object comprehension (Pyramid and Palm Trees Test: Howard & Patterson, 1992)
Score: 42/52 (control range 49–52)
Boston Naming Test (Kaplan et al., 1983)
1st administration: 14/60; 2nd administration: 13/60 (Control mean 55.8/60)

READING
Letter recognition I. Letter orientation (PALPA Battery: Kay et al., 1992)
Score: 36/36
Letter recognition II. Same–different judgement of letter strings (PALPA Battery: Kay et al., 1992)
Words: 27/30, Nonwords: 21/30
Visual lexical decision (PALPA Battery: Kay et al., 1992)
Words: 25/30, Nonwords: 30/30
Reading aloud (word naming – PALPA Battery: Kay et al., 1992)
Overall score: 27/80
High frequency, high imageability 8/20
High frequency, low imageability 6/20
Low frequency, high imageability 7/20
Low frequency, low imageability 6/20
Nonword reading (PALPA Battery: Kay et al., 1992)
Score: 5/24

SEMANTICS AND SENTENCE PROCESSING
Spoken word-to-picture matching (PALPA Battery: Kay et al., 1992)
Score: 30/40 (Control mean 39.3, range 35–40)
Written word-to-picture matching (PALPA Battery: Kay et al., 1992)
Score: 36/40 (Control mean 39.9, range 35–40)
Auditory synonym judgements (PALPA Battery: Kay et al., 1992)
Score: 36/60
Written synonym judgements (PALPA Battery: Kay et al., 1992)
Score: 41/60
Reversible sentence comprehension test (Byng & Black, 1999)
Overall score: 21/40
Action verbs: 8/10 (control range 8–10)
Non-action verbs: 3/10 (control range 6–10)
Adjectives: 4/10 (control range 7–10)
Prepositions: 6/10 (control range 8–10)

the same or different). That impairment may have been partly responsible for his tendency to classify nonwords as words in auditory lexical decision, though he only made six more errors than the control average on the nonwords, and performed within normal limits on the real words. Repetition of words was more impaired and was not significantly affected by the frequency or imageability of the words being repeated. It was, however, better than his nonword repetition, implying some residual lexical-semantic support for the repetition process. While MM classified 76/80 words as real words in auditory lexical decision, he could repeat only 40/80 of the same words, and he could repeat only 14/80 nonwords when he had correctly judged 70/80 to be nonwords in lexical decision. This contrast between his performance on auditory lexical decision and repetition tasks, and his phonological errors in naming, repetition, and reading aloud, suggests an output phonological impairment in addition to the auditory-phonetic deficit that may have compromised his performance on minimal pairs and auditory lexical decision.

Turning to orthographic processing, MM could discriminate letters in their correct orientation from mirror-reversed letters and could name most letters in upper and lower case, although he had some problems comparing strings of upper- and lower-case letters. Visual lexical decision was reasonably well preserved although he failed to recognise 5 of the 30 real words. But he could read aloud only 28/80 words and 5/24 nonwords. Overall, the results of the reading tests indicate a mild visual-orthographic problem allied to the same problem with output phonology that affected his repetition of words and nonwords.

There is clear evidence of semantic impairments in addition to any problems with orthographic and phonological processing. MM's low-level auditory-phonetic impairment could have contributed to his impaired performance on spoken word-picture matching, but six of his nine errors showed a degree of semantic relatedness to the target word. He scored slightly better on written word–picture matching, where three of his four errors were again to close semantic distractors. His lexical errors in sentence–picture matching and his poor scores on non-action verbs and adjectives are compatible with a semantic impairment (Byng & Black, 1999), as is his great difficulty with both spoken and written synonym judgements. His poor performance on the object decision task, where he recognised only 47 of the 64 real objects, and his difficulties with the all-picture version of the Pyramids and Palm Trees task (which involved making semantic decisions based on relations between pictured objects), suggest that his problems with spoken and written word–picture matching were not confined to comprehending words, but reflected an underlying semantic impairment that compromised his understanding of objects as well.

Five whole-word perseverations were observed in the mixed word and nonword repetition task. Part-word perseverations were also evident in the both repetition tasks. The word-reading task induced one whole-word and several part-word perseverations. Perseverative errors were seen in abundance in the Boston Naming Test (Kaplan, Goodglass, & Weintraub, 1983) where MM made 17 whole-word and 15 part-word perseverations on the first administration of the test, and 14 whole-word and 9 part-word perseverations on the second administration.

COMPARISON OF NAMING, REPETITION, AND READING ALOUD

MM was asked to name 140 object pictures taken from the Snodgrass and Vanderwart (1980) picture set in one session in May 2000. He repeated the same object names in one session in September 2000 and read the object names aloud in a session in March 2001. He read the object names for a second time in September 2001, named the object pictures again in October 2001, and repeated the names for a second time in November 2001. Responses in the three tasks were deemed correct if the target word was produced as the first substantive, stressed response (excluding ums and ers). Errors were recorded and analysed. The aims of this exercise were to gain further insights into the organisation of MM's lexical system and to elucidate the nature and origins of MM's perseverative errors by analysing those errors, and other error types, across the three tasks.

Comparing performance between and within the three tasks

Table 3 shows the number of items named, repeated, or read aloud correctly by MM on each administration of the three tasks. There were no significant differences between his performance on first and second administrations of each tasks, attesting to the stability of his condition at the time of testing. Each item in each task was given a score of 2, 1, or 0 according to whether he had responded correctly to that item twice, once, or not at all. Performance on the different tasks was compared using the Wilcoxon matched-pairs signed-ranks test. MM was significantly better at reading the object names aloud than repeating them ($z = 3.23$, $p < .01$). Reading and repetition were both significantly better than naming (reading vs naming: $z = 7.59$, $p < .001$; repetition vs naming: $z = 5.21$, $p < .001$).

When the same items are administered on two separate occasions it is possible to look at consistency of performance. Does a patient tend to get the same items correct or incorrect on the two administrations or do more random forces appear to be at work? Table 4 shows the consistency between his performance on the same items across the two administrations of the naming, repetition and reading tasks.

Naming. Picture naming was the task MM found most difficult. He scored around 20% correct on each of the two administrations (Table 3). This means that most items ($N = 91$) were responded to incorrectly on both occasions. However, there was little consistency in which items he named correctly on the two occasions. Of the 28 items named correctly on the first administration, only 6 were named correctly on

TABLE 3
Items named, repeated, or read aloud correctly in two administrations of the same items

	Number correct	*Percent correct*
Naming		
1st administration	28/140	20%
2nd administration	27/140	19%
Repetition		
1st administration	60/140	43%
2nd administration	65/140	46%
Reading aloud		
1st administration	88/140	63%
2nd administration	82/140	59%

TABLE 4
Consistency of performance between two administrations of the naming, repetition, and reading tasks

		1st administration	
		Correct	*Incorrect*
Naming			
2nd administration	Correct	6	21
	Incorrect	22	91
Repetition			
2nd administration	Correct	30	35
	Incorrect	30	45
Reading			
2nd administration	Correct	53	29
	Incorrect	35	23

the second administration. He named a further 21 items correctly on the second administration that he had failed to name correctly on the first administration. Cramer's contingency coefficient *C*, which measures the degree of association between performance on two separate occasions, was not significant ($C = 0.005$, *ns*).

Repetition. MM repeated about 45% of the words correctly on the two administrations. Of the 60 object names that he repeated correctly on the first administration, only 30 were repeated correctly on the second administration. He repeated a further 35 words correctly on the second administration that he had failed to repeat correctly on the first administration. Cramer's contingency coefficient was not significant ($C = 0.047$, *ns*).

Reading aloud. MM read about 60% of the words correctly on the two administrations. Of the 88 object names that he read correctly on the first administration, only 53 were read correctly on the second administration. He read a further 29 words correctly on the second administration that he had failed to read correctly on the first administration. Cramer's contingency coefficient was again not significant ($C = 0.029$, *ns*).

Predicting response accuracy in the three tasks

Norms are available for the 140 items used in the three tasks, which give measures for a range of properties of the pictures and their names (Morrison, Chappell, & Ellis, 1997; Quinlan, 1992; Snodgrass & Vanderwart, 1980). It is possible using multiple regression techniques to see if any of these characteristics of the items influenced whether or not MM could respond to them correctly in the three tasks (see Cuetos, Aguado, Izura, & Ellis, 2002; Ellis, Lum, & Lambon Ralph, 1996; Nickels & Howard, 1995). We employed five item properties in our analyses of MM's naming, repetition, and reading accuracy. Each of these factors has been found to exert an influence in some aphasic patients.

Object familiarity. This is a measure based on the degree to which people estimate that they come into contact with or think about a given object. The values were taken from Morrison et al. (1997).

Imageability. In the context of objects and their names, this is a measure of the ease with which the name of an object can evoke a mental image of the object. The values were taken from Morrison et al. (1997).

Word frequency. The combined frequency count from the CELEX database (Baayen, Piepenbroeck, & Van Rijn, 1993) was taken as the measure of the frequency of occurrence of the different object names in spoken and written British English. The values were log transformed to reduce skew.

Age of acquisition. The AoA75 measure from Morrison et al. (1997) gives the lowest age at which 75% of British children can name an object picture. The measure was square-root transformed to reduce skew. Studies of aphasic naming have found age of acquisition to be an important predictor of naming accuracy, with early-learned words tending to be better preserved than later-learned words (Cuetos et al., 2002; Ellis, 2006; Nickels & Howard, 1995).

Word length. For naming and repetition, word length was measured in syllables. For reading aloud, length was measures in terms of the number of letters in the written word.

Of the 140 items, 3 were outliers on one or other of the measures and were removed from the analysis. The results of the regression analyses of naming, repetition, and reading on the remaining 137 items are shown in Table 5. The combined predictors were unable to predict MM's naming scores to a significant degree, $F(5, 131) = 1.74$, *ns*, and none of the individual predictors reached significance. A similar result was found for repetition, $F(5, 131) = 1.18$, *ns*. Only in the case of reading aloud were the item properties able to predict performance to a significant extent, $F(5, 131) = 2.71$, $p < .05$. As Table 5 shows, this was because the number of letters in a word significantly affected MM's reading accuracy, with the probability of his being able to read a word correctly decreasing as the number of letters increased. None of the other predictors influenced his reading performance.

Error analyses

MM's errors in the three tasks were analysed. As with correct responses, only the first substantive responses were considered. If MM failed to respond to an item or said something like "I can't remember" or just "No", that was classified as a no-response error. The remaining errors were divided into those that involved producing a real-word response and those that involved producing a nonword response. Word errors were classed as semantic if they bore a clear similarity in meaning to the target. Word and nonword errors were classed as form related if they shared at least half the phonemes of the target name (naming and repetition) or at least half the letters of the target (reading). Word and nonword errors that showed no similarity to the target in either meaning or form were classed as unrelated.

Having made that initial classification, each error was analysed for whether it could also be classified as the perseveration of a whole word, a whole nonword, or part of a word or nonword. Whole-word perseverations were defined as the production of either a previous target or a previous whole-word response,

TABLE 5
Regression analyses

Variable	*B*	*Standard error of B*	*Beta*	*t*	*Significance*
Naming					
Object familiarity	.034	.071	.056	0.48	.635
Imageability	.067	.195	.034	0.35	.730
Word frequency	.173	.115	.172	1.51	.135
Age of acquisition	−.008	.043	−.019	−0.18	.861
Word length	−.053	.089	−.055	−0.60	.552
Repetition					
Object familiarity	−.008	.090	−.011	−0.09	.930
Imageability	.393	.248	.157	1.58	.116
Word frequency	.138	.146	.109	0.95	.346
Age of acquisition	.000	.055	.001	0.01	.991
Word length	.132	.114	.108	1.16	.248
Reading					
Object familiarity	.070	.086	.095	0.81	.418
Imageability	.200	.237	.081	0.85	.400
Word frequency	−.044	.137	−.035	−0.32	.749
Age of acquisition	.063	.052	.125	1.20	.232
Word length	−.139	.042	−.292	−3.34	.001

Results of regression analyses of MM's naming, repetition, and reading using combined scores across two administrations of the 140 items as the dependent variable.

reproduced in its entirety. A target may have been correctly responded to when it first appeared, or it may have elicited a no-response error, so that a perseveration could be a delayed "correct" response to a previous target, but an error to the current target. Part-word (or part-nonword) perseverations were defined as errors that were different from the previous response but contained at least 50% of the phonemes of the previous response. This is a relatively conservative definition in that it does not consider the possibility of parts of previous responses being perseverated across non-adjacent items. Although there were some quite convincing examples of this happening in MM's data, across a long sequence of items the probability that a later response may, by chance, contain phonemes that also appeared in some earlier response becomes high and impossible to control statistically. We opted, therefore, for the conservative definition.

The results are shown in Table 6. Because the analysis involves both first and second administrations of each 140-item test, the total number of correct responses and errors for each task is 280.

Naming. MM's rate of correct responding was lowest in the naming task. The most common form of error was unrelated word errors in which he produced a real word that bore no semantic or phonological relationship to the target in front of him. Such errors comprised 33% of all his responses, 41% of his errors, and 75% of his whole-word errors. Over half of MM's unrelated word errors (53/92) involved the perseveration of words that had occurred as previous targets, previous responses, or both. A further 14 of his unrelated word errors in naming involved perseverations of elements from the previous response.

Nonword errors accounted for 28% of MM's naming responses and 35% of his errors. About three-quarters (74%) of the nonword errors were unrelated to the target word (e.g., naming shoe as "birrow"). A substantial number of the unrelated nonword errors (21/58 = 36%) incorporated phonemes from the previous response perseverating into the current response. The remaining nonword errors were form related (e.g., naming a peacock as "peatot") and were less likely to include perseverated phonemes (3/20 = 15%). There was just one perseveration of a whole nonword: MM named hat as "humbrehat", a blend of the target word "hat" with a part-word perseveration on the word "umbrella". Seven items later he named house as "humbrehat", repeating the nonword in its entirety.

Repetition. MM's rate of correct responding in repetition was over twice as high as in the naming task. Whole-word errors accounted for 29% of his responses and 52% of his errors, with unrelated errors again the most common type (48/81 = 59% of word errors). Form-related errors accounted for a higher proportion of word errors in repetition (37%) than in naming. Semantic errors were rare.

Whole-word perseverations accounted for 23% of his unrelated word errors in repetition, but only 1 of his 30 form-related word errors was a whole-word perseveration. A further five of MM's unrelated word errors in repetition involved the perseveration of elements from the previous response. Nonword errors accounted for 20% of MM's responses in the repetition task, and 37% of his errors. Of the nonword errors made in repetition, 50% (33/57) were unrelated phonologically to the target word (e.g., "knife" repeated as "garf") while the remaining 42% (24/57) shared at least half the phonemes of the target (e.g., "dress" repeated as "gress"). There were very few part-word perseverations of phonemes from responses made on immediately preceding trials, and no perseverations of whole nonwords.

Reading. Of the three tasks, MM's accuracy was highest in reading aloud. Word errors accounted for 27% of his responses, and 68% of his errors. Unlike naming and repetition, form-related errors were more common than unrelated errors. Semantic errors were rare.

Of MM's 23 unrelated word errors in reading, 6 (26%) involved perseverations of previous words (e.g., reading *leg* as "book", having read *book* correctly six trials earlier). Only 8 of his 47 form-related word errors (17%) involved whole-word perseverations.

Nonword errors accounted for 12% of MM's reading responses, and 32% of his errors. Of the 35 nonword errors made in reading, 57% (20/35) were unrelated phonologically to the target word while the remaining 43% (15/35) shared at least half the phonemes of the target (e.g., *zebra* read as "zimba"). Again, there were only a few part-word perseverations of phonemes from responses made on immediately preceding trials. There was one perseveration of a complete nonword (when *balloon* was read as "camballoon" and the next target, *kangaroo*, was also read as "camballoon"). As with the nonword perseveration in naming, the initial error was a hybrid of part of the target ("balloon") and part of the previous target ("camel"). "Camballoon" is also phonologically related to the target "kangaroo" to which it was produced as a perseveration.)

TABLE 6
Distributions of correct responses and error types in naming, repetition, and reading based on two administrations of the 140 items

		Response type		Perseverations	
				Whole-word or whole-nonword	Part-word or part-nonword
		No.	%	No.	No.
Naming					
Correct		55	20%		
No response		25	9%		
Word error					
	Semantic	21	8%	6	0
	Form-related	9	3%	1	0
	Unrelated	92	33%	53	14
	Total	122	44%	60	14
Nonword error					
	Form-related	20	7%	1	3
	Unrelated	58	21%	0	21
	Total	78	28%	1	24
Repetition					
Correct		125	45%		
No response		17	6%		
Word error					
	Semantic	3	1%	2	0
	Form-related	30	11%	1	3
	Unrelated	48	17%	11	5
	Total	81	29%	14	8
Nonword error					
	Form-related	24	9%	0	1
	Unrelated	33	11%	0	2
	Total	57	21%	0	3
Reading					
Correct		169	60%		
No response		1	0.4%		
Word error					
	Semantic	5	2%	2	0
	Form-related	47	17%	8	3
	Unrelated	23	8%	6	2
	Total	75	27%	16	5
Nonword error					
	Form-related	15	5%	1	3
	Unrelated	20	7%	0	4
	Total	35	12%	1	7

DISCUSSION

The nature of MM's aphasia

The cognitive neuropsychological battery indicated the presence of more than one impairment in MM. The difficulty making same–different judgements to spoken nonwords in the minimal pairs task suggested a possible auditory input problem, although auditory lexical decision was only mildly impaired. Repetition was much worse than auditory lexical decision for the same words, and nonword repetition was worse than word repetition, indicating the presence of additional phonological output problems. Difficulties in making same–different judgements to pairs of words and nonwords, one written in UPPER CASE, the other in lower case, suggested some visual-orthographic problems, as did the decline in reading accuracy with word length, although visual lexical decision was again reasonably good. Reading aloud was worse than visual lexical decision for words, and nonwords were read less accurately than real words. That pattern is compatible with the suggestion of a phonological output deficit that would affect reading aloud as well as repetition. MM made phonological errors in naming, repetition, and reading, so that form-related word and nonword errors together accounted for 13%, 35%, and 56% respectively of his errors in naming, repetition, and reading of the 140 objects and their names.

Although auditory and visual lexical decision were reasonably good, synonym judgements to spoken or written word pairs were at or close to chance, suggesting a more profound semantic impairment. The same semantic impairment was probably responsible for at least part of MM's problems with sentence–picture matching, which matched the profile given by Byng and Black (1999) for patients with semantic deficits. His low level of performance on object decision and semantic judgements to object pictures implies that the semantic impairment extended beyond words and sentences to objects and concepts.

Object naming (20% correct) was worse than repetition of the same object names (45% correct) which in turn was worse than reading aloud the object names (60% correct). Other patients have been reported who were prone to perseveration and whose naming was worse than their reading and/or repetition (Gotts, Incisa della Rocchetta, & Cipolotti, 2002; Moses et al., 2004; Papagno & Basso, 1996; Santo Pietro & Rigrodsky, 1982). It is usually assumed that there is only one cognitive "route" that will allow an object to be named. That route involves perceiving the object (or object picture), recognising it as familiar, accessing stored semantic knowledge about the object, then using the semantic knowledge to access the object's name (Ellis & Young, 1988). In contrast, repetition and reading aloud are supported by additional routes from input to output that are not available for naming. In repetition, those additional routes include processes for converting auditory inputs to spoken outputs that can be used to repeat unfamiliar words or invented nonwords that have no lexical or semantic representations. In reading, they include processes for converting letters to sound (so-called grapheme–phoneme conversion processes) that can be used to read aloud unfamiliar words or invented nonwords. In repetition and reading, there is therefore the possibility that these non-lexical mechanisms may assist the operation of lexical-semantic processes to boost performance on those tasks compared with naming (Miceli, Capasso, & Caramazza, 1994; Miceli, Giustolisi, & Caramazza, 1991). MM managed to repeat around 20% of nonwords correctly and to read aloud a similar proportion. A contribution from these defective but not abolished nonlexical processes could go some way towards explaining why he was better at repetition and reading than at naming, but could not explain why his reading aloud was better than his repetition (given that nonword repetition and reading were of similar accuracy). It may be that the source of the difference between reading and repetition lay in better preservation of input processing of written compared to spoken input. Another possibility is that a spoken word for repetition lasts for only a fraction of a second, and then is gone. In contrast, a written word in a reading task is usually presented for as long as is required for the patient to make a response. MM therefore had more time to process the written words in reading than the spoken words in repetition, which may account for better reading than repetition. Hirsh's (1998) patient CJ, who was unusual in being as poor at reading aloud as object naming, was a deep dyslexic who was unable to read any nonwords (Hirsh, 1992). The assumption in this instance would be that CJ lacked any non-semantic support for reading aloud, and that reading aloud used the same associations between semantics and phonology that were used for naming, with the result that performance was similar on the two tasks. MM's performance on naming, repetition, and reading was characterised by a high degree of inconsistency. Although his overall accuracy levels were similar when he performed a task on two separate occasions, there was no consistency regarding which particular items he got right or wrong. It is not surprising, therefore, that properties of the individual items such as their familiarity, frequency, and age of acquisition had no detectable effect on whether he named, read, or repeated them correctly or incorrectly on a given occasion. Table 2 also presents the results of tests in which MM failed to show any effect of word frequency or imageability on his repetition or reading aloud. The only significant determinant of performance accuracy we could discern in MM was a tendency to read shorter words more accurately than longer words.

In all three tasks, MM's errors involved a mixture of no-response errors, whole-word errors, and nonword errors. Although the absolute numbers of nonword errors varied across tasks, they constituted similar proportions of his errors in the three tasks (35% in naming, 37% in repetition, and 31% in reading). Thus, if MM was unable to respond correctly to an item, there was a roughly one in three chance that his error would involve the production of a nonword, irrespective of the task. What varied across tasks was the ratio of no-response errors to word errors. In naming and repetition, MM made very similar proportions of word errors (54% in naming; 52% in repetition) and no-response errors (11% in both tasks). In reading, he made a higher proportion of word errors (68%) and a very low proportion of no-response errors (less than 1%). The difference between reading and repetition may reflect either better preservation of input processes for reading compared to repetition, or the fact that in the reading task written words remained available until a response was made, whereas spoken words whereas in the repetition task the spoken target word was only fleetingly available.

In naming, most of MM's whole-word errors (75%) were unrelated to the target item, as were the majority of his nonword errors (74%). Taken together with his no-response errors, these imply that on 63% of naming trials the stimulus picture induced too little relevant activation in MM's semantic system to generate a response which showed any indication that he had recognised the object or understood what it was. A total of 17% of his whole-word errors were semantically related to the target item. These could be construed as occasions when partial activation of the semantics of the pictured object led to the selection of the name of an incorrect but semantically similar object.

In repetition, unrelated errors were again the commonest form of word error (59%) and nonword error (58%). Combined with MM's no-response errors, these imply that on 35% of repetition trials there was too little activation of either semantics or output phonology to generate a response that was related in meaning or form to the target. However, form-related errors were more common in repetition than in naming, comprising 37% of word errors and 42% of nonword errors. The activation of output phonology by auditory input using non-semantic routes may be responsible for this higher proportion of form-related errors in repetition. Better activation of target phonology in repetition may also be the reason why semantic errors (whose phonology is usually quite different from that of the target) were rare (just 4% of word errors).

In reading, form-related errors were the largest category of whole-word errors (60%), followed by unrelated errors (31%), with semantic errors again being uncommon (7%). There were relatively few nonword errors (12% of all responses, compared with 28% in naming and 20% in repetition), with 57% being unrelated and 43% form-related. As with repetition, non-semantic routes from input to output of the sort that could sustain nonword reading were available to a degree, although their functioning was well below normal levels. The ability of such routes (e.g., grapheme–phoneme conversion) to activate output phonology directly from orthographic input may be responsible, at least in part, for the higher rate of correct responding in reading, the higher proportions of form-related errors, and the low proportions of no-response errors and semantic errors.

In fact, MM made just three semantic errors in repetition, and five in reading. The words used in the three tasks were the names of familiar objects and therefore inevitably come from a restricted set of semantic categories (animals, clothing, household objects, etc). Most of MM's word errors in all three tasks were other object names. When that is the case, a word produced in error stands a non-trivial chance of being semantically related to the stimulus word purely by chance (Ellis & Marshall, 1978; Hirsh, 1998). The rates of semantic errors in repetition and reading were so low that there are no real grounds for suggesting that these were anything more than the products of chance relationships between target words and responses that were actually unrelated word errors. MM's rather higher rate of semantic errors in naming (17% of word errors) probably indicates some genuine contribution of the meaning of the target object on error responses, but even here we must acknowledge that some of the errors classed as semantic will actually be unrelated errors that bore a coincidental similarity in meaning to the target. Moses et al. (2004) argued that the influence of semantic relatedness might have been overestimated in previous studies of perseveration, a view with which we are inclined to agree.

Perseveration in MM's naming, repetition, and reading

Hirsh (1998) reported what she considered to be four characteristics of perseveration in aphasia. They were (a) that whole words are the commonest unit for perseveration, but parts of words and whole nonwords may also perseverate, (b) that a response need not have been correct in the first instance for it to be perseverated: both errors and correct responses can be perseverated, as can items presented as targets that were not responded to correctly in the first instance, (c) that a word can appear as a perseveration to the item that immediately follows it, but it is also common for one or more other items to intervene before the perseveration occurs, and (d) that perseverating words may be semantically or phonologically related to the target word that evokes them, but are often unrelated. As we have seen, all of those things were true for MM.

Perseverations accounted for 49% of MM's whole-word errors in naming, 17% in repetition, and 21% in reading. They were particularly prominent among his unrelated word errors in naming, where they accounted for 56% of errors. Form-related whole-word errors were rare in naming, but more common in repetition and reading. Whole-word perseveration played only a small part in the generation of such errors: just 17% (8/47) of MM's word errors in reading involved word perseveration, and a mere 3% (1/30) of his word errors in repetition. Semantic errors were at chance levels in repetition and reading, though more common in naming, where whole-word perseveration accounted for a lower proportion (29%) than for unrelated word errors. The tendency for perseverations to be particularly common among unrelated word errors was also true of Hirsh's (1998) patient CJ, the patients of Papagno and Basso (1996), and two of Martin et al.'s (1998) three cases. Perseveration of complete nonwords were noted by Hirsh (1998) and Basso (2004), but MM was only observed to make two such errors across the naming, repetition, and reading tasks. More common was the situation where a nonword error contained a perseverating fragment from the previous response. This was more apparent in naming than in repetition or reading. In naming, such perseverations contributed to the production of 14 unrelated word responses and 21 unrelated nonword responses. They contributed to none of the semantic or form-related word responses, and to only three form-related nonword responses. Perseverations of fragments therefore contributed more to unrelated than to related responses in naming, just as perseverations of whole words did.

Martin and Dell (2007 this issue) present a theory of perseverative errors in aphasia, the starting point of which is a well-established computational model of word retrieval that involves semantic, lexical, and phonological representations (Dell, 1986; Dell, Burger, & Svec, 1997a). Word retrieval is initiated within the model by activating the semantic features of a word. When the model is functioning normally, those semantic features activate the lexical entry for the target word, which in turn activates the appropriate output phonemes. But the model can be "lesioned" by disrupting the connections between the different representations, thereby impairing its performance. Considerable progress has already been made in simulating forms of aphasic naming breakdown using this approach (Dell, Schwartz, Martin, Saffran, & Gagnon, 1997b; Dell, Lawler, Harris, & Gordon, 2004). Martin and Dell (2007 this issue) show how the model can be extended to provide an account of perseverative errors.

Martin and Dell argue that the same mechanisms that cause non-perseverative aphasic errors also cause perseverative errors. There is no need on this view to invoke additional error-generating mechanisms to explain perseverations (e.g., an impairment specifically affecting inhibitory mechanisms). Errors are caused by weak activation of the target word in the context of competition from other words. That may be competition from other words that are similar in meaning or sound to the target, or from words that have been activated recently and which therefore retain some level of residual activation. Martin and Dell show that weakening the connections between semantics and the lexicon in their model gives rise to some no-response errors; also to whole-word errors, both non-perseverative and perseverative. Weakening the connections between semantics and the lexicon can also give rise to nonword ("phonological") errors, although such errors are induced to a greater extent by weakening the connections between the lexicon and phonological output units. The reason why phonological errors can be induced by weakening connections between semantics and the lexicon may be that this has the knock-on effect of reducing the amount of activation passing from the lexicon to the phonological units. Once again, however, non-perseverative and perseverative errors go hand in hand: anything that increases the number of non-perseverative phonological errors also increases the number of perseverative phonological errors,

MM produced both whole-word errors and phonological (nonword) errors. Martin and Dell's model would probably simulate his pattern of errors by weakening both the connections between semantics and the lexicon and the connections between the lexicon and phonological output units. That would not be unreasonable, given the independent evidence for both semantic and phonological output impairment. Whole-word errors, and whole-word perseverations, could certainly be explained in terms of reduced semantic input to lexical retrieval. We might want to use the evidence of conceptual-semantic impairment on all-picture tasks to argue that the damage was to MM's semantic system itself rather than the links between it and lexical representations, but that is a minor aspect of the way Martin and Dell's model works. Phonological (nonword) errors, including perseverations, might require an additional weakening of lexical to phonological connections, but we have noted that Martin and Dell's model makes phonological errors even when only the links between semantics and the lexicon are damaged. There were clear word-level influences on MM's nonword errors. Part-word perseverations were only seen in MM's naming when the whole word from which the part was derived had been produced in full. That is, syllables and phonemes could perseverate from one item to the next, but only when the whole word that acted as the source of the fragments had been produced first. In addition, some of MM's nonword errors had the quality of blends between real words. For example, having named items 41 (pelican) and 42 (stethoscope) of the naming test correctly, he responded "peliscope" to a picture of a pyramid (item 43). "Peliscope" is a nonword that would seem to be a blend of the two previous responses "pelican" and "stethoscope". It may or may not be a coincidence that it shares the initial phoneme of the target "pyramid". The point is that a phonological error that incorporates fragments of previous responses can be construed as a product of the reactivation of previous lexical responses rather than being a product of residual activation at the phoneme level. These observations, along with the extreme scarcity of perseverations of whole nonwords, argue for a lexical involvement in MM's phonological perseverations that could result from reactivation of words exciting some but not all of their component phonemes, with those phonemes being incorporated into the response along with phonemes that may have been activated by the target or through other processes.

These aspects of MM's aphasia and of his perseverations can be accommodated readily within the Martin and Dell theory. However, there are two predictions of that theory that do not seem to fit MM. The predictions are also made by the theory of Gotts and Plaut (2004), which therefore has similar problems with MM's data. The first prediction is that perseverative word errors in naming, like non-perseverative word errors, should tend to be related in meaning and/or form to the target item that induced them. Martin et al. (1998) argued that this was the case, although others have reported a predominance of unrelated word errors among their aphasic perseverations (Hirsh, 1998; Moses et al., 2004; Papagno & Basso, 1996). We have seen that about three-quarters of MM's whole-word perseverations (and a similar proportion of his nonword perseverations) were unrelated to the target item, and that perseverations contributed much more to unrelated errors than to related errors in naming, repetition, and reading. Thus, perseveration was more strongly associated with unrelated than with related word errors. The same was true of nonword errors.

The second prediction of the Martin and Dell framework (and of the Gotts & Plaut, 2004, framework) that does not fit MM is the expectation that error words, including those featuring in whole-word perseverations, will tend to be of higher frequency than that the target words that induce them. We have seen that MM's errors were completely inconsistent from one administration to another (which they would not be if factors like word frequency were influencing the vulnerability of words on each occasion) and that there was no detectable influence on MM's naming of word frequency or any of the other variables that have been implicated as determinants of naming accuracy in aphasia. Some studies have reported effects of frequency in aphasic patients prone to perseverative errors (Hirsh, 1988; Gotts et al., 2002; Santo Pietro & Rigrodsky, 1982), but other studies were unable to find an effect (Halpern, 1965; Martin et al., 1998). Our observations with MM add strength to the claim that aphasic patients may show large numbers of perseverative errors without showing effects of word frequency or other lexical variables.

It seems to us that MM's overall pattern is better accommodated by Cohen and Dehaene's (1998) proposal that perseverations are particularly likely to happen when a stimulus generates virtually no activity within the patient's language systems; that is, on trials when the semantic and phonological systems are effectively "de-afferented", receiving no input that might constrain their output. One thing that could happen on such occasions is that the patient may be unable to generate any form of output and therefore make a no-response error. But there may also be an endogenously driven reactivation of the semantic and/or phonological representations of words and phonemes that have been activated in the recent past. The resulting perseverative responses fill the void left by a lack of effective input (see Moses et al., 2004). Because the target item has made no impression on the system, those perseverative responses will tend to be unrelated to the target. The inconsistency of MM's responses and the absence of effects of word frequency, age of acquisition, and similar factors, suggests that in him at least, temporary deafferentation struck at random moments, periodically depriving his semantic and phonological systems of input they could work on and leaving the way clear for perseverations to occur.

REFERENCES

Albert, M. L., & Sandson, J. (1986). Perseveration in aphasia. *Cortex*, *22*, 103–115.

Allison, R. S., & Hurwitz, L. J. (1967). On perseveration in aphasics. *Brain*, *90*, 442–448.

Baayen, R. H., Piepenbroeck, R., & Van Rijn, H. (1993). *The CELEX lexical database (CD-ROM)*. Philadelphia: University of Pennsylvania, Linguistic Data Consortium.

Basso, A. (2004). Perseveration, or the Tower of Babel. *Seminars in Speech and Language*, *25*, 375–389.

Buckingham, H. (1985). Perseveration in aphasia. In S. Newman & R. Epstein (Eds.), *Current perspectives in dysphasia* (pp. 113–154). Edinburgh, UK: Churchill Livingstone.

Buckingham, H., Whitaker, H., & Whitaker, H. A. (1979). On linguistic perseveration. In H. A. Whitaker & H. Whitaker (Eds.), *Studies in neurolinguistics, vol. 4* (pp. 329–352). New York: Academic Press.

Byng, S., & Black, M. (1999). *The Reversible Sentence Comprehension Test*. Oxford, UK: Winslow Press.

Cohen, L., & Dehaene, S. (1998). Competition between past and present: Assessment and interpretation of verbal perseverations. *Brain, 121*, 1641–1659.

Cuetos, F., Aguado, G., Izura, C., & Ellis, A. W. (2002). Aphasic naming in Spanish: Predictors and errors. *Brain and Language, 82*, 344–365.

Dell, G. S. (1986). A spreading activation theory of retrieval in sentence production. *Psychological Review, 93*, 283–321.

Dell, G. S., Burger, L. K., & Svec, W. R. (1997a). Language production and serial order: A functional analysis and a model. *Psychological Review, 104*, 123–147.

Dell, G. S., Lawler, E. N., Harris, H. D., & Gordon, J. K. (2004). Models of impaired lexical access in speech production. *Journal of Memory and Language, 43*, 182–216.

Dell, G. S., Schwartz, M. F., Martin, N., Saffran, E. M., & Gagnon, D. A. (1997b). Lexical access in aphasic and nonaphasic speakers. *Psychological Review, 104*, 801–838.

Ellis, A. W. (2006). Word finding in the damaged brain: Probing Marshall's caveat. *Cortex, 42*, 817–822.

Ellis, A. W., Lum, C., & Lambon Ralph, M. A. (1996). On the use of regression techniques for the analysis of single case aphasic data. *Journal of Neurolinguistics, 9*, 165–174.

Ellis, A. W., & Marshall, J. C. (1978). Semantic errors or statistical flukes? A note on Allport's "On knowing the meaning of words we are unable to report". *Quarterly Journal of Experimental Psychology, 30*, 569–575.

Ellis, A. W., & Young, A. W. (1988). *Human cognitive neuropsychology*. Hove, UK: Psychology Press.

Goodglass, H., Kaplan, E., & Weintraub, S. (1983). *The Revised Boston Naming Test*. Philadelphia: Lea & Febiger.

Gotts, S. J., Incisa della Rocchetta, A., & Cipolotti, L. (2002). Mechanisms underlying perseveration in aphasia: Evidence from a single case study. *Neuropsychologia, 40*, 1930–1947.

Gotts, S. J., & Plaut, D. C. (2004). Connectionist approaches to understanding aphasic perseverations. *Seminars in Speech and Language, 25*, 323–334.

Halpern, H. (1965). Effect of stimulus variables on verbal perseveration in dysphasic subjects. *Perceptual and Motor Skills, 20*, 421–429.

Hirsh, K. W. (1992). *Word production and comprehension in aphasia*. Unpublished doctoral thesis, University of York, UK.

Hirsh, K. W. (1998). Perseveration and activation in aphasic speech production. *Cognitive Neuropsychology, 15*, 377–388.

Howard, D., & Patterson, K. E. (1992). *The Pyramids and Palm Trees test*. Bury St. Edmunds, UK: Thames Valley Test Corporation.

Kaplan, E., Goodglass, H., & Weintraub, S. (1983). *The Boston Naming Test*. Philadelphia: Lea & Febinger.

Kay, J., Lesser, R., & Coltheart, M. (1992). *PALPA: Psycholinguistic Assessments of Language Processing in Aphasia*. Hove, UK: Lawrence Erlbaum Associates Ltd.

Martin, N., & Dell, G. S. (2007). Common mechanisms underlying perseverative and non-perseverative sound and word substitutions. *Aphasiology, 21*, 1002–1017.

Martin, N., Roach, A., Brecher, A., & Lowery, J. (1998). Lexical retrieval mechanisms underlying whole-word perseveration errors in anomic aphasia. *Aphasiology, 12*, 319–333.

Miceli, G., Capasso, R., & Caramazza, A. (1994). The interaction of lexical and sublexical processes in reading, writing and repetition. *Neuropsychologia, 32*, 317–333.

Miceli, G., Giustolisi, L., & Caramazza, A. (1991). The interaction of lexical and non-lexical processing mechanisms: Evidence from aphasia. *Cortex, 27*, 57–80.

Morrison, C. M., Chappell, T. D., & Ellis, A. W. (1997). Age of acquisition norms for a large set of object names and their relation to adult estimates and other variables. *Quarterly Journal of Experimental Psychology, 50A*, 528–559.

Moses, M. S., Nickels, L. A., & Sheard, C. (2004). "I'm sitting here feeling aphasic!" A study of recurrent perseverative errors elicited in unimpaired speakers. *Brain and Language, 89*, 157–173.

Nickels, L., & Howard, D. (1995). Aphasic naming: What matters? *Neuropsychologia, 33*, 1281–1303.

Papagno, C., & Basso, A. (1996). Perseveration in two aphasic patients. *Cortex, 32*, 67–92.

Quinlan, P. T. (1992). *The MRC Psycholinguistic Database*. London: Oxford University Press.

Riddoch, M. J., & Humphreys, G. W. (1993). *The Birmingham Object Recognition Battery (BORB)*. Hove, UK: Lawrence Erlbaum Associates Ltd.

Sandson, J., & Albert, M. L. (1984). Varieties of perseveration. *Neuropsychologia, 22*, 715–732.

San Pietro, M. J., & Rigrodsky, S. (1982). The effects of temporal and semantic conditions on the occurrence of the error response of perseveration in adult aphasics. *Journal of Speech and Hearing Research*, *25*, 184–192.

San Pietro M., J., & Rigrodsky, S. (1986). Patterns of oral-verbal perseveration in adult aphasics. *Brain and Language*, *29*, 1–17.

Snodgrass, J. G., & Vanderwart, M. (1980). A standardized set of 260 pictures: Norms for name agreement, image agreement, familiarity, and visual complexity. *Journal of Experimental Psychology: Human Learning and Memory*, *6*, 174–215.

Yamadori, A. (1981). Verbal perseveration in aphasia. *Neuropsychologia*, *19*, 591–594.

APHASIOLOGY, 2007, 21 (10/11), 1039–1078

Psychology Press
Taylor & Francis Group

Perseveration and conversation in TBI: Response to pharmacological intervention

Tali Frankel and Claire Penn

University of the Witwatersrand, Johannesburg, South Africa

Background: Perseveration is a frequently encountered characteristic of individuals with organic brain involvement, including individuals with traumatic brain injury (TBI). Current theory implicates disordered executive functioning, particularly deficient inhibitory control, in the manifestation of perseverative phenomena (McNamara & Albert, 2004). To date, no work has been published related to conversational data despite numerous allusions in the literature to the presence of perseveration during conversational discourse. Existing research indicates that pharmacological approaches to reduction of verbal perseveration may be effective, although no full-scale clinical trial of any pharmacological agent targeted specifically at reducing perseveration has been conducted (McNamara & Albert, 2004).

Aims: This study examines conversational correlates of perseveration in TBI, the accompanying executive functioning profiles in relation to Barkley's hybrid model of executive functioning and self-regulation (1997) and responses to pharmacotherapy (Ritalin).

Methods & Procedures: Two participants, in chronic stages following TBI with prefrontal and sub-cortical damage, participated in parallel case studies with a quasi-experimental research design. Baseline, active, placebo, and withdrawal phases were included as well as double blind and randomisation precautions. Conversational data were generated using Conversation Analysis. Neuropsychological data were generated following a full battery of tests investigating behavioural inhibition, nonverbal working memory, internalisation of language, regulation of affect, and reconstitution.

Outcomes & Results: Conversational data demonstrated disturbed topic management as a result of verbal perseveration. Participant AA demonstrated recurrent perseveration while PB demonstrated stuck-in-set perseveration, which influenced their conversations in highly specific ways. These findings were accompanied by discrete profiles indicating unique disruptions of executive functioning, particularly in relation to behavioural inhibition. Deficits in attention impacted profoundly on self-regulating functions, in particular nonverbal working memory and reconstitution. Improvements were noted during active drug phases related to improved behavioural inhibition and subsequent amelioration of perseverative manifestations with some evidence of improved topic shift and contribution and greater capacity for reconstitution and working memory tasks. Context was found to exert significant effects in relation to perseveration and its conversational manifestations.

Address correspondence to: Tali Frankel, University of the Witwatersrand, Private Bag 3, Wits 2050, Johannesburg, South Africa. E-mail: tdfranky@absamail.co.za

The first author would like to acknowledge the donors of the Medical Faculty Research Endowment Fund, University Council Scholarship, and the University of the Witwatersrand Postgraduate Merit Award, as well as Novartis South Africa for their generous grants that helped finance this project.

This paper was presented at the 10th International Aphasia Rehabilitation Conference, South Africa, June 2002, as well as the British Aphasiology Conference, UK, September 2003.

http://www.psypress.com/aphasiology DOI: 10.1080/02687030701198395

Conclusions: Perseveration co-exists with marked deficits in behavioural inhibition, which differentially affects executive functioning abilities, resulting in discrete cognitive profiles with corresponding conversational outcomes. Positive responses to pharmacotherapy present optimistic potential for future treatment, while context variables highlight the need for individualised, data-driven intervention programmes with an emphasis on continuous conversational interaction to preserve and improve communicative skills in individuals with chronic TBI.

Perseveration is probably the most frequently encountered characteristic of people with organic brain involvement (Eisenson, 1973) and one of the most common behaviours that disrupt communication in these populations (Aten, 1994). This paper addresses the manifestation of perseveration at a conversational level in two individuals with traumatic brain injury (TBI). It also looks at the hypothesis that individuals with varying profiles of executive functioning deficit—secondary to deficits in inhibition—present with unique manifestations of perseveration commensurate with those profiles.

Perseveration has been described as "a tendency to repeat a behavior pattern over and over irrespective of the context or stimulus … in all modalities…' (Code, 1982, p. 166). One of the more prevailing taxonomies, considered by some to represent perseverative typology in general (Christman, Boutsen, & Buckingham, 2004), is that proposed by Sandson and Albert (1984). These authors described three forms, including recurrent, continuous, and stuck-in-set subtypes, each with its own neuroanatomic and neuropharmacological underpinnings. Recurrent perseveration is the inappropriate recurrence of a previous response following an intervening production or subsequent stimulus. Continuous perseveration refers to the inappropriate prolongation or continuation of behaviour without cessation. Finally, stuck-in-set reflects the inappropriate maintenance of a framework or category across tasks (see Christman et al., 2004, for a thorough review). Perseveration occurring in aphasia has received the most attention although it occurs in numerous clinical populations, including individuals with head injury, the population that forms the focus of this paper.

Furthermore, there is a prevalence of observations made during structured, closed-ended activities. In fact many of the theories postulated were derived from data collected during naming tasks (Lundgren, Helm-Estabrooks, Magnusdottir, & Emery 1994). While other descriptions come from clinical observations in more open-ended contexts (Bryant, Emery, & Helm-Estabrooks, 1994), the assessment and subsequent management of perseveration appear to be restricted to tightly structured interactions. Even those researchers who acknowledge the need to investigate perseveration in a variety of language tasks adopt tools like picture naming, oral reading, and verbal repetition that do not reflect spontaneous interaction (Moses & Sheard, 2001).

The significance of investigating perseveration in more spontaneous day-to-day interactions, as in conversation, is emphasised by the acknowledgement that decreased ability to participate in conversation is one of the principal factors accounting for the devastation experienced by patients with neurological involvement (Lock, Wilkinson, Bryan, Maxim, Edmundson, Bruce, 2001). In addition to the role that conversation plays in terms of social functioning and identity, Penn (2000) has also pointed out that conversational breakdown in individuals with brain injury offers a window onto the processes and mechanisms prerequisite for this interaction. This is because the ability to converse efficiently rests on a finely tuned coordinated and adaptive system for processing and responding to continuous symbolic information.

PERSEVERATION AND EXECUTIVE DYSFUNCTION

Predominantly, perseveration has been viewed wholly or partly to be associated with disorders related to executive functions such as response inhibition, working memory, conceptual change, and control of emotions and motivational drives (Blanken, Dittmann, Grimm, Marshall, & Wallesch, 1993; Hauser, 1999). Consequently the frontal lobe, and specifically the prefrontal cortex and its various connections, particularly to the striatum and basal ganglia, are most frequently implicated (Fuster, 1997). In this light, the paucity of research involving clinical populations suffering from frontal dementias and traumatic brain injury (TBI) is particularly significant.

This study investigated the manifestations of perseveration in the TBI population, as their loss of executive functioning is often cited as the most disabling of all its outcomes (Adamovich & Henderson, 1992). Despite the number of theories that account for perseverative phenomena by proposing limitations in executive functioning, few studies have shown empirically that deficits in the executive functions cited co-exist with perseverative phenomena. Also, in spite of the frequency with which executive dysfunction is cited, the terms used in conjunction with such notions are rarely defined.

BARKLEY'S MODEL OF EXECUTIVE FUNCTIONING

Theories of perseveration that implicate disturbed inhibition have interesting implications for other areas of higher-order executive processes. This is because behavioural inhibition appears to represent a form of attention. According to Pashler (1998), the most prominent conception associated with attention is perceptual selectivity, the ability to choose one object from among many for awareness, memory, and control of action. This is particularly significant in light of the dominant role attention plays in cognitive processing and without which no higher-order processing can occur (Watt & Penn, 2000).

In order to explore this contention, Barkley's hybrid model of self-regulation and executive functioning (1997) was utilised. It describes functions related to the frontal lobe and specifically the prefrontal cortex (PFC), including the connections to the striatum and caudate nuclei. Significantly, as a result of its anterior position in the brain, the PFC is one of the areas of the brain most susceptible to brain damage resulting from TBI (Newcombe, 1997). Given that the prefrontal cortex is crucial for inhibitory control, it is not surprising that resistance to interference and attentional switching have also been linked to prefrontal systems (McNamara & Albert, 2004). The theory therefore takes into account the neuroanatomical links of the relevant sites implicated previously in perseveration (Fuster, 1997). Space constraints do not allow as detailed a description of this model and its links as it deserves. Rather functions and relationships that were deemed to be particularly relevant to perseveration and conversation in TBI are highlighted for discussion. Readers are therefore referred to Barkley (1997) for a complete description of the original model.

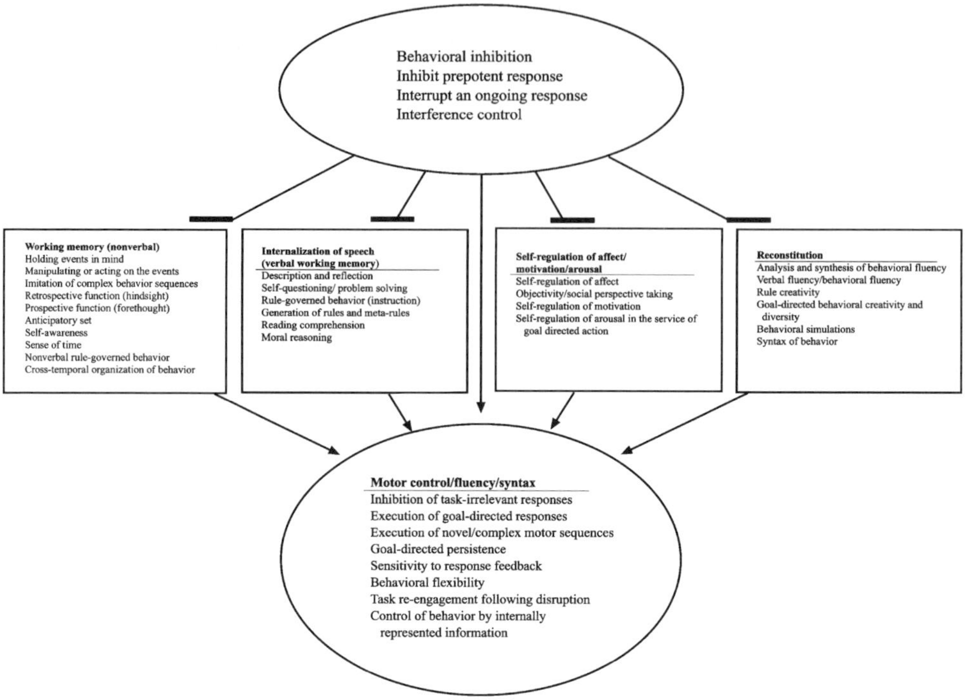

Figure 1. Diagram illustrating the complete hybrid model of executive functions (boxes) and the relationship of these four functions to the behavioral inhibition and motor control systems. From Barkley (1997). Copyright 1997 by the Guilford Press. Reprinted by Permission.

As depicted in Figure 1, Barkley's model sets forth a linkage between behavioural inhibition and four executive functions that depend on such inhibition for their own effective performance (working memory, internalised speech, regulation of affect, and reconstitution). The inhibitory functions exert a direct controlling influence over the motor system, depicted by a direct downward arrow between behavioural inhibition and motor control-fluency-syntax. Inhibition does not directly cause the four intermediate executive functions but merely provides the opportunity for them to occur. This relationship is represented by four blunted lines connecting inhibition to those four executive functions. However, because the executive functions produce direct and causal effects on motor control, arrows connect the executive functions with motor control (Barkley, 1997).

Three key concepts are central to the understanding of Barkley's model. These relate to behavioural inhibition, self-regulation, and executive functions, and are defined in the following way:

Behavioural inhibition

Behavioural inhibition refers to three interrelated processes. These include (a) the inhibition of the initial prepotent response to an event (the prepotent response is defined as that response for which immediate reinforcement is available or has been previously associated with that response); (b) stopping of an ongoing response; and (c) interference control through the protection of this period of delay from disruption by competing events and responses. As a result of effective inhibition self-directed actions are protected, as is the execution of goal-directed responses.

Self-regulation

Self-regulation refers to self-directed activity, which functions to change the self; it is future and not moment directed. It involves a special form of temporal and sequential memory and values delayed consequences as opposed to current ones. In terms of the model, self-regulation is said to be achieved when an individual is able to utilise response inhibition in order to engage the four executive functions to influence motor output.

Executive functions

Executive functions refer to the mainly private (cognitive) self-directed actions that contribute to self-regulation. The term is meant to incorporate the following attributes: (a) self-directed actions; (b) the organisation of behavioural contingencies across time; (c) the use of self-directed speech, rules, or plans; (d) deferred gratification; and (e) goal-directed, future-oriented, purposive, or intentional actions. Specifically, the four executive functions are encapsulated by the following systems: (nonverbal) working memory, internalisation of speech, self-regulation of affect-motivation-arousal, and reconstitution.

EXTENSION OF THE MODEL TO TBI, PERSEVERATION, CONVERSATION

As noted previously, the PFC (its structure and function as well as its networks with other brain regions) is one of the areas most susceptible to damage in TBI (Newcombe, 1997). Barkley's model predicts that deficiency in behavioural inhibition, (often leading to perseverative behaviour), diminishes the effective deployment of the four executive abilities that subserve self-control and goal-directed behaviour. This inhibitory deficit thereby indirectly disrupts the control of goal-directed motor behaviour by its influence on these executive functions. Specifically we were interested in how deficits in behavioural inhibition would affect conversational manifestations of perseveration and whether or not amelioration of this deficit (treated pharmacologically), would be echoed by a decrease in perseveration. A brief review of the evidence that supports the view of perseveration in TBI as a deficit in behavioural inhibition and the executive functions, together with predictions of how conversation may be affected, follows.

Deficient inhibition

Evidence of poor inhibition in TBI comes from studies that used motor inhibition tasks such as go–no-go paradigms and stop signal tasks (Stuss, Kaplan, Benson, Weir, Chiulli, & Sarazin, 1982). Poor behavioural inhibition is also evident when a task requires stopping an ongoing response when feedback suggests that the response is ineffective or maladaptive. Failure to do so results in behaviour that is either impulsive or perseverative, as observed in the TBI population (Prigatano & Fordyce, 1986).

Evidence for poor behavioural inhibition in conversation has been observed in individuals with TBI who have been rated as talking too much (Coelho, Liles, & Duffy 1991), holding the floor for inappropriately long periods of time (Gillis, 1996), and interrupting others during a conversation (Linscott, Knight, & Godfrey, 1996).

Deficient interference control

Evidence for poor interference control in patients with TBI comes from several sources. First, individuals with TBI take more time and make more errors than normals on the Stroop Colour Word Interference Test (Golden, 1978). The capacity to maintain performance towards a task despite distraction also serves as an indicator of poor interference control. Studies have indicated that individuals with TBI often present as distractible with poor sustained attention to internal representations and behavioural or mental tasks (Stuss & Benson, 1986). These individuals fatigue easily, and have impaired selective attention and scanning, and poor shifting of attention back and forth (Hartley, 1995). Such attention deficits manifest in social conversations—particularly during group interaction—where tracking meaning becomes particularly taxing (Godfrey & Shum, 2000). This may account for difficulty in staying on topic and a tendency to stray to a preferred point of reference, which is then repeated continually and perseverated.

Deficient (nonverbal) working memory

Barkley (1997) refers to nonverbal working memory as the capacity to hold an event in mind across a temporal delay, in order to guide a future response. In addition, working memory refers to the ability to manipulate that which is held in mind in order to integrate it with prior knowledge in preparation for use in a range of tasks (Barkley, 1997). The model predicts that poor inhibition should lead to secondary deficiencies of working memory and its sub-functions, which are specified in the model in Figure 1. Not all of these are addressed in the discussion below due to space constraints.

Working memory deficits in individuals with TBI have been assessed in neuropsychological research with the following tasks (among others) (Lezak, 1995; Spreen & Strauss, 1998): retention and oral repetition of digit spans (particularly in the reversed order), mental arithmetic, locating stimuli within spatial arrays of information that must be held in memory, and holding sequences of information in memory to properly execute a task as in self-ordered pointing tasks.

Storage and recall of complex information that must be held in mind over lengthy delay periods also presents difficulty. When strategies are required for organising material so as to remember it more effectively, those with TBI perform less well. Therefore patients with TBI may have an inability to imitate lengthy sequences of goal-directed behaviours demonstrated by others, as they cannot hold in mind the sequence of orchestration of their execution.

Studies that look at discourse in TBI such as the organisation of sequential material in the retelling of stories also imply organisational difficulty (Ulatowska, Freedman-Stern, Doyel, Macaluso-Haynes, & North, 1983). Conversation with others has been shown to include fewer references to concepts related to time, past, and especially the future (Mentis & Prutting, 1987). In terms of social skills, the implications memory deficits have for patients with TBI are profound. As the deficit typically involves the inability to recall new information, or maintain and manipulate current information in working memory, patients who cannot hold recently stated information might lose the thread of social interactions in that they cannot integrate new utterances with a previously stated one (Schapiro & Sacchetti, 1993). This inability means that patients lose the facility for developing coherence, and conversations may become difficult to follow and meaningless as they represent disembodied texts that have no prior mention or orientation. In a study analysing conversational performance, individuals with TBI used incomplete cohesive ties, and different proportions of referential, elliptical, conjunction, and lexical ties, as compared to controls (Mentis & Prutting, 1987).

Deficient internalisation of speech (verbal working memory)

Self-direction and internalisation of speech, and the profound control they may exert on the individual's behaviour, are important. Self-directed speech is also believed to provide a means for reflection, description, and self-questioning through language, creating an important source of problem-solving ability as well as a means of formulating rules and plans. Eventually rules about rules (meta-rules) can be generated into a hierarchically arranged system that resembles the concept of meta-cognition. (These functions are listed separately in Figure 1 under internalisation of speech.)

Rule-governed behaviour appears to provide a means of sustaining behaviour across large gaps in time. By formulating rules the individual can construct novel, complex, and prolonged behavioural chains. Control of behaviour is shifted to internally represented information (rules). The motor execution of such verbal rules appears to be partially dependent on the capacity to retain them in working memory and to inhibit prepotent or irrelevant responses that compete with the rule. Therefore the processes that would be affected, leading to perseveration as discussed previously in relation to deficient working memory and inhibition, apply here.

Patients with TBI have difficulty developing strategies to organise material to be memorised and therefore display difficulty with rote learning and short-term memory deficits (Prigatano & Fordyce, 1986). An impairment of abstract attitude is also evident, showing the lack of sophistication related to language use that would allow for the development of meta-thought. So individuals with TBI may interpret verbal messages literally instead of symbolically, thus impairing understanding of the subtle innuendo that often characterises emotional aspects of conversation (Schapiro & Sacchetti, 1993).

Deficient self-regulation of affect, motivation, arousal

According to Barkley (1997) the regulation of affect or motivation and arousal are closely connected. Emotions, once elicited, come to be moderated or regulated by self-directed executive actions. Included in this component of the model is the self-generation of drive or motivational and arousal states that support the execution of goal-directed actions and persistence towards the goal (Barkley, 1997).

Lang (1995) argued that the array of human emotions can be reduced to a two-dimensional model, of which one dimension is motivation (reinforcement and punishment) and the other level of arousal. Therefore the ability to self-regulate and even induce emotional states as needed in the service of goal-directed behaviour may also involve the ability to regulate and induce motivation, drive, and arousal states in support of such behaviour. When images are separate to motivation, one cannot guide or direct behaviour. Therefore, even when one is able to hold information, when there is a disconnection between that information and its motivational properties, one cannot act on that information.

Emotional changes secondary to frontal lobe injury can be grouped into three types of disturbance: (a) disorders of drive or motivation; (b) subjective emotional experience (mood); and (c) emotional expression (for a more thorough review that looks at the neuroanatomical correlates of each of these three disorders refer to Stuss, Gow, & Hetherington, 1992).

In terms of drive disorders, Luria (1980) described a loss of or weakness in drive, interest, and motivation in patients with frontal lobe damage. The apathy and indifference to surroundings represent disorders of self-activation. As a result these patients with TBI demonstrate increased helplessness and therefore a greater dependence on others. During conversational interactions, individuals with TBI may only produce restricted or minimal output (which may appear perseverative in nature because of its limited repertoire), placing a greater burden on their conversational partner to carry the responsibility for the interaction (Ylvisaker & Szekeres, 1994).

Several mood disorders are related to TBI, the most common of which is depression, which can immobilise the patient and lead to indifference and social withdrawal (Prigatano, 1986). Other mood disorders related to TBI are increased anxiety, anger and hostility, emotionally lability, and lack of awareness of their own impact on others (Prigatano & Fordyce, 1986). These manifestations conform to the predictions made by the Barkley model.

Reconstitution

According to Barkley (1997), reconstitution reflects the ability to create novel behaviour and is composed of two functions, analytic and synthetic. These functions allow individuals to take apart units of behaviours and recombine them, in a type of internalised play during which the contents of working memory are manipulated to enable the individual to produce flexible, generative behaviour. The specific functions resulting from this executive function are listed in Figure 1.

In TBI the ability to unfold motor programs and analyse them in terms of their component parts is often disrupted (Stuss & Benson, 1986). Evidence for decreased abilities in this area comes from a variety of sources. Performance on verbal fluency tasks, which demand the accurate and efficient communication of information, is diminished in TBI, with increased perseveration (Prigatano & Fordyce, 1986).

Confrontational story narratives and responses to direct questions or requests for information in both speech and writing are limited in terms of both amount and organisation of content. Phrases and ideas tend to be repeated over and over again, tending towards perseverative responding. Joint peer communication tasks and other situations or tasks that demand accurate and efficient communication of information are frequently disrupted (Barkley, 1997).

Breakdown in the processes governing reconstitution is also evident in nonverbal behaviour and in problem-solving tasks requiring complex and novel motor sequences or goal-directed creativity. Reduced capacity for interpretive statements such as deriving a moral from a story has also been demonstrated in these patients

(Ulatowska et al., 1983), indicating a diminished capacity to analyse components and interpret them meaningfully.

Creation of multiple novel complex alternative response sequences, whether in language or motor behaviour such as in gestural or drawing fluency, is often impaired in patients with damage to frontal lobes (Stuss & Benson, 1986). As a result behavioural flexibility is restricted, and perseverative tendencies dominate, as behaviours selected and executed come from a smaller pool of possibilities. The ability to initiate new topics of conversation as well as contribute to ongoing topics of conversation by engaging in topic maintenance and shift may also be impaired (Hartley, 1995).

Deficient motor control, fluency, syntax

The result of successful inhibition and engagement with the four executive functions results in the production of motor behaviour that is controlled, fluent, and structured. Inhibition and the executive functions contribute greater timing, persistence, flexibility, novelty, complexity, and syntax to motor actions that are goal directed (Fuster, 1997). Therefore, deficits in behavioural inhibition should lead to insensitivity to errors and to a loss of behavioural flexibility (Milner, 1995). These assertions are consistent with the theory of perseveration which suggests that perseveration is essentially a failure of inhibition of normally inhibited memory traces or a failure to resist interference from activation of these normally inhibited memory traces (Sandson & Albert, 1984). Current neural network models of verbal and other forms of perseveration are consistent with these suppositions (McNamara & Albert, 2004).

PERSEVERATION AND PHARMACOLOGY

These prefrontally based cognitive processes are modulated primarily by catecholaminergic (noradrenergic and dopamine) activity (McNamara & Albert, 2004). Pharmacotherapeutic trials targeted specifically towards the reduction of verbal perseveration are few and far between. Those specifically investigating dopaminergic or noradrenergic effects on verbal perseveration are even scarcer. One study using bromocriptine reported a reduction in cognitive and verbal perseverations in vascular and degenerative dementia (McNamara & Albert, 2004). Levadopa has been associated with reduced verbal perseveration in Parkinson's disease (see McNamara & Albert, 2004, for a more detailed review). McNeil, Small, Masterson, and Fossett, (1995) and Walker-Batson (1998) reported some amelioration of perseveration in aphasic clients when treated with a combination of amphetamines and behavioural therapy. Given these preliminary results, McNamara and Albert (2004) suggest that dopaminergic D2 agonists should be more intensely investigated as a potential pharmacological treatment for verbal perseveration. This study explored the treatment benefits of methylphenidate (Ritalin), a member of the amphetamine family and a drug that has gained increasing prominence in the literature surrounding treatment of TBI (Holmes, 1995).

There are several rationales for the use of psychostimulants in TBI. First, they are known to improve symptoms of ADHD (Gualtieri & Evans, 1988). Many patients with TBI have similar symptoms of inattention, distractibility, disorganisation, impulsivity, and emotional lability. These symptoms tend to be ameliorated with stimulant medication in low and moderate doses (Holmes, 1995).

Another rationale for the use of stimulants in brain injury comes from the area of restorative neurology. Animal studies have suggested that amphetamine enhances cortical recovery by shortening recovery time in lesioned animals (Feeney & Sutton, 1993). Psychostimulants have been prescribed for the treatment of depression and apathy as well as behavioural disorders such as aggression, secondary to TBI (Rao & Lyketsos, 2000). In addition, the positive effects of drugs such as methylphenidate (Ritalin) are apparent within days of optimal dosage, making improvements easy to track. Side effects are not difficult to monitor and negative reactions are often amenable to changes in dosage or prescription (Gualtieri, 1991).

PERSEVERATION AND CONVERSATION

Studies that examine the pharmacological treatment of perseveration may also help to redress the problem of limited treatment options for perseveration in functional settings. Existing therapy suggestions have only been related to tightly structured interactions, such as alerting the client to an upcoming change in activity or monitoring the rate of test stimulus presentation, increasing time allowed for a response, or changing modalities (Bryant et al., 1994). This stance and the broader perception of therapeutic intervention in which it is embedded, have been increasingly challenged by studies evaluating the congruence of formal communication assessment with functional aims and outcomes (Penn, 1999). Alternative methods have sought to achieve ecological validity by assessing communication within the social context in which it takes place and to acknowledge the collaborative nature of human interaction (Perkins, Whitworth, & Lesser, 1998). One such method is the assessment of conversational ability using Conversation Analysis as both a research tool and as a supplement to clinical measures. The application of Conversation Analysis within a clinical setting has been well documented for patients with aphasia (Booth & Perkins, 1999; Laakso & Klippi, 1999; Perkins, Crisp, & Walshaw, 1999; Wilkinson, 1999). The benefits of using Conversation Analysis as a tool, and its usefulness within the communication assessment and therapy framework, have been well highlighted. Although it seems likely that conversation would be affected by perseveration, relevant conversational correlates have yet to be formally investigated, identified, and specified. As McNamara and Albert (2004) point out, some forms of perseveration such as stuck-in-set perseveration are less likely to be detected in sentences and words than in longer samples of discourse that reflect conceptual content. Careful observations of the conversational components that are compromised as a result of perseveration in TBI may provide more informative and comprehensive hypotheses of underlying neural functioning than other observational devices.

AIMS OF THE STUDY

Specifically, the primary aim of the study was to explore conversational correlates of perseveration as they manifested in two individuals with TBI. Possible explanations for perseveration were explored with reference to neuropsychological profiles provided by the application of Barkley's model of self-regulation and executive functioning. Discrete profiles were expected because of the complexities in the phenomena under study. Finally, the study investigated the response of perseveration to pharmacological treatment as measured by conversational ability and executive functioning.

METHOD

Research design

Two individuals with TBI, AA and PB, participated in single-subject, experimental research. Experimental and placebo conditions were included to ensure validity (Parloff, 1986). Further, random assignment by an external researcher to each of the treatment conditions took place, as well as a double blind precaution. All participants in the research, including the primary researcher, the participants and their conversational partners, were blind to which phase of the study the participants were in until after all the results had been analysed.

As the key focus of the research related to the manifestation of perseveration in everyday communication, Conversation Analysis was employed. This method allows the transition from description to applications for therapeutic interventions to be authentic, as analysis occurs at the level at which intervention is ultimately targeted (Perkins et al., 1998).

Participants

Two participants with TBI were identified, AA and PB, both permanent residents of a local nursing home. Recruitment procedures complied with Medical Ethics Board as stipulated by the University of the Witwatersrand. The participants were diagnosed as having suffered frontal lobe injuries as a result of TBI in initial medical reports and by a consulting neurologist. According to clinical observations as well as previous clinical therapy reports from the local university administered therapy services, neither participant was aphasic. However, both presented with behaviours associated with TBI including anomia, paucity of output, and abstract language deficits for AA, and slowed speech initiation and reduced rate of speech, anomia, and abstract language deficits for PB. Both participants were considered to be perseverative on the basis of a Conversation Analysis conducted by the researcher, as well as meeting criteria for perseveration on the Wisconsin Card Sorting Test (Paolo, Axelrod, & Troster, 1996). For the Conversation Analysis, participants were videotaped with a familiar caregiver and were considered perseverative if they displayed repetition, recurrence, or continuation of an earlier response uttered in syllables, words, sentences, or ideas in the face of changing contextual demands. Both participants had reliable primary caregivers, in the form of nurses who were assigned to care for them on almost a daily basis. Neither had a history of chronic alcohol or toxic substance abuse or treatment for psychiatric conditions or mood disorders prior to onset, although PB was being treated with anti-depressants secondary to his reaction to his head injury. Salient information is presented in Table 1.

Test battery

Communicative behaviours. Conversational data were analysed using Conversation Analysis. Data were generated by video-recording naturally occurring interactions in

TABLE 1
Salient participant information

Characteristic	*AA*	*PB*
Age at onset	30	40
Time since onset	10 years	9 years
Age at time of study	40 years	49 years
Sex	Male	Male
First language	English	Bilingual – English/Afrikaans
Pre-injury education	12 years plus 1 year technical diploma	12 years
Pre-injury employment	Photocopier technician	Self-employed, business manager
Laterality	Left-handed	Right-handed
Aetiology	TBI from motor vehicle accident	TBI from motor vehicle accident
Length of coma	3 months	6 weeks
Current medication	Rivotril (spasticity)	Amitryptiline (anti-depressant)
Reading ability	Intact	Intact
Colour-naming ability	Recognises, matches, and names colours accurately	Recognises, matches, and names colours accurately
Visual and hearing acuity	Responds to conversational loudness levels, visual acuity normal – see neurological findings	Responds to conversational loudness levels, visual acuity normal – see neurological findings
Conversation Analysis – Verbal perseveration	Perseverates on sentences, e.g., "I live in Durban.", "What day is it?", "Is this Joburg?"	Perseverates on ideas, e.g., returns to topic once subject has been closed
Wisconsin Card Sorting Test – Nonverbal perseveration	85 errors, 4 standard deviations above mean	27 errors, 2 standard deviations above mean
Preliminary neurological findings	Sub-cortical lesions, affecting left more than right as a result of shearing forces associated with TBI	Sub-cortical lesions as a result of shearing forces associated with TBI

the absence of the researchers (Ten Have, 1999). A 10-minute segment of each recording, depicting 10 minutes of continuous interaction at least 10 minutes into the video recording, was chosen for transcription (Lesser & Perkins, 1999) and later analysed for both verbal and nonverbal behaviours. Three characteristics of conversation were analysed: turn taking, topic management, and repair. These were selected for their ability to set the context for more micro-level behaviours (Lesser & Milroy, 1993) as well as because a wide range of typical performance literature exists in relation to these components. It was therefore assumed that, were turn taking, topic management, or repair affected by perseveration, they would be observable in relation to normative, typical performance for each area. Guidelines proposed by

TABLE 2
Conversational interactions recorded for the participants

Phase of the study	*AA – 1 hour after lunch or breakfast*	*PB – 2 hours after breakfast*
Baseline	Day nurse, in AA's room	Researcher, lounge
Active	Student therapist, in therapy room	Group workshop, sun-room,
Placebo	Student therapist, in therapy room	Group workshop, sun-room
Withdrawal	(1) Day nurse, in AA's room (2) Student therapist, in therapy room	Group workshop, sun-room

TABLE 3
The neuropsychological battery

Construct measured		*Task*
Behavioural Inhibition	Interference control	The Stroop Colour Word Test
	Response inhibition	Echopraxia Tasks
Executive Functioning	Nonverbal Working Memory	The Face Recognition Task The Self Ordered Pointing Test
	Internalisation of Speech / Verbal working memory	Verbal Paired Associates Word Lists
	Regulation of Affect	The Neuropsychology Behavior and Affect Profile (NBAP)
	Reconstitution	Controlled Oral Word Association Test (COWA) Category Naming

Sacks, Schegloff, and Jefferson (1974) and Schegloff, Jefferson, and Sacks (1977) were referred to in this regard. Table 2 summarises the interactions recorded for each of the participants at every phase of the study.

For AA, all interactions with the exception of the first were recorded with a speech therapy student. In the baseline phase, he was recorded with a day nurse, while in the withdrawal phases conversations with both his student therapist as well as a day nurse were recorded. Interactions took place at similar times for each recording. PB was recorded with a group workshop run by a social worker during all phases except for the baseline phase, during which he was recorded with the researcher.

Neuropsychological functioning. The Scales of Cognitive Ability in Traumatic Brain Injury (SCATBI) (Adamovich & Henderson, 1992) was administered to both participants in order to measure common aspects of cognition: Perception and Discrimination (Attention); Orientation; Organisation; Recall and Reasoning. Performance ranges in terms of normal functioning were obtained for each of the participants, providing a context within which to interpret and discuss research findings as well as a source of triangulation (Appendix A and B). Table 3 lists the other neuropsychological tasks, selected for their correspondence with Barkley's model, and the corresponding construct measured (Appendix C provides a table with the rationale for choosing the tests listed). Parallel versions of the tests were used wherever possible so that the stimuli presented at each stage of the study would be novel, and would counter practice and institutionalisation effects.

Procedure

Caregiver training. Nurses, social workers, and the matron were formally enlisted and trained for administration of The Neuropsychology Behavior and Affect Profile (NBAP).

Preparation and administration of the drug. The consulting neurologist prescribed 25 mg of methylphenidate (Ritalin) daily for 2 weeks to be administered as follows: 15 mg in the morning (8:00 am), 5 mg at lunch time (12:00 pm), and 5 mg at tea time

(3:30 pm). To ensure this, identical opaque coloured capsules were used. Capsules containing the active drug were divided into two groups. Group A contained a full 10 mg tablet, while Group B contained half a tablet (5 mg) in order to make up the prescribed dose (25 mg/daily). The capsules were then filled with lactose powder, an inert, non-reactive substance that further weighted the capsules and disguised their contents. Placebo capsules contained only lactose powder. A randomisation procedure was then carried out in order to determine whether the participants entered the drug or placebo stage first.

Data were collected over approximately a 6-week period, with 2 weeks given to the active, placebo, and withdrawal phases, and data being collected towards the end of the second week of each of those phases. This time frame was felt sufficient owing to the nature of the medication, which is rapidly and almost completely absorbed, with peak plasma concentrations 1–2 hours after administration. In addition, effects last only for as long as the medication is within the system, after which the dose is excreted. Neuropsychological data were collected by a psychometrist who randomised the order of tests to further control for practice effects. Testing as well as video recording always occurred 1–2 hours after ingestion of the drug, after breakfast or lunch.

At each phase of testing, the complete battery of all neuropsychological tests (as stipulated in Table 3) were administered and conversational data recorded (baseline, active, placebo, and withdrawal phases). The conversational data were transcribed by the first author using CA conventions. Portions of the transcripts were then submitted to an external researcher for verification of interpretation.

RESULTS AND DISCUSSION

Primary findings indicated that each of the two participants demonstrated unique expressions of perseveration affecting topic management. While AA's data were consistent with recurrent perseveration in terms of perseverative topic initiation, PB's were more consistent with stuck-in-set perseveration manifesting at topic boundaries. Both AA and PB demonstrated intact turn-taking and repair skills. The discussion below illustrates these findings by highlighting significant communication and neuropsychological findings for both cases.

Profile 1: Recurrent perseveration in AA

Recurrent perseveration refers to the inappropriate occurrence of part or all of a previous response after a different intervening response (Sandson & Albert, 1984) and best describes AA's verbal perseveration during conversation. AA's tendency to perseverate impacted on all aspects of topic management including topic bias, initiation, maintenance, and shift. All his topic initiations were perseverative and consisted of requests for orientation to time and place. Example 1 below is typical of AA's interactions. AA was also significantly distractible and was unable to maintain a topic without reverting to perseverative utterances. He was generally unable to contribute to topic shift.

Example 1
[N = Nurse]
1. **AA**: Day?

2. **N**: Day is Sunday I told you
3. **AA**: Day date?
4. **N**: 26th
5. **AA**: Month?
6. **N**: August
7. **AA**: Year?
8. **N**: Is (.) 2000
9. **AA**: Ch- (.) Jo- (.) Joburg?
10. **N**: mm is Joburg
11. **AA**: I live in Durban
12. (1.4)
13. **AA**: What city of accident?
14. **N**: Is Pretoria
15. **AA**: What day's today?

Analysis of the conversational data between AA and his nurses compared to interactions with his student therapist revealed the significant impact of interlocutor style and therefore context on AA's communication. As depicted in Figure 2, there are notably fewer perseverative utterances in interactions with the student therapist than during interactions with his nurses. This finding was more notable than drug effects for AA, although subtle changes in topic shift ability were noted during the active phase.

It appeared that the success of interactions with AA depended to a large extent on the interlocutor's skill in securing new topics of conversation. The nurses tended to offer closed-ended questions that were often not linked to prior conversational content. In contrast the student therapist offered a greater number of topics with broad scopes, which she introduced in more open-ended ways. Thus the possibility for discussion over a greater number of turns with topic shift, which the student mediated for AA, increased. The student therapist also appeared to consistently ignore AA's perseverations, instead re-orienting him to the topic at hand, while the nurses more often than not responded to perseverative utterances.

The fact that AA's turn-taking skills were intact (Example 2 below) was surprising given his significantly poor ability to resist interference and high levels of distractibility. Previous research and predictions from Barkley's model suggested that interruptions and overlaps would be expected (Gillis, 1996). Yet the data

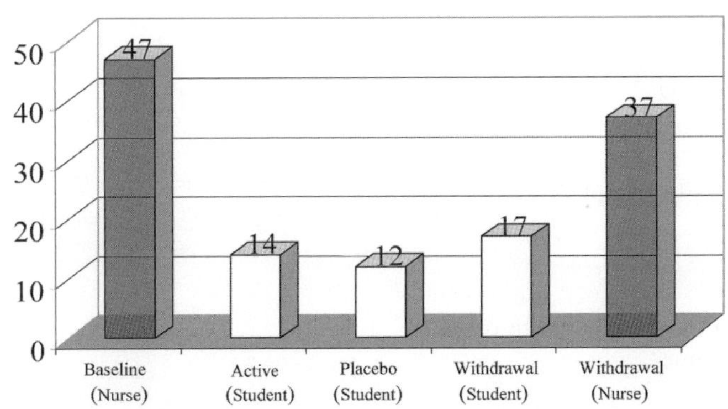

Figure 2. Total number of perseverations per conversation for AA with different conversational partners.

indicated that overlaps and interruptions were not characteristic of his conversation and when they occurred, reflected normal conversational practice. Analyses further revealed that AA was able to take up his turn promptly, responding appropriately to questions and statements put to him (line 2), when he was directly selected as the next speaker, thus managing the split-second timing of turn handovers in conversation. In addition, he appeared sensitive to lapses in the conversation and inserted utterances during these silences when his interlocutor, his nurses in this instance, did not provide an alternative as demonstrated in lines 5 (lapse) and 6 (topic initiation) below. However he also showed an ability to tolerate silences when he had asked a question and was waiting for a response (line 8 – question, line 9 – long pause, line 10 – response from nurse; similar sequence in lines 11–13).

Example 2
1. **N**: Is it painful?
2. **AA**: Very sore
3. (1.5)
4. **AA**: very sore
5. (3.3)
6. **AA**: Is this Joburg?
7. **N**: Ja
8. **AA:** What day?
9. (2.6)
10. **N**: Tuesday love =
11. **AA**: = Date?
12. (2.6)
13. **N**: It's the last day of the month. What's the last day tell me.

In addition, AA demonstrated intact repair abilities. He showed instances of self-initiated self-repair as demonstrated in Example 3 line 2. He also initiated a number of repair trajectories by accurately interpreting silence or facial expression as an indication that his interlocutor had not understood him (Example 3 lines 4–6). At these times he used a number of strategies including repetitions of utterances (Example 4 lines 6 and 8), partial repeats (Example 5 lines 8–10), as well as changes of some words (Example 4 lines 8–10) and changes in stress or loudness (Example 5 line 12) as described by Schegloff et al. (1977).

Example 3
1. **N**: What were you doing before you get an accident?
2. **AA**: I was fixix (0.9) I fixed photocopy machines
3. **N**: You what?
4. **AA**: Photostat machines
5. (1.2)
6. **AA**: I fixed photocopiers
7. **N**: Where?

Example 4
1. **AA**: I didn't go to the beach often.
2. **T**: How come?
3. (1.4)
4. **AA**: I didn't like the surf.
5. **T**: You didn't like to surf OK

6. **AA**: I didn't surf at all
7. **T**: Pardon?
8. **AA**: I didn't surf at all.
9. (1.5)
10. **AA**: I never surfed
[ ]
11. **T**: Oh
12. you didn't surf at all OK
13. **AA**: No

Example 5

1. **N**: Did you like going to the beach?
2. **AA**: Ja sure
3. (1.8)
4. **AA**: Good talent
5. **N**: mm?
6. **AA**: I look at – I look at the talent
7. **N**: I beg your pardon?
8. **AA**: I look at the talent on the beach
9. **N**: You look at?
10. **AA**: Talent
11. **N**: You have a good talent for the beach?
12. **AA**: (hhh) I LOOK at the talent
13. (0.6)
14. **N**: You look at the what?
15. **AA**: The females
16. **N**: The FEMALES (0.7) A I cannot believe this A I'm going to tell Caroline
[ ] [ ]
17. **AA**: Ja Ja (hhh)
18. (hhh)
19. **N**: Should I tell her?
20. **AA**: No
21. **N**: Hey?
22. **AA**: No
23. **N**: That you go to the beach to look at the females now A

Despite his profound distractibility, AA was able to remain focused and attentive during repair trajectories for significant lengths of time and remained committed to resolution of trouble spots as long as his interlocutor was also committed to repairing the breakdown. Example 5 above is an excellent demonstration of this. Interestingly, during this lengthy exchange, AA did not initiate a single perseverative utterance, despite the fact that the situation required sustained attention. Perhaps this finding can be explained in terms of current neural network models of verbal perseveration.

Cohen and Dehaene (1998) proposed a model in which cognitive representations exist at relatively high activation levels for some time following initial activation. In healthy people, persistence is suppressed through a competitive process between a new stimulus and the initial one when the new stimulus is presented. When brain damage degrades the inhibitory powers of the frontal lobes, representations persisting in activity are not always effectively suppressed, resulting in perseveration. Gotts, della Rocchetta, and Cipolotti (2002) point out that this model predicts that perseveration will increase, as a weak current stimulus will be less likely to override a persistent initial stimulus. Perseveration will also become less likely as the number of intervening stimuli increases presumably because the activation level of the initial stimulus weakens over time, thereby making it more vulnerable to being overridden by the current stimulus and frontal lobe inhibition.

This model explains AA's ability to respond to repair, which represents a strong current stimulus that has the potential to override the initial stimulus. It further explains why, during interactions with the student therapist, perseverations decreased, as she failed to respond to perseverated utterances, instead reinforcing the newer, current stimulus. As intervening stimuli (various topics of conversation or topic shifts) increased, the tendency towards reverting to the initial stimulus decreased, resulting in fewer perseverations. It is possible that the nurses, by responding to the perseverated utterances, kept those stimuli primed, and therefore less susceptible to being overridden by more appropriate forms of exchange.

The neuropsychological data gathered fit well with the conversational data to form a coherent profile. AA's performance on the Scales of Cognitive Ability in traumatic brain injury suggested that he would present with difficulties related to attention, orientation, and recall (Appendix A), which triangulated well with the neuropsychological data, presented in Table 4 (Appendices D – K provide scores).

AA presented with deficits in behavioural inhibition in terms of poor interference control as well as all of the executive functions assessed—nonverbal working memory, internalisation of speech (verbal working memory), regulation of affect, and reconstitution. Scores for functions highlighted in bold in Table 4, normalised or

TABLE 4
Neuropsychological findings for AA

Construct	*Test used*	*Level of baseline performance*	*Changes with Ritalin*
Interference Control	**The Stroop Colour Test**	**Below mean**	**Interference score normalized during active phase**
Response Inhibition	Echopraxic Tests	Could not perform	No change
Nonverbal working memory	Face Recognition	Below mean, contaminations in scoring, leading to elevated scores as a result of response perseveration	No change
	Self Ordered Pointing Test	Below mean	No change
Internalisation of speech/Verbal working memory	**Verbal Paired Associates**	**Below mean**	**Qualitative change during active phase**
	Word Lists	Below mean	No change
Regulation of Affect	Neuropsychology Behavior and Affect Profile (NBAP)	Inappropriateness and Pragnosia identified	No change
Reconstitution	**Controlled Oral Word Association (COWA)**	**Below mean High percentage of perseverative responses**	**Improvement in performance during active phase**
	Category Naming	**Below mean High percentage of perseverative responses**	**Perseveration decreased during active phase**

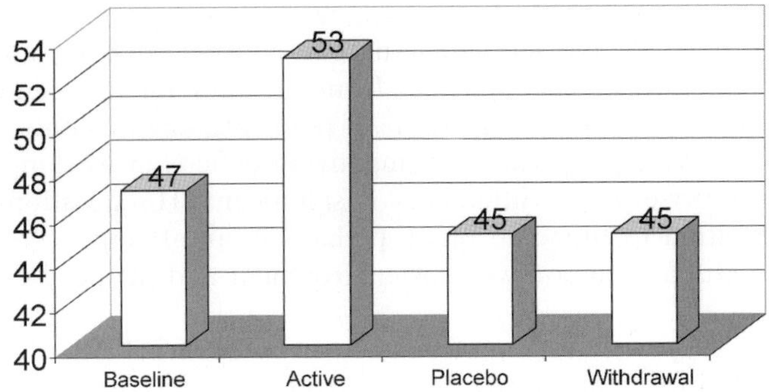

Figure 3. AA's interference t-scores on the Stroop Colour Word Test (normal = 50).

improved during the active drug phase. Some qualitative improvements were seen for the Verbal Paired Associates task but were not reflected in scores.

Interference control. Poor interference control as measured by the Stroop Colour Word Test is consistent with diffuse brain injury and perseverative tendencies, and is suggestive of poor attentional inhibition and set-switching behaviour (Golden, 1978). The finding also implies generally limited attentional resources and reduced speed of information processing (Ponsford & Kinsella, 1992). This finding is significant because it demonstrates a relationship between poor interference control and the presence of perseveration. This finding is consistent with recent research that links perseverative errors to failure to inhibit a prepotent response (Spencer & Schutte, 2004). For a comprehensive discussion of the relationship between interference control and the prepotent response, the reader is referred to Barkley (1997). The normalisation of the interference score during the active phase (see Figure 3) signifies improved resistance to distraction with improved sustained attention capacities (Appendix D).

The impact of depleted inhibition skills is clearly reflected in AA's inability to resist distraction. The inability to sustain attention to internal representations or tasks has been implicated in difficulty with topic management in discourse (Stuss & Benson, 1986).

Nonverbal working memory. AA's consistently poor long-term recall as measured by Faces (nonverbal memory) (Appendix E) and poor performance on the Self Ordered Pointing Test (nonverbal working memory) (Appendix F) suggests poor working and strategic memory (Spreen & Strauss, 1998) as well as a more long-term learning deficit (Adamovich & Henderson, 1992). As Faces is a task of recognition, the interpretation of the results is complex. Recognition tasks are not purely testing a working memory construct and long-term memory ability also impacts on performance (see Levin, Goldstein, Williams, & Eisenberg, 1991 for a more in-depth review).

AA's poor performance on both Faces and the Self Ordered Pointing Test is significant in terms of the ability to demonstrate the co-occurrence of perseveration and working memory deficits. These findings were anticipated by the Scales of Cognitive Ability in traumatic brain injury results, which indicated a severe deficit in orientation for AA. Lezak's comments on the disorienting effect of poor working memory are highly pertinent. As context can never be integrated due to poor short-term span of attention, the individual becomes displaced from any meaningful contact with the world as well as from meaningful communication with conversational partners. Given this profile of poor interference control and extreme distractibility and the unsurprising accompanying deficits in working memory, the content of AA's perseverated utterances is significant. His questions all reflect a desire for orientation to time and place, perhaps in an attempt to re-engage some form of meaningful association with his environment and the people in it.

Internalisation of speech. AA's performance on both Verbal Paired Associates and Word Lists remained consistently weak throughout the study indicating poor immediate memory span (Appendix G and H). However, qualitatively AA's performance differed during the drug phase from that in the other stages of the study for Verbal Paired Associates. During the drug phase, AA was able to draw from the pool of target words to create associations, despite the fact that his matches were mostly incorrect. During the other phases, he relied solely on semantic memory associations and failed to recall any of the target words. His difficulties are indicative of reduced memory span where verbal information is lost rapidly and transmission to a more permanent store cannot take place (Lezak, 1995). It is possible that the improvements seen in AA's interference score on the Stroop Colour Word Test as a result of improved resistance to distraction can account for the qualitative changes seen in this subtest.

Taking into account AA's poor working memory (nonverbal as well as verbal) as measured by the neuropsychological tests, it is not surprising that he struggled to contribute meaningfully to topic shift. These contributions rely heavily on the ability to integrate previously stated information in order to generate novel responses that are relevant to exchanges (Molloy, Brownell, & Gardner, 1990). In order to accomplish this integration, one must be able to resist distractions and remain attentive (Barkley, 1997; Hartley, 1995). Therefore the clinical deficits of poor topic selection, maintenance, relevance, and quantity in individuals with TBI (Milton, Prutting, & Binder, 1984), as well as reduced amount of content and further limitations in efficiency and connectivity in discourse (Wyckoff, Jensen, & LaPointe, 1984), can be linked to executive factors.

Regulation of affect. The Neuropsychology Behavior and Affect Profile mean scores indicated that AA's caregivers consistently viewed him as displaying "Indifference" across all four phases of the study (Appendix I). The impairment of drive or motivation is a significant factor in the manifestation of perseveration. This disturbance in particular would result in dissociation between information and the drive to act on it, thus presenting as behavioural inflexibility or perseveration (Luria, 1980).

Reconstitution. For both Category Naming and the Controlled Oral Word Association test, AA's performance initially demonstrated low scores with a significant number of perseverative utterances. On the Controlled Oral Word Association test, the decrease in perseverative responses was more pronounced, with a notable improvement in descriptive rating for performance during the active phase, as demonstrated in Figure 4 (also Appendix J). On Category Naming, although the total number of perseverations decreased significantly during the active phase, standard scores remained low (Appendix K).

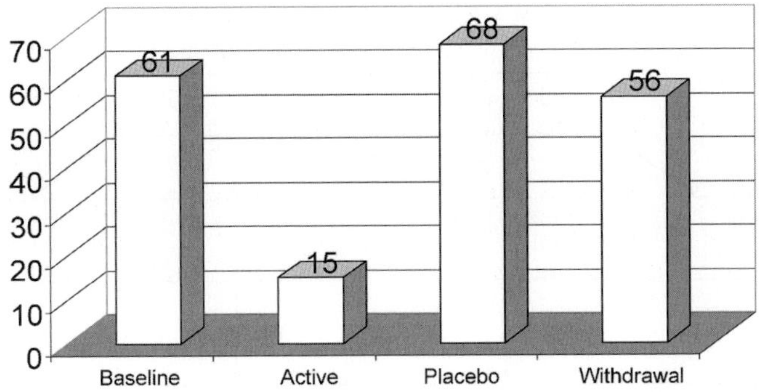

Figure 4. Percentage of perseverative responses for AA on the COWA.

The integrated nature of the category naming task requires a number of abilities supported by the frontostriatal circuits. It is well accepted that these functions are supported by information-processing systems (Raskin, Sliwinski, & Bond, 1992) as well as attention and working memory factors (Van Zomeren & Brouwer, 1994). Lesions to the prefrontal cortex, affecting these systems, result in the inability to analyse and synthesise material in a flexible manner, therefore resulting in impairment in the ability to create multiple, novel, and complex response sequences, thus giving rise to perseveration (Barkley, 1997). It is therefore significant that the number of perseverative responses decreased so substantially for AA during the drug phase. Improvements in the ability to resist interference therefore allowed for more consistent deployment of attention resources, which could better support some of the functions needed for performance of this task. Most notably, it would seem that increased temporary storage of stated items occurred, so that items were not repeated as often, indicating again the impact of attention on working memory and consequently behavioural flexibility.

The Controlled Oral Word Association appeared to be more sensitive to the administration of pharmacotherapy than Category Naming, which may be accounted for by differences in the processes required for semantic and phonemic activation, the latter requiring more effortful processing and greater allocation of attentional recourses (Gathercole & Baddeley, 1993). The benefit of pharmacotherapy, leading to subtle changes in resistance to distraction and resulting ability to remain engaged in a task with greater capacity for voluntary attention and better organisation of that activity towards a specific purpose, would therefore be most noticeable.

Summary of AA. In summarising AA's profile, Barkley's model is revisited with specific reference to AA's unique manifestations of perseveration at a conversational level (see Figure 5). AA's conversation was characterised by recurrent perseveration, affecting topic management. He had significant difficulty maintaining and initiating topics and generally was unable to contribute meaningfully to topic shift. On the neuropsychological battery, AA presented with a significant interference control deficit with poor resistance to distraction. Failure to remain focused and pursue goal-directed behaviour results in permanent disruption of working memory processes. In AA's conversation, the chain of questions requesting orientation to time and place are consistent with predictions from the literature (Gillis, 1996; Hartley, 1995). This profile not only fits comfortably with current theories of

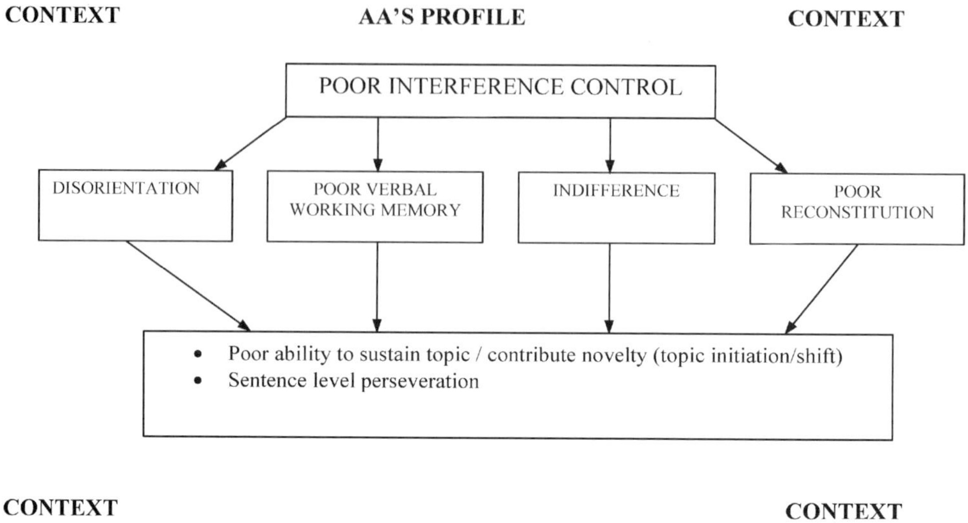

Figure 5. AA's profile of perseveration and behavioural inhibition/executive functioning deficits.

perseveration in terms of disordered response inhibition but also accounts for the cascade effect on other areas of executive functioning, particularly the ability to generate novel responses. A further possible contribution to AA's perseveration may be a disorder of motivation or drive, as demonstrated by the identification of "Indifference" on the Neuropsychological Behavior and Affect Profile. AA responded positively to pharmacological intervention, showing a normalisation of the interference score on the Stroop Colour Word Test and subsequent improvements in reconstitution and working memory. Conversational context was found to be a highly significant factor, with interlocutor input significantly affecting the proportion of perseverative utterances per conversation. This factor makes it difficult to interpret what, if any, effects the drug itself had on the manifestation of perseveration in AA's conversation.

Profile 2: Stuck-in-set perseveration in PB

Like AA, PB demonstrated intact turn-taking and repair skills with impaired topic management skills. Unlike AA, however, the nature of this disturbance was not traceable to poor sustained attention, rather to difficulty in changing or shifting topics, reflecting what has traditionally been called "stuck-in-set" perseveration (Sandson & Albert, 1984). This is the inappropriate maintenance of a framework of response after introduction of a new task. PB demonstrated adequate inter-topic management skills. He was able to initiate meaningful topics (Example 6 line 1), contribute and respond to shift (Example 6 lines 8–13), and maintain topics over significant lengths of time. However, he demonstrated difficulty disengaging with a topic and therefore inter-topic boundaries presented a problem for him. PB had a tendency, once engaged with a topic, to perseverate on the content, after the topic has been closed. It took a number of turns, before he was able to disengage and engage with a new subject (Example 7 lines 13 and 46–53). At times, this perseveration interfered with the conversation and PB interrupted others (Example 8 lines 11 and 17–20). PB's conversational data correspond directly to the neuropsychological testing, which revealed adequate sustained attention and ability to resist distraction as measured by the Stroop Colour Word Test but poor set-switching abilities as indicated by performance on echopraxia tasks. There is precedence in the literature, linking topic maintenance, perseveration, and performance on echopraxia tasks (Watt & Penn, 2000).

Example 6
[R = researcher]
1. **PB**: de Klerk is getting out of politics (.) is it because he changes the politics?
2. **R**: no, well remember he also cheated on his wife
3. **PB**: (hhh) ahah oo that's bad
4. **R**: Ja that's very bad
5. **PB**: very bad hu I didn't know that
6. **R**: Ja it was all in the newspapers
7. **PB**: Oh and I remember him I didn't know that that is a t- a really v-bad
8. **R**: It's a bad thing to do (0.8) ja sure
9. **PB**: very bad
10. **R**: his poor wife
11. **PB**: Ja not at that age =
12. **R:** = Not at <u>any</u> age
13. **PB**: You can not do that mm I fully disagree with that

Example 7
[E = Social worker running the group]
1. **E**: Did you have any pets?
2. (1.4)
3. **PB**: Only a dog geh- geh- E
4. **E:** What sort of dog?
5. **PB**: Bull terrier
6. **E:** Oooh did you have a terrier?
7. **PB**: and we and we called him PV
8. (1.2)
9. **PB**: PW Botha

[The group laughs]

10. **E**: (hhh) Oh did you? (hhh)
11. (6.5)
12. **E**: Did he look like him?
13. **PB**: (hhh) we just called him that (.) it was- we called him PV (.) we called him PV
14. **E**: What colour was it?

[…]

[The conversation shifts to talking about how strong bull terriers are and what good guard dogs they make. Then E turns her attention to other members of the group who in turn discuss their pets. The conversation comes to a conclusion when one of the occupational therapists interrupts to talk about hand writing with one of the participants, and E and several members of the group talk about hand-writing skills and the practice they do during the first part of the workshop. The occupational therapist leaves]

46. **PB**: We called it PV
47. (4.5)
48. **PB**: Ja huh
49. (2.2)

50. **PB**: We called him PW. We liked to call him PW Botha. We gave him the name PW huh
51. **E**: Very original
52. (7.6)
53. **PB**: PV
54. **E**: Right R (.) it's your turn

Example 8

[S = member of the group]

1. **E**: Did you ever play (.) cowboys and Indians or anything like that?
2. **PB**: Cowboys, cowboys and crooks
[ ]
3. **E**: Crooks
4. gangsters. Did you S?
5. **S**: Because you had lots of trees and things
[ ]
6. **PB**: Correct ja =
7. **E**: = Because they lived in the country.
8. (1.0)
9. **E**: What did you used to play (0.7) S?
10. **S**: I told you hopscotch
[ ]
11. **PB**: Cowboys and crooks
12. **E**: OK
13. **S**: and learning to ride a bike =
14. **E**: = Oh yeah
(1.2)
16. **E**: Did you used to dress up?
[ ]
17. **PB**: We used to
18. (1.2)
19. **PB**: to call them cowboys and crooks ja
20. **E**: Cowboys and crooks

In terms of turn taking, PB demonstrated an ability to handle split-second timing of handovers in both individual and group settings (Example 7 lines 5 and 7). This ability was compromised only when new topics were introduced (Example 7 lines 1–3). This finding again may relate to attention shift or the interruption of an ongoing response. This deficit was only evident in the group context, highlighting the challenges that are not always evident in less demanding interactions.

Repair skills remained intact for PB over the course of the study and he was competent at initiating repair (Example 7 lines 7–9), self-correcting (Example 6 line 7), and requesting clarification during trouble spots (Example 9 below).

Example 9

1. **R**: I think the aviary is lovely
2. (2.3)
3. **PB**: What was that?
4. **R**: I love the aviary (.) with the birds

For PB, subtle difficulties with orientation and recall were indicated on the Scales of Cognitive Ability in traumatic brain injury (Appendix B); findings that

TABLE 5
Neuropsychological findings for PB

Construct	*Test used*	*Level of baseline performance*	*Changes with Ritalin*
Interference Control	The Stroop Colour Word Test	Within average range	Incremental improvements indicative of learning effects
Response Inhibition	**Echopraxic Tests**	**6 errors per minute, indicative of poor motor inhibition**	**0 errors during active phase**
Nonverbal Working Memory	Face Recognition	Within average range	Incremental improvements indicative of learning effects
	Self Ordered Pointing Test	Below mean	Incremental improvements indicative of learning effects
Internalisation of Speech/Verbal working memory	Verbal Paired Associates	Below mean	Incremental improvements indicative of learning effects
	Word Lists	**Below mean, intrusions from previous test noted**	**Improvement in active phase with significant decrease in percentage of intrusions**
Regulation of Affect	Nuropsychology Behavior and Affect Profile (NBAP)	No area of difficulty identified	No change
Reconstitution	**Controlled Oral Word Association (COWA)**	**Below mean**	**Improvement in performance in terms of descriptive rating during active phase**
		High percentage of perseverative responses	**Perseveration decreased substantially during active phase**
	Category naming	Below mean	No change, perseveration decreased slightly during active phase.

triangulated well with his neuropsychological data summarised in Table 5. Significantly, PB presented with normal interference control but poor behavioural inhibition, which normalised during the active phase of the study. He further presented with poor reconstitution, which also showed some improvement with drug therapy. His affect profile indicated normal presentation. Nonverbal and verbal working memory abilities on the selected tasks showed incremental improvements over the course of the study, suggesting learning effects, despite the fact that control measures had been put into place.

Behavioural inhibition. PB demonstrated poor scores for all test conditions, including colour naming, word reading, and naming of discongruent ink colour and, as with AA, these findings are consistent with diffuse brain injury and perseverative tendencies (Golden, 1978). However, his interference scores fell within normal limits during all stages of the study (Appendix L). Thus for PB, although his overall poor performance is consistent with perseverative tendencies, his good interference score implies that his perseveration is not linked to interference control problems. Therefore, slow rate of information processing and poor set-switching behaviour are more pertinent factors affecting his performance. This finding was confirmed by his performance on the echopraxia tasks where he manifested difficulties in all phases except the drug phase (Appendix M). During the drug phase, although PB's response times were slow, no errors were present (see Figure 6). Errors during the other phases of the study were significant in terms of reflecting poor motor inhibition (Spreen & Strauss, 1998).

Barkley's model (1998) differentiates between behavioural inhibition and interference control. In PB it is possible to see how one may be affected but not the other. The result is an ability to sustain attention and withstand interference, but difficulty with set switching or disengaging from an ongoing stimulus to another when the contextual demands change. These findings seem to fit with the conversational data and provide sound explanations for their occurrence. The echopraxic tasks proved to be especially sensitive to improvements in response inhibition in relation to PB.

Nonverbal working memory. PB initially presented with a moderate difficulty with nonverbal working memory as measured by his performance on Faces, which remained fairly consistent over the study (Appendix N). His performance on the Self Ordered Pointing Test, showed incremental improvements (Appendix O). For PB a

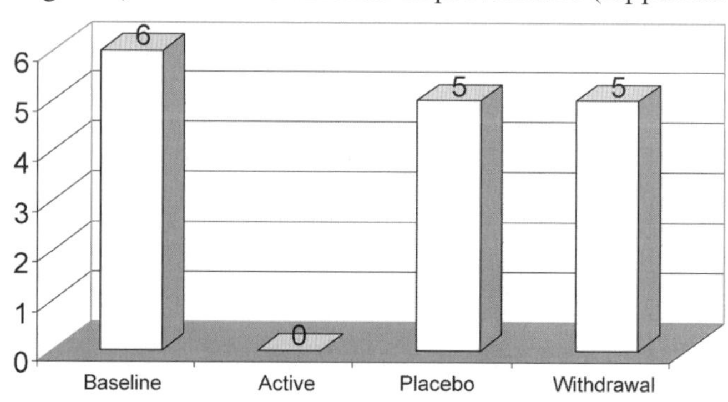

Figure 6. Total number of errors per minute for PB during echopraxic tests.

clear discrepancy was noted between recognition and free recall abilities, the former being better preserved than the latter. This performance is often characteristic of individuals with prefrontal lesions (Lezak, 1995). While PB does not appear to present with a disorder of the memory system itself, he does not use context spontaneously to facilitate recall, i.e., he has a working memory deficit. This finding was echoed in the verbal working memory subtests.

Internalisation of speech. On Verbal Paired Associates, PB's performance showed gradual incremental changes across the four phases of the study, implying increasing familiarity with task requirements (Appendix P). However, notable improvement was seen in performance on Word Lists (Appendix Q) in the active phase, which could be related to improved ability to interrupt or inhibit an ongoing or prepotent response (Barkley, 1997). In addition, during baseline, placebo, and withdrawal phases PB demonstrated high degrees of intrusion from the previously administered Verbal Paired Associates Test.

In Verbal Paired Associates, successful performance relies on the ability to engage the articulatory rehearsal process to maintain the associations in memory and then later retrieve them from a more permanent store. During administration of the latter task, inadvertent rehearsal of previously practised items continued, accounting for their intrusion in PB's performance of the second task, Word Lists. With regard to perseveration, several authors refer to the possibility of uninhibited augmentation of facilitatory activity for creation of new memory or uninhibited retention of information in working memory (Blanken et al., 1993; Gathercole & Baddeley, 1993). This may also explain why across the four stages of the study, PB's performance on the test that was administered first (Verbal Paired Associates), showed steady and consistent improvement, while his performance on Word Lists did not.

PB's demonstration of a practice or learning effect for most of the tasks used in the battery, despite the use of parallel versions of the tests to control for this factor, was significant. PB thus demonstrated a spontaneous ability to adjust to test requirements, substantially improving his performance over a relatively brief period of time. This capacity for learning reveals a high degree of potential that essentially remains untapped in this particular institutionalised setting. Extension of cognitive and communicative abilities therefore appears possible for PB.

Regulation of affect. PB's caregivers did not identify any of the five constructs relating to affect regulation as being compromised (Appendix R). Whereas AA's profile of perseveration may involve contributions from drive and motivation disorders, PB's appears to be more localised to attention shifting factors.

Reconstitution. On the Controlled Oral Word Association test, PB's performance also showed improvements, with his performance approximating normal during the active drug phase (Appendix S). PB also demonstrated high levels of perseveration above the norm for all phases of the study, but these were at their lowest during the active phase. This observation provides support for the effects of attention and hence flexibility in conversational discourse. His performance on Category Naming did not improve as well. His scores remained consistently poor, reflecting limited mental flexibility and recall impairments (Appendix T). While the number of perseverations was also lowest during the active phase for PB, this finding was not as robust in relation to his other scores for this task.

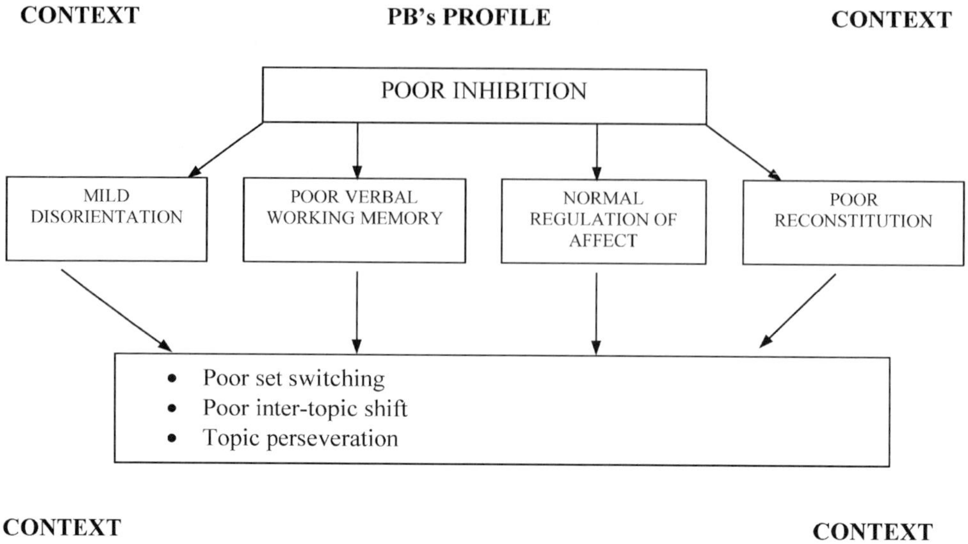

Figure 7. PB's profile of perseveration and behavioural inhibition/executive functioning deficits.

Summary of PB. PB's profile highlights stuck-in-set perseveration manifesting with problems of inter-topic management. While PB was able to initiate, maintain, and shift topics adequately, his ability to disengage with the old topic and shift attention to a new one was significantly compromised during all but the drug phase of the study. These findings are further associated with significant results on the echopraxic tasks, which clearly demonstrated a problem with behavioural inhibition, for all phases except the drug phase of the study. Accompanying normalisation of inter-topic management and performance on the echopraxia tasks was an improvement on the reconstitution tasks with decreased perseveration. Finally, PB showed learning effects, demonstrating greater potential for cognitive and communicative achievement than his current level of functioning suggests. Figure 7 demonstrates the relevant areas of Barkley's model affected and the resulting profile of perseveration for PB.

GENERAL CONCLUSIONS AND IMPLICATIONS

This study has demonstrated that perseveration appears to have differing underlying explanations, which manifest in unique ways in conversation. For AA, recurrent perseveration was associated with deficits in interference control and inability to initiate, maintain, or shift topics. While for PB stuck-in-set perseveration was observable at topic boundaries and co-existed with deficits in behavioural inhibition.

The necessity of aspects of attention to all cognitive functions, as supported by the prefrontal cortex and its related circuits, appears to suggest a directional link between inhibition and executive functions, with deficits in the former anticipating deficits in the latter, as predicted by Barkley (1997). In particular, working memory functions are integrally related to communication outcomes with a further impact on reconstitution and generative language skills.

These findings give credence to current theories of perseveration that postulate just such disturbances of the fundamental processes of inhibitory control, including resistance to interference and attentional switching. Relationships between the role of the prefrontal cortex in accomplishing inhibitory control and the modulation of such cognitive processes by the catecholaminergic networks suggest that perseveration is amenable to pharmacological intervention, as was modestly demonstrated in this investigation by PB's data. The fact that both individuals demonstrated observable change is significant given that both were so chronic and have been institutionalised for so long, and suggests that further investigation into the usefulness of psychostimulants in the TBI population is warranted. Participant variables that require further investigation include: time since onset, severity of injury, interactions with other medication and, significantly, place and conditions of residence. Variables related to the drug itself include dosage and length of treatment. Pharmacotherapy represents a promising, optimistic option as a treatment for perseveration by stabilising behavioural inhibition, particularly in light of the scarcity of effective treatments currently available.

Third, perseveration is sensitive to contextual and environmental factors, which can either exacerbate or minimise the effects of perseveration on conversation. This was particularly true in AA's case, where interlocutor style and skill, by carefully structuring conversational input variables, reduced the number of perseverations and overall competence of AA's interactions. While the influence of environment on communication outcomes is intuitively clear, its place in theories of perseveration is not explicit. Yet contextual variables seem to play a key role in the perpetuation or amelioration of perseveration. Social isolation, reduced opportunities for communication, perceptions of incompetence, and the caregivers' difficulties coping with communicatively impaired individuals, all contribute to a negative spiral (Lubinski, 1991). The difficulties outlined are exacerbated in institutional settings where caregivers are burdened with long hours and heavy workloads, which are intensified with demanding patients, less than optimal knowledge of communication disorders, and frequently unsatisfying work conditions.

The need to manage contextual and environmental factors to reduce verbal perseveration should be guided by theoretical inferences and comprise individualised programmes that reflect the unique manifestations and underlying deficits of perseveration in a particular individual. For AA the strategies that may be useful include: ignoring perseverative utterances, reorientating to the current topic, taking responsibility for the introduction of new topics to the interaction, and making gradual topic shifts, providing alternatives for AA when he is unable to contribute a novel response, and making use of broad, open-ended themes, rather than closed-ended ones.

For PB, the clinical strategies may differ slightly. It may be worthwhile to signal the ends of activities or topics, emphasising a shift in framework and thereby assisting PB to orient more quickly to a new mindset, as suggested by Bryant et al. (1994). The fact that PB demonstrated practice effects has significant implications for intervention. While Lezak (1995) cautions that practice effects are common in individuals who have difficulty developing or shifting to a new set, PB's improvements are meaningful because of the fact that this variable was controlled for. Practice with different tasks encouraged PB to approach these tasks more efficiently and with greater skill. Thus, his potential for learning appeared to be disproportionate to his current level of functioning. Paradigms that focus on the ability to learn novel information and promote memory functioning may therefore present good therapy options for PB. One such approach is Errorless Learning, which could be used in conjunction with other learning principles (Landauer & Bjork, 1978). Expanding these strategies into everyday functional contexts may allow PB to acquire new types of knowledge that will allow him to function in more creative, novel, and complex ways.

For both individuals, conversation training is a possibility. Such training should be dynamic, occurring in a variety of settings, within a group context, and may include the use of techniques such as frequency counts, and video or audio recordings (Gillis, 1996). In addition, role-play and clinician modelling can be used, as well as simulations of a variety of situations with facilitators providing specific and descriptive feedback (Hartley, 1995). Giles and Clark-Wilson (1993) describe a number of techniques that are based on behaviour principles. Most important though is the fact that individuals are provided with the opportunity to interact frequently with a variety of people for a number of different purposes.

Finally, the use of Barkley's model proved useful in providing operational and descriptive definitions of constructs under investigation. Attention, working memory, and short-term memory interactions are clearly highlighted. In further evaluating Barkley's model (1997) it should be noted that language is addressed only in as much as it is represented by verbal working memory and higher-order comprehension and reasoning skills. However, the location of language is not addressed directly in the model, as it assumed that this executive function is more closely associated with working memory. Although cognitive deficits have a complex and intricate relationship with communicative outcomes, they cannot encompass or account for all of language functioning. In addition, the model looks at a one-way interaction in terms of the effects that executive functions have on language performance, and might be extended by showing how self-regulating systems work in conjunction with language processes and what the impact of language deficits (found in conditions such as aphasia) have on the performance of cognitive tasks.

We are still in the infant stages of improving our understanding of how the complex processes of cognitive executive functioning interacts with speech and language processing. As McNamara and Albert (2004) suggest, results from theoretical modelling of verbal perseveration should be brought to bear on the design of future pharmacological studies in order to improve this understanding and identify targets for pharmacological intervention.

REFERENCES

Adamovich, B., & Henderson, J. (1992). *Scales of Cognitive Ability for Traumatic Brain Injury*. New York: The Riverside Publishing Company.

Aten, J. L. (1994). Functional communication treatment. In R. Chapey (Ed.), *Language intervention strategies in adult aphasia* (3rd ed.). Baltimore: Williams & Wilkins.

Barkley, R. A. (1997). Behavioural inhibition, sustained attention and executive functions: Constructing a unifying theory of ADHD. *Psychological Bulletin, 121*(1), 65–94.

Benton, A. L., & Hamsher, K. D. E. S. (1976). *Multilingual Aphasia Examination*. Iowa City: University of Iowa.

Blanken, G., Dittmann, J., Grimm, H., Marshall, J. C., & Wallesch, C. W. (1993). *Linguistic disorders and pathologies: An international handbook*. Berlin: Walter de Gruyter.

Booth, S., & Perkins, L. (1999). The use of conversation analysis to guide individualized advice to carers and evaluate change in aphasia: A case study. *Aphasiology, 13*(4–5), 259–282.

Bryant, S. L., Emery, P. A., & Helm-Estabrooks, N. (1994). Management of different forms of perseveration in severe aphasia. *Seminars in Speech and Language*, *15*(1), 71–84.

Christman, S. S., Boutsen, F. R., & Buckingham, H. W. (2004). Perseveration and other repetitive verbal behaviors: Functional dissociations. *Seminars in Speech and Language*, *25*(4), 295–307.

Code, C. (1982). Recurrent utterances and automatisms in aphasia. In C. Code (Ed.), *The characteristics of aphasia*. London: Taylor & Francis.

Coelho, C. A., Liles, B. Z., & Duffy, R. J. (1991). Analysis of conversational discourse in head injured adults. *Journal of Head Trauma Rehabilitation*, *6*, 92–98.

Cohen, L., & Dehaene, S. (1998). Competition between past and present: Assessment and interpretation of verbal perseverations. *Brain*, *121*, 1641–1659.

Eisenson, J. (1973). *Adult aphasia: Assessment and treatment*. New York: Appleton Century Crofts.

Feeney, D., & Sutton, R. L. (1993). Pharmacotherapy for recovery of functions after brain injury. *CRC Critical Review in Neurobiology*, *3*, 135–197.

Fuster, J. M. (1997). *The prefrontal cortex: Anatomy, physiology and neuropsychology of the frontal lobe*. New York: Raven Press.

Gathercole, S. E., & Baddeley, A. D. (1993). *Working memory and language*. Hove, UK: Lawrence Erlbaum Associates Ltd.

Giles, M., & Clark-Wilson, J. (1993). *Brain injury rehabilitation: A neurofunctional approach*. London: Chapman & Hall.

Gillis, R. J. (1996). *Traumatic brain injury rehabilitation for speech-language pathologists*. Boston: Butterworth-Heinemann.

Godfrey, H. P. D., & Shum, D. (2000). Executive functioning and the application of social skills following traumatic brain injury. *Aphasiology*, *14*(4), 433–444.

Golden, J. C. (1978). *Stroop Color and Word Test*. Chicago: Stoelting Company.

Gotts, S. J., della Rocchetta, A. I., & Cipolotti, L. (2002). Mechanisms underlying perseveration in aphasia: Evidence from a single case study. *Neuropsychologia*, *40*, 1930–1947.

Gualtieri, C. G. (1991). Psychostimulants in traumatic brain injury. In L. L. Greenhill & B. B. Osman (Eds.), *Ritalin: Theory and patient management*. New York: Liebert.

Gualtieri, C. G., & Evans, R. W. (1988). Stimulant treatment for the neurobehavioural sequelae of TBI. *Brain Injury*, *2*, 273–290.

Hartley, L. L. (1995). *Cognitive communicative abilities following brain injury: A functional approach*. San Diego, CA: Singular Publishing.

Hauser, M. D. (1999). Perseveration, inhibition and the prefrontal cortex: A new look. *Current Opinion in Neurobiology*, *9*, 214–222.

Holmes, V. F. (1995). Medical use of psychostimulants: An overview. *International Journal of Psychiatry in Medicine*, *25*(1), 1–19.

Laakso, M., & Klippi, A. (1999). A closer look at the 'hint and guess' sequences in aphasic conversation. *Aphasiology*, *13*(4–5), 259–282.

Landauer, T. K., & Bjork, R. A. (1978). Optimum rehearsal patterns and name learning. In M. M. Gruneberg, P. E. Morris, & R. N. Sykes (Eds.), *Practical aspects of memory*. London: Academic Press.

Lang, P. J. (1995). The emotion probe: Studies of motivation and attention. *American Psychologist*, *50*, 372–385.

Lesser, R., & Milroy, L. (1993). *Linguistics and aphasia: Psycholinguistics and pragmatic aspects of intervention*. London: Longman Group Ltd.

Lesser, R., & Perkins, L. (1999). *Cognitive neuropsychology and conversation analysis in aphasia: An introductory casebook*. London: Whurr Publishers.

Levin, H. S., Goldstein, F. C., Williams, D. H., & Eisenberg, H. M. (1991). The contribution of frontal lobe lesions to the neurobehavioural outcome of closed head injury. In H. S. Levin, H. M. Eisenberg, & A. L. Benton (Eds.), *Frontal lobe function and dysfunction*. New York: Oxford University Press.

Lezak, M. D. (1995). *Neuropsychological Assessment* (3rd ed.). New York: Oxford University Press.

Linscott, R. L., Knight, R. G., & Godfrey, H. P. D. (1996). The profile of functional impairment in communication (PFIC): A measure of communication impairment for clinical use. *Brain Injury*, *10*, 397–412.

Lock, S., Wilkinson, R., Bryan, K., Maxim, J., Edmundson, A., & Bruce, C. et al. (2001). Supplement. Supporting partners of people with aphasia in relationships and conversation (SPPARC). *International Journal of Language and Communication Disorders*, *36*, 25–30.

Lubinski, R. (1991). Learned helplessness: Application to communication of the elderly. In R. Lubinski (Ed.), *Dementia and communication*. Philadelphia: B. C. Decker, Inc.

Lundgren, K., Helm-Estabrooks, N., Magnusdottir, S., & Emery, P. (1994). Exploring mechanisms underlying recurrent perseveration: An aphasic naming study. *Brain and Language*, *47*(3), 370–373.

Luria, A. R. (1980). *Higher cortical functions in man*. New York: Basic Books.

McNamara, P., & Albert, M. L. (2004). Neuropharmacology of verbal perseveration. *Seminars in Speech and Language*, *25*(4), 309–321.

McNeil, M. R., Small, S. L., Masterson, R. J., & Fossett, T. (1995). Behavioural and pharmacological treatment of lexical-semantic deficits in case of primary progressive aphasia. *American Journal of Speech Language Pathology*, *4*, 76–87.

Mentis, M., & Prutting, C. A. (1987). Cohesion in the discourse of normal and head-injured adults. *Journal of Speech And Hearing Research*, *30*, 88–98.

Milner, B. (1995). Aspects of human frontal lobe function. In H. H. Jasper, S. Riggio, & P. S. Goldman-Rakic (Eds.), *Epilepsy and the functional anatomy of the frontal lobe*. New York: Raven Press.

Milton, S., Prutting, C., & Binder, G. (1984). Appraisal of communicative competence in head injured adults. In R. Brookshire (Ed.), *Clinical Aphasiology Conference proceedings*. Minneapolis: BRK Publishers.

Molloy, R., Brownell, H. H., & Gardner, H. (1990). Discourse comprehension by right hemisphere stroke patients: Deficits of prediction and revision. In Y. Joanette & H. H. Brownwell (Eds.), *Discourse ability and brain damage*. New York: Springer-Verlag.

Moses, M., & Sheard, C. (2001). *When is a camel a candle? Towards an understanding of recurrent perseverative errors in aphasia*. British Aphasiology Society Biennial Conference, Exeter, UK.

Nelson, L. D., Drebing, C., Satz, P., & Uchiyama, C. (1998). Personality changes in head trauma: A validity study of the Neuropsychology Behavior and Affect Profile. *Archives of Clinical Neuropsychology*, *13*, 549–560.

Nelson, L. D., Satz, P., & D'elia, L. F. (1994). *Neuropsychology behavior and affect profile*. Palo Alto, CA: Mind Garden.

Newcombe, F. (1997). Frontal lobe disorders. In R. Greenwood, M. P. Barnes, T. M. McMillan, & C. D. Ward (Eds.), *Neurological rehabilitation*. Hove, UK: Psychology Press.

Paolo, A. M., Axelrod, B. N., & Troster, A. I. (1996). Test–retest stability of the Wisconsin Card Sorting Test. *Assessment*, *3*, 137–143.

Parloff, M. B. (1986). Placebo controls in psychotherapy research: A sine qua non or a placebo for research problems? *Journal of Consulting and Clinical Psychology*, *54*, 79–87.

Pashler, H. (1998). *Attention*. Hove, UK: Psychology Press.

Penn, C. (1999). Pragmatic assessment and therapy for persons with brain damage: What have clinicians gleaned in two decades? *Brain and Language*, *68*, 535–552.

Penn, C. (2000). Paying attention to conversation. *Brain and Language*, *71*(4), 185–189.

Perkins, L., Crisp, J., & Walshaw, D. (1999). Exploring conversation analysis as an assessment tool for aphasia: The issue of reliability. *Aphasiology*, *13*(4–5), 259–282.

Perkins, L., Whitworth, A., & Lesser, R. (1998). Conversing in dementia: A conversation analytic approach. *Journal of Neurolinguistics*, *11*, 33–53.

Ponsford, J., & Kinsella, G. (1992). Attentional deficits following closed head injury. *Journal of Clinical and Experimental Clinical Neuropsychology*, *14*, 822–838.

Prigatano, G. P. (1986). Personality and psychosocial consequences of brain injury. In G. P. Prigatano (Ed.), *Neuropsychological rehabilitation after brain injury*. Baltimore: The Johns Hopkins University Press.

Prigatano, G. P., & Fordyce, D. J. (1986). Cognitive dysfunction and psychosocial adjustments after brain injury. In G. P. Prigatano (Ed.), *Neuropsychological rehabilitation after brain injury*. Baltimore: The Johns Hopkins University Press.

Rao, V., & Lyketsos, C. (2000). Neuropsychiatric sequelae of traumatic brain injury. *Psychosomatics*, *41*, 95–103.

Raskin, S. A., Sliwinski, M., & Bond, J. C. (1992). Clustering strategies on tasks of verbal fluency in Parkinson's disease. *Nuropsychologia*, *30*(1), 95–99.

Sacks, H., Schegloff, E. A., & Jefferson, G. (1974). A simplest systematics for the organisation of turn-taking for a conversation. *Language*, *50*(4), 696–735.

Sandson, J., & Albert, M. L. (1984). Perseveration in behavioural neurology. *Neurology*, *37*, 1736–1741.

Schachar, R. J., Tannock, R., Marriott, M., & Logan, G. D. (1995). Deficient inhibitory control in attention deficit hyperactivity disorder. *Journal of Abnormal Child Psychology*, *23*, 411–438.

Schapiro, S. R., & Sacchetti, T. S. (1993) In S. Mandel, R. T. Sataloff, & S. R. Schapiro (Eds.), *Minor head trauma: Assessment, management and rehabilitation*. New York: Springer-Verlag.

Schegloff, E. A., Jefferson, G., & Sacks, H. (1977). The preference for self-correction in the organisation of repair in conversation. *Language*, *53*(2), 361–382.

Spencer, J. P., & Schutte, A. R. (2004). Unifying representations and responses: Perseverative biases arise from a single behavioural system. *Psychological Science*, *15*(3), 187.

Spreen, O., & Strauss, E. (1998). *A compendium of neuropsychological tests: Administration, norms and commentary (2nd ed.)*. New York: Oxford University Press.

Stuss, D. T., & Benson, D. F. (1986). Frontal lobe lesions and behavior. In A. Kertesz (Ed.), *Localization neuropsychology*. New York: Academic Press.

Stuss, D. T., Gow, C. A., & Hetherington, C. R. (1992). "No longer Gage": Frontal lobe dysfunction and emotional changes. *Journal of Consulting and Clinical Psychology*, *60*, 349–359.

Stuss, D. T., Kaplan, E. F., Benson, D. F., Weir, W. S., Chiulli, S., & Sarazin, F. F. (1982). Evidence for the involvement of orbitofrontal cortex in memory functions: An interference effect. *Journal of Comparative Physiological Psychology*, *96*, 913–925.

Ten Have, P. (1999). *Doing conversation analysis*. London: Sage Publications.

Ulatowska, H. K., Freedman-Stern, R., Doyel, A. W., Macaluso-Haynes, S., & North, A. J. (1983). Production of narrative discourse in aphasia. *Brain and Language*, *19*, 317–334.

Van Zomeran, A. H., & Brouwer, W. H. (1994). *Clinical neuropsychology of attention*. New York: Oxford University Press.

Walker-Batson, D. (1998). Pharmacotherapy in the treatment of aphasia. In L. B. Goldstein (Ed.), *Restorative neurology: Advances in pharmacotherapy for recovery after stroke*. New York: Futura Publishing.

Watt, N., & Penn, C. (2000). Predictors and indicators of return to work following traumatic brain injury in South Africa: Findings from a preliminary experimental database. *South African Journal of Psychology*, *30*(2), 27–37.

Wechsler, D. (1997). *Wechsler Memory Scale* (3rd ed.). San Antonio, TX: The Psychological Corporation.

Wilkinson, R. (1999). Sequentiality as a problem and resource for intersubjectivity in aphasic conversation: Analysis and implications for therapy. *Aphasiology*, *13*(4–5), 259–282.

Wyckoff, L. H., Jensen, P. J., & LaPointe, L. (1984). *Narrative and procedural discourse following closed head injury*. Technical Paper presented at ASHSA Convention: San Francisco, California.

Ylvisaker, M., & Szekeres, S. F. (1994). Communication disorders associated with closed head injury. In R. Chapey (Ed.), *Language intervention strategies in adult aphasia* (3rd ed.). Baltimore: Williams and Wilkins.

APPENDIX A

Composite Scales of Cognitive Ability for Traumatic Brain Injury (SCATBI) scores for AA

Composites	*Attention SS*	*Orientation SS*	*Organisation SS*	*Recall SS*	*Reason SS*	*Sum std score*	*PR*	*Std score*
Lower function	85	80	88	–	–	253	12	82
Higher function	–	–	–	77	93	170	14	84
SCATBI Total	85	80	88	77	93	423	12	82

SCATBI Severity = 6 (Severe disability).

APPENDIX B

Composite Scales of Cognitive Ability for Traumatic Brain Injury (SCATBI) scores for PB

Composites	*Attention SS*	*Orientation SS*	*Organisation SS*	*Recall SS*	*Reason SS*	*Sum std score*	*PR*	*Std score*
Lower function	95	91	98	–	–	284	27	91
Higher function	–	–	–	93	96	189	32	93
SCATBI Total	95	91	98	93	96	473	27	91

SCATBI Severity = 8 (Moderate disability)

APPENDIX C

TEST	*RATIONALE*	*DESCRIPTION*
The Stroop Colour Word Test (Golden, 1978)	Breakdown on this task signifies difficulty in warding off distractions	Participants read names of colours printed in black ink; then name colour names printed in corresponding ink. Finally they state the colour a word is printed in, when the printed word does not match the colour of the ink.
Echopraxia Tasks (Schachar, Tannock, Marriot, & Logan, 1995)	Sensitivity of the stop signal paradigms to the ability to inhibit or interrupt an ongoing response has been demonstrated.	Participants engage in a primary task and occasionally and unpredictably are presented with a signal that instructs them to withhold their motor response or produce a different one.
The Face Recognition Task (Wechsler, 1997)	This assesses the capacity to store and retrieve information during a delay period. Interference items are presented in this task, consistent with research testing working memory.	The participant is shown a series of faces and asked to remember each one. A new series is shown and the participant has to identify those that were previously seen.
The Self-Ordered Pointing Test (Petrides & Milner, 1982, cited in Spreen & Strauss, 1998)	This test has been shown to assess nonverbal working memory	The same set of stimulus items are arranged in varying layouts on different pages. Examinees are required to point to a different item on each page, the sole restriction being that they are not allowed to point to a stimulus already chosen.
Verbal Paired Associates (Wechsler, 1997)	This assesses the ability to hold, organise, and retrieve information over time delays.	The examinee is read a list of eight word pairs. The first word of each pair is read and the examinee is asked to provide the second word. This procedure is repeated another three times, with the words presented in a different order each time. For the delayed trial, the list is presented once in the same manner as presented previously. Then a recognition task is presented where a list of word pairs is read and the participant must indicate whether or not the items were presented previously.
Word Lists (Wechsler, 1997)	This assesses the ability to hold, organise, and retrieve information over time delays as well as measure learning capacity.	The participant is read a list of words and asked to recall them in any order. Delayed recall and recognition tasks are also administered.
The Neuropsychology Behaviour and Affect Profile (NBAP) (Nelson, Satz, & D'Elia, 1994)	This is an affect inventory, developed specifically for use with neurologically involved individuals, (Nelson, Drebing, Satz, & Uchiyama, 1998).	A caregiver reads the questionnaire and marks agree or disagree for each item.
Controlled Oral Word Association Test (COWA) (Benton & Hamsher, 1976)	Word fluency is a sensitive indicator of brain dysfunction and in particular of frontal lobe pathology.	In the Benton and Hamsher (1976) version of this test, norms for the letters CFL and PRW are provided. The participant must name as many words as possible in 1 minute, beginning with each of the letters provided.
Category Naming (Lezak, 1995)	It has been shown that individuals with mild, moderate, and severe head injuries show decreased ability to generate word lists in semantic categories.	The participant is given 1 minute to provide as many words as possible within a given semantic category (Lezak, 1995)

APPENDIX D

Results of Stroop Word Colour Test for AA in *t*-scores (construct: Interference control)

Test phase	*Baseline*	*Active phase*	*Placebo phase*	*Withdrawal*
Words	< 20	< 20	< 20	< 20
Colours	< 20	< 20	< 20	< 20
Colour-Word	< 20	< 20	20/22	< 20
Interference score	47	53*	46	46

* Average = *t*-score of 50

APPENDIX E

Results of Faces for AA with raw score (standard score) (construct: Nonverbal Working Memory)

	Baseline	*Active phase*	*Placebo phase*	*Withdrawal*
Immediate recall	34(8)	21(4)	26(5)	23(4)
Delayed recall	30(6)	25(4)	24(4)	24(4)

APPENDIX F

Results of Self Ordered Pointing Test for AA (construct: Nonverbal Working Memory)

	Baseline	*Active phase*	*Placebo phase*	*Withdrawal*
Total number of errors ($x = 15.2$; $SD = 6.22$)	55	67	55	65
Standard deviations below the mean	6	8	6	8

APPENDIX G

Results of Verbal Paired Associates for AA with raw scores (standard scores) (construct: Internalisation of speech)

	Baseline	*Active phase*	*Placebo phase*	*Withdrawal*
Immediate recall	1(2)	1(2)	1(2)	1(2)
Delayed recall	0(3)	0(3)	0(3)	0(3)

APPENDIX H

Results of Word Lists for AA with raw scores (standard scores) (construct: Internalisation of speech)

	Baseline	*Active phase*	*Placebo phase*	*Withdrawal*
Immediate recall	11(1)	9(1)	6(1)	6(1)
Delayed recall	0(5)	0(5)	0(5)	0(5)
Delayed recognition	9(1)	15(1)	14(1)	14(1)

APPENDIX I
Results of the Neuropsychological Behavior and Affect Profile (NBAP) for AA (construct: regulation of affect)

Scale	*Rater 1*	*Rater 2*	*Rater 3*	*Rater 4*
Baseline				
Indifference: X = 1.59 (2.48)	9*	9*	9*	7*
Inappropriateness: X = 2.60 (2.72)	3	3	1	0
Pragnosia: X = 2.06 (2.87)	7*	9*	6*	6*
Depression: X = 2.55 (3.05)	1	2	2	1
Mania: X = 5.36 (4.44)	4	1	2	2
Active phase				
Indifference: X = 1.59 (2.48)	9*	10*	6*	6*
Inappropriateness: X = 2.60 (2.72)	4	2	1	2
Pragnosia: X = 2.06 (2.87)	10*	8*	4	4
Depression: X = 2.55 (3.05)	1	2	1	0
Mania: X = 5.36 (4.44)	5	1	0	2
Placebo phase				
Indifference: X = 1.59 (2.48)	9*	10*	5*	2*
Inappropriateness: X = 2.60 (2.72)	3	4	2	1
Pragnosia: X = 2.06 (2.87)	7*	7*	6*	1
Depression: X = 2.55 (3.05)	1	2	1	0
Mania: X = 5.36 (4.44)	1	1	3	0
Withdrawal				
Indifference: X = 1.59 (2.48)	9*	11*	6*	1
Inappropriateness: X = 2.60 (2.72)	2	2	1	0
Pragnosia: X = 2.06 (2.87)	7*	9*	4	2
Depression: X = 2.55 (3.05)	1	2	1	0
Mania: X = 5.36 (4.44)	2	0	2	0

* Exceeds mean.

APPENDIX J
Results of Controlled Oral Word Association (COWA) for AA (construct: Reconstitution)

	Baseline	*Active phase*	*Placebo phase*	*Withdrawal*
Percentile rank	1	4	1	1
Rating	Seriously deficient	Deficient	Seriously deficient	Seriously deficient
Perseverative responses	61	15	68	56

APPENDIX K
Results of Category Naming for AA (construct: Reconstitution)

	Baseline	*Active phase*	*Placebo phase*	*Withdrawal*
Total number	11	22	16	22
Perseverative responses	50	11	60	56
X = 19.8 (4.2)				

APPENDIX L

Results of Stroop Word Colour Test for PB in T-scores (construct: Interference Control)

Test phase	*Baseline*	*Active phase*	*Placebo phase*	*Withdrawal*
Words	22/24	34	32/34	26/28
Colours	28/30	26	26/28	30
Colour-Word	32	36	40	42
Interference score	74/76	76/78	78	78

* Average = T-score of 50

APPENDIX M

Results of Echopraxia Tests for PB (construct: Response Inhibition)

	Baseline	*Active phase*	*Placebo phase*	*Withdrawal*
Total number of errors per minute	6	0	5	5

APPENDIX N

Results of Faces for PB with raw score (standard score) (construct: Nonverbal Working Memory)

	Baseline	*Active phase*	*Placebo phase*	*Withdrawal*
Immediate recall	32(8)	35(4)	34(8)	38(11)
Delayed recall	33(8)	33(8)	33(8)	34(9)

APPENDIX O

Results of Self-Ordered Pointing Test for PB (construct: Nonverbal Working Memory)

	Baseline	*Active phase*	*Placebo phase*	*Withdrawal*
Total number of errors (x = 21.67; *SD* = 5.58)	33	29	21	16

APPENDIX P

Results of Verbal Paired Associates for PB with raw scores (standard scores) (construct: Internalisation of speech)

	Baseline	*Active phase*	*Placebo phase*	*Withdrawal*
Immediate recall	4(5)	7(7)	12(9)	13(9)
Delayed recall	1(5)	1(5)	4(8)	5(9)

APPENDIX Q

Results of Word Lists for PB with raw scores (standard scores) (construct: Internalisation of Speech)

	Baseline	*Active phase*	*Placebo phase*	*Withdrawal*
Immediate recall	19(4)	24(6)	16(3)	15(2)
Delayed recall	0(5)	3(8)	0(5)	0(5)
Delayed recognition	15(3)	23(11)	15(3)	19(6)

APPENDIX R

Results of the Neuropsychological Behavior and Affect Profile (NBAP) for PB (construct: Regulation of Affect)

Scale	*Rater 1*	*Rater 2*	*Rater 3*	*Rater 4*
Baseline				
Indifference: X = 1.59 (2.48)	3	1	4	1
Inappropriateness: X = 2.60 (2.72)	1	0	0	1
Pragnosia: X = 2.06 (2.87)	6*	2	4	0
Depression: X = 2.55 (3.05)	2	1	1	0
Mania: X = 5.36 (4.44)	1	0	3	0
Active phase				
Indifference: X = 1.59 (2.48)	1	4	1	0
Inappropriateness: X = 2.60 (2.72)	0	1	0	2
Pragnosia: X = 2.06 (2.87)	1	5*	0	0
Depression: X = 2.55 (3.05)	2	2	1	2
Mania: X = 5.36 (4.44)	0	0	1	0
Placebo phase				
Indifference: X = 1.59 (2.48)	0	6*	0	2
Inappropriateness: X = 2.60 (2.72)	0	1	0	0
Pragnosia: X = 2.06 (2.87)	3	2	0	0
Depression: X = 2.55 (3.05)	1	2	0	0
Mania: X = 5.36 (4.44)	0	0	1	0
Withdrawal				
Indifference: X = 1.59 (2.48)	4	2	0	1
Inappropriateness: X = 2.60 (2.72)	0	1	0	0
Pragnosia: X = 2.06 (2.87)	2	1	0	0
Depression: X = 2.55 (3.05)	2	0	0	0
Mania: X = 5.36 (4.44)	0	0	0	1

* Exceeds mean.

APPENDIX S

Results of Controlled Oral Word Association (COWA) for PB (construct: Reconstitution)

	Baseline	*Active phase*	*Placebo phase*	*Withdrawal*
Percentile rank	9	43	34	10
Rating	Borderline	Average	Average	Borderline
Perseverative responses	33	18	29	29

APPENDIX T
Results of Category Naming for PB (construct: Reconstitution)

	Baseline	*Active phase*	*Placebo phase*	*Withdrawal*
Total number	10	12	15	8
Perseverative responses	9	8	12	27
X = 19.8 (4.2)				

APHASIOLOGY, 2007, 21 (10/11), 1079–1113

Psychology Press
Taylor & Francis Group

Verbal perseveration as the initial symptom in a case of Creutzfeldt-Jakob disease

Jacqueline Stark

Austrian Academy of Sciences, Vienna, Austria

Wolfgang Kristoferitsch and Martin Graf

Social Medical Center (SMZ)-East, Vienna, Austria

Ellen Gelpi and Herbert Budka

Medical University of Vienna, Austria

Background: In the literature on cortical degenerative processes and primary progressive aphasia, language disorders have been discussed as the initial sign of higher cortical dysfunction. Verbal perseveration has also been cited to precede the occurrence of other cortical signs. In this paper we present language data from an autopsy-confirmed case of Creutzfeldt-Jakob disease (CJD) who exhibited profound verbal perseveration as the initial symptom.

Aims: This case report aims to provide a description of the extent and pattern of verbal perseveration in a client with the rapidly progressing fatal CJD. Language test data and medical data, i.e., EEG and neuropathology—which confirm the diagnosis of CJD—are presented.

Methods & Procedures: Language testing was performed with our patient to determine the nature of the language disorder at a time when the diagnosis of CJD had not yet been made. The tape-recorded sessions were transcribed and the language data analysed.

Outcomes & Results: The pervasive perseverative behaviour mirrors the underlying language-processing difficulties and the magnitude of the progression of the disease process. Perseverative errors account for between 87% and 95% of the language-processing errors on the various language tasks. In general, the first items of each task were responded to correctly, indicating that our client was trying to meet the various test demands and at the time of testing was still able to process language, albeit in a very restricted manner.

Conclusions: The rapid deterioration of language functions in our case and in other reported cases necessitates acting quickly without delay. Immediate recognition and analysis of the language disturbance and verbal perseverative behaviour may provide relevant information for differentially diagnosing clients presenting with various cortical degenerative diseases at an early stage.

Address correspondence to: Jacqueline Stark PhD, Department of Linguistics and Communication Research, Austrian Academy of Sciences, Kegelgasse 27 3rd Floor, A-1030 Vienna, Austria. E-mail: jacqueline-ann.stark@univie.ac.at

The authors would like to thank Karin Geisler, Maura Bayer, and Caroline Brew for their critical reading of this paper, and the colleagues who provided the two reviews of this manuscript for their constructive comments and suggestions.

http://www.psypress.com/aphasiology DOI: 10.1080/02687030701198403

In the literature on cortical degenerative processes and primary progressive aphasia, language disturbance and/or isolated aphasia are cited as one of the initial symptoms (see Kirshner, Webb, Kelly, & Wells, 1984; Wechsler, 1977, etc.). Based on an autopsy-confirmed case report of a patient with isolated aphasia and Creutzfeldt-Jakob disease (CJD), Mandell, Alexander, and Carpenter (1989) extend the list of diseases with language disorders to include CJD (Hillis & Selnes, 1999; see also Cohen, Kutluay, Edwards, Peltier, & Beydoun, 2004). CJD disease is a rare and fatal neurodegenerative disease. The incidence for this disease is 0.5 to 1.0 cases per million per year. From the initial signs to death, the duration ranges from several weeks or months to a year. In the literature on CJD two main types are distinguished: sporadic and familial. In 10% to 15% of the CJD cases, a familial origin has been discerned. In contrast, in 85% to 90% of the cases a sporadic origin has been assumed. Descriptions of sporadic CJD cases refer to an onset age of between 50 and 70 years, although younger cases (26 years old) have been reported (see Cohen et al., 2004). Among its causes, the viral hypothesis and the prion theory (abnormal protein = prion) have been put forward. The clinical features include rapidly progressive dementia that begins focally, startle myoclonus, and rigidity, and a characteristic EEG pattern showing progressive periodic discharges may occur. Neuropathological examination reveals cortical spongiform change, hence the term “spongiform encephalopathy” (Gálvez, Dörr-Zegers, & Cartier, 1982; Matthews, 1985; Yamanouchi, Budka, & Vass, 1986), neuronal loss, and gliosis.

In a handbook article on CJD, Matthews (1985) addresses the neurological symptoms as follows: “The commonest clearly focal initial abnormality of higher cerebral function is dysphasia. This often occurs suddenly, with confusion of speech, or inability to understand the written word. Occasionally the initial speech disorder can be recognized as dysarthria” (p. 290). In a recent case report, Sowman, Robinson, O’Riordan, Connolly, and O’Neill (2006) document these and other features in a case of probable sporadic CJD presenting with rapidly deteriorating speech and language. Verbal perseveration[1] has also been cited as one of the first indicators of brain dysfunction in aphasia and in progressive brain disease. Even in the classical literature the relevance of the symptom of perseveration for early diagnosis of progressive degenerative diseases was noted. Heilbronner (1906) stresses that in progressive processes, perseverative responses should be anticipated as one of the first indicators of a focal lesion (p. 343) (cf. Stark, 2007 this issue). With regard to perseveration, Kleist (1934) states that, in certain cases, perseveration also precedes the occurrence of other cortical symptoms. Based on his clinical cases he discusses two developments of the symptoms—one with a favourable and the other with an unfavourable outcome. In the case of an unfavourable development, the initial minor perseveration increases in accordance with the exacerbation of the disease processes. Rosenberg (1912) discusses a patient demonstrating an unfavourable outcome, namely a patient who had suffered two mild strokes and who exhibited moderate dementia and apractic symptoms in which “... the perseveration, at first not so striking, comes to the fore of the symptoms with increasing severity of the dementia, so that finally, due to massive perseveration, an adequate response is hardly possible” (p. 123).

[1] Perseveration is defined as the unintentional production of a previously spoken, heard, written, or read linguistic form/language unit or action unit.

In more recent group studies on perseveration in patients exhibiting various types of degenerative diseases affecting language and cognitive functions, perseverative responses have been classified and their patterns of performance compared to those of people with aphasia and elderly controls. In these studies, the frequency of occurrence of perseverative responses in selected language and cognitive tasks, the differential diagnostic power of the various types of perseveration in differentiating among dementia types, and the possible underlying mechanisms have been investigated (see, for example, Bayles, Tomoeda, Kasniak, Stern, & Eagans, 1985; Nagahama, Okina, Nabatome, & Matsuda, 2006; Possin et al., 2005; Shindler, Caplan, & Hier, 1984). The results from these group studies with mixed clinical populations are not conclusive and they diverge in terms of correlations with types of dementia, neuroanatomical data, and degree of severity of the dementing illness.

In an analysis of perseverations and intrusions produced by dementia patients of varying aetiology, Shindler et al. (1984) discuss the rate of occurrence and genesis of the two response types based on data from a battery of language and cognitive tasks. Perseverative responses are defined as the immediate inappropriate repetition of a prior response, whereas intrusion errors are the inappropriate repetition of prior responses after intervening responses(= [recurrent] perseverative responses). Intrusions did not correlate with dementia severity. With regard to perseverative responses, the correlation between dementia severity and number of perseverations was not statistically significant. Since low correlations between intrusions and perseverations were found, Shindler et al. (1984) assume separate neuropsychological mechanisms for the two response types. They consider perseveration to be the result of a two-stage event: "… [1] the subject fails to change mental set or to recognize that a new stimulus has been presented and then [2] fails to suppress the incorrect perseverative response". In contrast, in accounting for intrusion errors they assume a four-stage process: [1] "… the subject presumably initiates an unsuccessful search through long term memory for the correct word or phrase, [2] he then selects from short-term memory a recently heard word or phrase, and then [3] after failing to inhibit the incorrect word or phrase [4] the incorrect word is emitted" (p. 156).

In another study using a verbal descriptive discourse task, Bayles et al (1985) confirm Rosenberg's (1912) aforementioned case study description regarding perseveration. They found an increase in perseveration to be associated with the progression of the severity of dementia. When severity was controlled for, dementia patients of different aetiologies did not differ significantly in their rates. Bayles et al. assert that the severity of the dementing illness is "… a more potent determinant of perseveration than etiology" (p. 113). These two group studies (Bayles et al., 1985; Shindler et al., 1984) demonstrate the importance of quantitative and qualitative analysis of perseverative responses. However, single cases presenting with an interesting pattern of perseverative responses allow an in-depth analysis of perseverative responses within the context of a subject's overall language-processing abilities and deficits.

In this paper we report on an autopsy-confirmed case of sporadic CJD in a 56-year-old female, AP, who revealed the initial symptom of verbal perseveration in the context of impaired language processing in various tasks—both production and comprehension. The initial symptoms progressed so rapidly that extensive language testing was not possible. AP died of pneumonia within 2 months after the first language symptoms were observed. We discuss AP's language performance and the impact of perseveration on her overall language performance in terms of language functions. Sowman et al. (2006) highlight the importance of detailed descriptions of language functions to enable differential diagnosis of the language disorders observed in patients presenting with cortical degenerative diseases. Hillis and Selnes (1999) also stress the need for clinicians "... to be aware of the diverse aetiologies of aphasia, neglect, and other 'focal' cognitive deficits". Moreover, they maintain that the implication of comprehensive case descriptions is that "... the rapid decline within one or more domains of cognition may raise the suspicion of CJD and permit early diagnosis" (Hillis & Selnes, 1999, p. 753).

When first contacted to assess AP's language functions, it was not at all foreseeable that she was suffering from CJD and that her condition would deteriorate so rapidly. On the contrary, it was thought that her condition would stabilise and that she would receive neuro-rehabilitation as soon as a diagnosis based on extensive language testing had been made. With hindsight, the lesson from this and other cases discussed in the literature is that when striking or specific symptoms are evident, no time should be lost before performing a comprehensive language evaluation. After recognising the initial symptoms, responding very quickly with an extensive battery of language and neuropsychological tests, and performing follow-up tests at small intervals, would provide valuable information on how the language system progressively breaks down; i.e., on the process of language deterioration in probable CJD. Thus, extensive case reports would provide relevant data for a better understanding of the mechanisms of disease. In the case of CJD, early differential diagnosis would make the decision-making process easier, in that comprehensive evaluation and not rehabilitation would be recommendable.

Bearing in mind the importance of characterising language impairments in degenerative diseases, this case report is relevant for at least two reasons. It provides:

1. A description of a further case of autopsy-confirmed CJD presenting with the initial symptom of language impairment and, in particular, verbal perseveration.
2. An analysis of the complex phenomenon of verbal perseveration, which in this case was the first symptom of brain dysfunction from the outset and remained the predominant symptom.

PATIENT DATA SUMMARY

AP, a 56-year-old single female with 9 years of schooling, lived and worked on her sister's farm in the country not far from Vienna, Austria. Her relatives stated that she was healthy prior to the onset of a rapidly progressive language impairment, the most striking symptom of which was verbal perseveration. Her main hobby was playing the church organ for Masses and weddings. Relatives reported that she was very active in her free time and that other hobbies included knitting and crocheting.

AP was transferred to a neurological unit in a Viennese hospital from a general hospital near Vienna due to her "abnormal" language. Upon admittance to the unit, her niece was present to provide the neurologist with relevant information regarding AP's illness. Friends and relatives had noticed sudden changes in her behaviour, mainly with regard to her language production—"she spoke in a strange manner"—and the way she carried out her job of harvesting crops. AP had complained of a severe headache; however, a few weeks elapsed before she was admitted to the hospital. On admission to the hospital, neurological examination revealed the following: In addition to her verbal perseveration she presented with a slight right-sided drooling. No other neurological signs were present. All laboratory tests including virology and serology tests were negative, i.e., within the normal range. Results from a duplex scan of the carotid arteries, a cranial CT scan, and MRI, as well as analysis of her cerebrospinal fluid (CSF), were without pathological findings. However, an EEG revealed a focal left frontotemporal constant activity of delta waves in the form of a rhythmic pattern of steep waves and peaks in second intervals. A PAO–SPECT examination with radioactive technetium also revealed a reduced left frontotemporal tracer activity. (This test result was obtained on the same day that the third language session was carried out.) Based on the changes in the EEG and the scintigraphy examinations in the context of normal CT, MRI, and cerebrospinal fluid results, AP was suspected of having CJD.

The further course of the disease showed a rapid progression. Two weeks after admission, AP developed a right hemiparesis and pronounced frontal signs. After another 2 weeks, AP lapsed into an akinetic mutistic state and had to be fed artificially. Two months after the first symptoms were observed, AP died of pneumonia.

LANGUAGE ASSESSMENT

Beginning 2 days after AP's admission to the neurology unit, four sessions of language testing were carried out on October 17th (first), 18th (second), 26th (third), and the 29th (fourth).[2] Language data from the first three test sessions are considered in this case report. It should be stressed that when the language testing was carried out, the examiner had no idea that AP was suffering from probable CJD. For this reason, a week's interval between the second and third session was not thought to be crucial. However, on October 29th language testing was discontinued due to her poor overall condition: Eye contact was only possible after she was called by name two to three times. On this occasion she was very echolalic or she turned away from the examiner. It was also noted that AP held on tightly to the armchair on which she was sitting for the test session and suddenly for no overt reason she tried to stand up in a quick movement.

Due to the rapid progression of the disease, only the following language tests were carried out:

All subtests of the *Aachener Aphasia Test* (AAT) (Huber, Poeck, Weniger, & Willmes, 1983) were administered in the first and second test sessions on two consecutive days:[3]

- Interview (first and second test sessions; conversation in the third and fourth test sessions).
- Token Test (second test session).
- Repetition (phonemes, words, sentences) (first test session).

[2] AP was tested by a psychologist 2 days after the third language testing session. The results from this session were briefly summarised by the psychologist as follows: AP received a score of 7 on the Mini Mental State Exam. She was disoriented for time and location. (For the language interview (first test session) she was able to supply her address and town.) Her short-term memory was mildly to moderately impaired. However, her long term memory (recall) and retrieval of information was more severely affected. Her visual-motor coordination was not impaired. She could name a few common everyday objects. On a functional psychosis scale she showed a mild clouding of consciousness and she revealed marked frontal signs.

[3] In the hospital where AP was a patient, speech therapists from the Speech Clinic also performed the AAT with AP two days after we tested her. Very similar scores were obtained on all the subtests.

- Written Language: reading aloud, word and sentence assembly (first test session), writing to dictation (second test session).
- Naming of visually presented drawings of objects and activities (targets: simple nouns, colours, compound nouns and sentences) (second test session).
- Comprehension (auditory/written) (second test session).

Other language tasks that were carried out (i.e., attempted) included:

- Picture description (Cookie Theft from the *Boston Diagnostic Aphasia Exam* (Goodglass & Kaplan, 1983) (third test session).
- Object confrontation naming (first 20 items of the *Boston Naming Test* (Kaplan, Goodglass, & Weintraub, 1983) (third test session).
- Word repetition (third test session).
- Fluency: animals (first test session).
- Automatised sequences: days of the week, months, and numbers (one to ten) (third test session).

All the language tasks were tape recorded and the recordings were transcribed. The last test session was also videotaped. All analyses are based on the transcriptions.

RESULTS FROM MEDICAL EXAMINATION

Electroencephalogram

In the first electroencephalogram (EEG) there was marked regional slowing over left frontal (F3) to temporal (T3) and central (C3) areas with triphasic waves in a quasiperiodic manner, most prominent over left frontal areas. Over the right hemisphere there was moderate diffuse slowing (Figure 1).

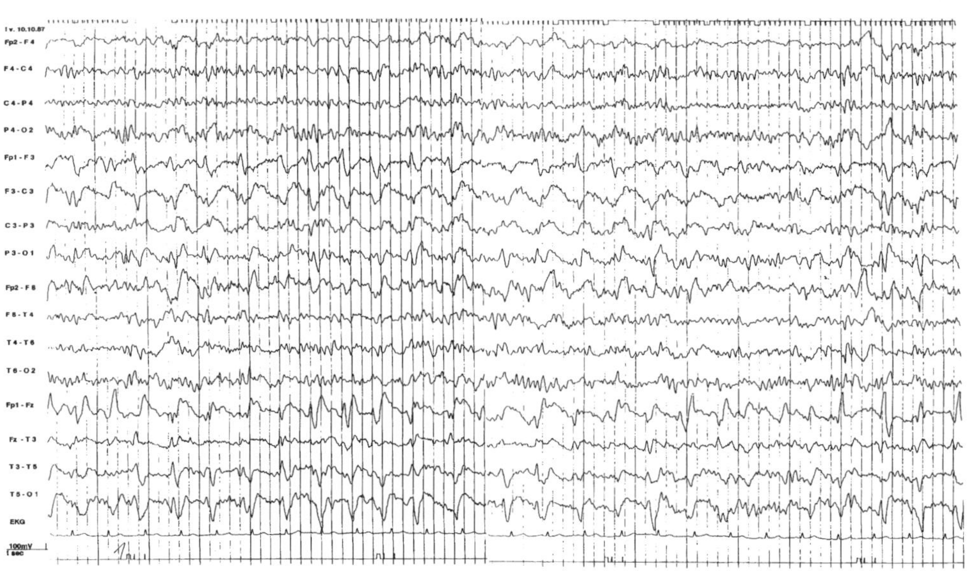

Figure 1. First electroencephalogram.

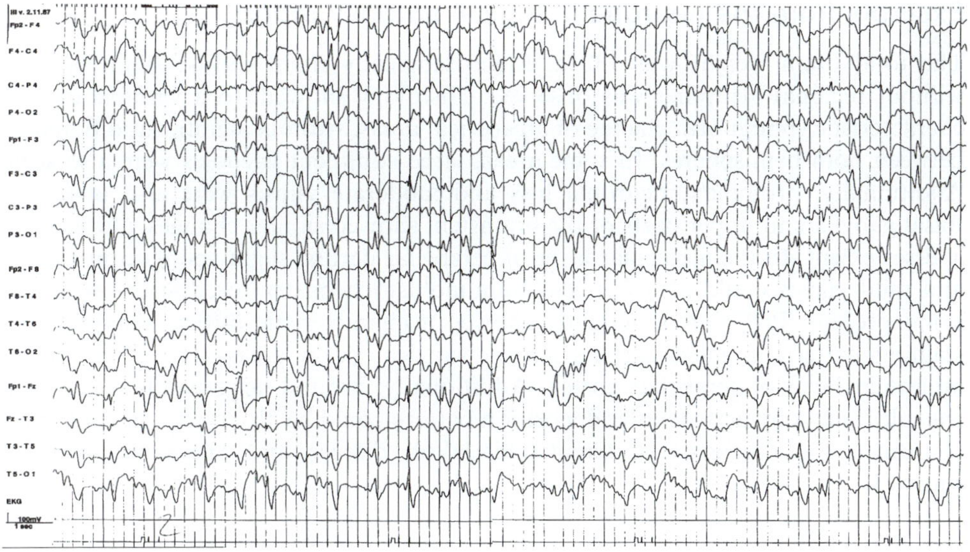

Figure 2. Second electroencephalogram, 3 weeks later.

After 3 weeks, the EEG showed marked diffuse slowing over both hemispheres and triphasic sharp components over the left hemisphere with a left mid-temporal (T3) maximum. There were brief stretches of diffuse suppression (Figure 2).

PAO-SPECT with technetium

A PAO-SPECT examination performed with technetium revealed a reduced tracer distribution in the left frontotemporal region (Figure 3).

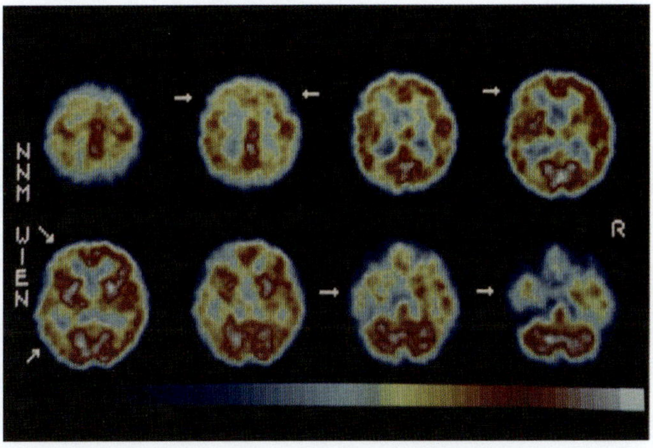

Figure 3. PAO-SPECT examination.

Excerpts from the neuropathological autopsy report

The total brain weight was 1325g. Macroscopically slight diffuse brain oedema without regional atrophies was observed. Histology showed, to a variable degree, characteristic spongiform change of all cortical areas, without significant differences between both hemispheres. In some areas, large confluent vacuoles were also seen. Additionally, prominent neuronal loss and moderate gliosis were also observed. Basal ganglia and upper parts of the brainstem showed similar changes, although to a lesser extent. In the molecular layer of cerebellar cortex, slight spongiform change and mild gliosis could also be seen. Immunohistochemistry for disease-associated prion protein (PrP^d) predominantly showed a characteristic diffuse synaptic type staining pattern in most cortical and subcortical brain areas, as well as in the molecular layer of cerebellar cortex. Additionally, around large confluent cortical vacuoles, a patchy perivacuolar deposition pattern could be observed. These findings confirmed the diagnosis of Creutzfeldt-Jakob disease and are summarised in Figure 4.

Language test data

At the first and second testing, AP's spontaneous speech was fluent, echolalic, and perseverative. She had word-finding difficulties and her overall spoken language production conveyed little information—apart from that in the perseverated utterances. She gave the impression of understanding the questions asked by the examiner. AP's verbal production revealed numerous break-offs with ensuing new starts. Her articulation became slightly dysarthric over the 2 weeks in which she was tested. All symptoms increased in intensity during the test period (test one to test

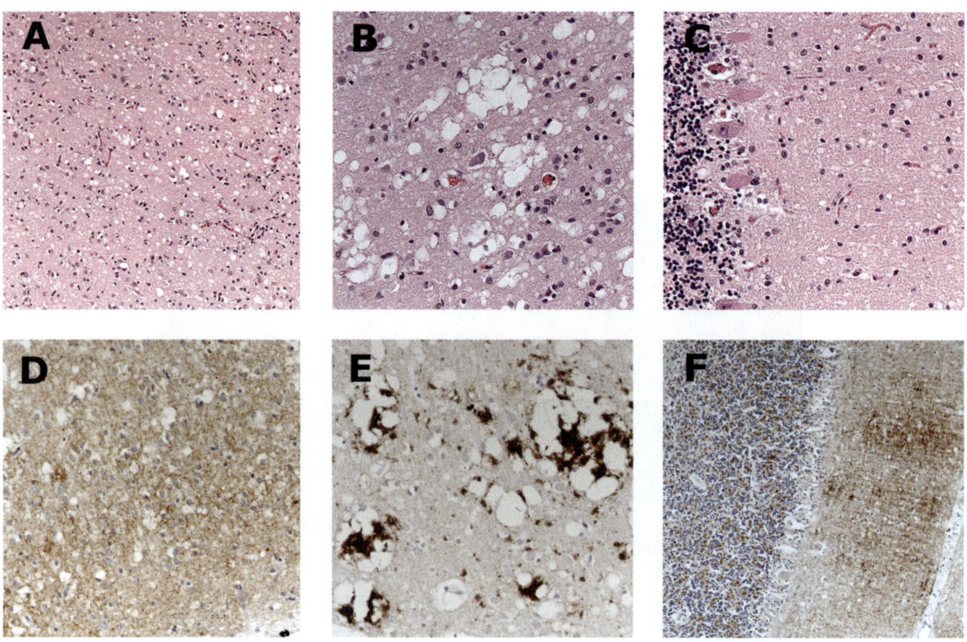

Figure 4. Selected microscopic findings.

TABLE 1
Results from the AAT repetition subtests

Subtest: Repetition *Repetition of:*	*Items correct*	*Raw score*	*Perseverative errors*
Phonemes	5/10§	23/30	2
One-syllable nouns	8/10	24/30	2
Foreign/Borrowed nouns	7/10	25/30	4
Compounds/Derived nouns	4/10*	15/30	5
Sentences	3/10	9/30	7
Total Repetition	27/50	96/150	20/23 (87%)

§ Three phonemes were not clearly articulated.
* For one stimulus item 50% was correctly repeated and 50% was deleted.

three). At times of persistent perseveration her speech tempo slowed down, and her intonation changed and became monotonous. Drawing a strict distinction among the symptoms echolalia, perseveration, and palilalia is at times difficult.[4] Although several authors surveyed by Lebrun (1993) stress that the speed of language production in palilalia usually increases with each repetition, Lebrun remarks that speech tempo can increase or slow down. With regard to AP, her spontaneous speech production is not considered to be palilalic.[5] With regard to AP, she did repeat phrases and sentences while responding to various task stimuli; however, it appears that the whole process became laboured for her in these passages and thus her speed of language production slowed down (cf. the description of her accompanying performance while carrying out the writing to dictation task). The phonemic structure of the produced responses was intact. The syntactic structure of her produced utterances was relatively intact until perseveration was observed.

The results for the various subtests of the AAT are given in Table 1 for repetition, Table 2 for the written language subtests, Table 3 for naming, and Table 4 for language comprehension.

Based on the AAT results, AP was diagnosed by the computer program for the AAT (Alloc Classification) as presenting with Wernicke''s aphasia. The overall results of the AAT and the profile for the subtests are given in Figure 6 and Figure 7 in Appendix A.

[4] Moen's (1993) definitions of echolalia and palilalia are cited here for the reader unfamiliar with the distinctions: "*Echolalia*: "the automatic and compulsive repetition of words by the patient in the absence of the understanding of their meaning" *Brain*, 1965, p. 105); "a reflex automatism of verbal response, providing an empty, stereotyped quality to speech" (Hecaen & Albert, 1978, pp. 74/75); "repetition of the investigator''s utterances with or without mild changes in position and choice of words" (Huber, Poeck, & Weniger, 1982, p. 80)."

Palilalia: "the involuntary repetition two or more times of a terminal word, phrase or sentence" (Critchley, 1970, p. 201); "a disorder of speech characterized by compulsive repetition of a phrase or word that the patient reiterates with increasing rapidity and with descrescendo of voice volume" (Boller, Boller, Denes, Timberlake, Zieper, & Albert, 1973, p. 1117)." These definitions are quoted from Moen (1993, p. 2). Critchley (1927–1928) describes the term palilalia as "… a variety of reiteration, whereby the patient repeats many times a word, phrase or sentence which he has just spoken. In addition the speech tends to be uttered more and more quickly and with less distinctness" (p. 23). Seven cases presenting with palilalia are discussed in his report.

[5] Wallesch (1990) provides a comprehensive discussion of verbal repetitive behaviour including the phenomena: echolalia, palilalia, and perseveration.

TABLE 2
Results from the AAT written language subtests

Subtest: Written Language *Task:*	*Items correct*	*Raw score*	*Perseverative errors*
Reading aloud*	8/10	28/30	1
Word composition of dictated stimuli#	5/10	19/30	2
Word and sentence dictation	3/10	15/30	7
Total	16/30	62/90	10/14 (71%)

* One foreign word is not accurately read aloud and one third of another item is deleted.
\# See text for a description of AP's perseverative behaviour while performing this task.

TABLE 3
Results from the AAT naming subtests

Subtest: Naming *Naming of:*	*Items correct*	*Raw score*	*Perseverative errors*
Objects (simple nouns)	5/10	17/30	5
Colours*	4/10	18/30	5
Objects (compound nouns)	0/10	0/30	10
Situations in sentence form	0/10	2/30	10
Total Naming	9/40	37/120	30/31 (97%)

*One error consists of a blend of two related colours: "vila".

TABLE 4
Results from the AAT language comprehension subtests

Subtest: Language Comprehension *Auditory presentation:*	*Items correct*	*Raw score*	*Perseverative errors*
Word-level	4/10	12/30	6
Sentence-level	1/10	3/30	9
Written presentation:			
Word-level	3/10	10/30	7
Sentence-level	0/10	0/30	10
Total Comprehension	8/40	25/120	31/32 (97%)

Spontaneous speech

Spontaneous speech excerpts from the interview (translated from German by the author) document AP's pattern of perseveration:

> Ex.: What do you do in your leisure time? (Ger.: "Was machen Sie in Ihrer Freizeit?")
> AP: Yes, in the leisure time, perhaps in the leisure time, what I do in the leisure time perhaps leisure time, what I do then. I do not know exactly what I do then (Ger.: "Ja, in der Freizeit vielleicht in der Freizeit, was ich in der Freizeit mache. Vielleicht Freizeit, was ich da mache. Da weiß ich eigentlich nicht, was ich da mache ↗"[6])

[6] The symbol ↗ denotes that AP ends the phrase with a rising intonation.

Ex.: Do you like to watch TV? (Ger.: "Sehen Sie gern Fernsehen?")
AP: Yes certainly I gladly TV or something like that what I do then (Ger.: "Ja, sicher gern Fernsehen oder so was, was ich da mache.")
Ex.: What do you like to watch on television? (Ger.: "Was schauen Sie gern an? – Im Fernsehen?")
AP: Perhaps television or something like that perhaps, that I like to do that (Ger.: "Vielleicht Fernsehen oder so was vielleicht, dass ich das gern mache↗")
Ex.: And which programmes do you like to watch? (Ger.: "Und welche Programme schauen Sie gern an?")
AP: That I do not know what I like to do (Ger.: "Das weiß ich nicht, was ich da gerne mache.")
Ex.: Do you watch the news? (Ger.: "Schauen Sie die Nachrichten an?")
AP: Perhaps that yes perhaps that I like to do that in the leisure time (Ger.: "Vielleicht das schon. Vielleicht, dass ich das gern mache- in der Freizeit")
Ex. Do you like to knit? (Ger.: "Tun Sie gern stricken?")
AP: Yes, perhaps like to// leisure time, that I like to do leisure time (Ger.: "Ja, vielleicht gern- Freizeit, dass ich das gern Freizeit mache.")
Ex.: And what else do you do? (Ger.: "Und was machen Sie so . sonst?")
AP: In the leisure time that is perhaps like to do leisure time (Ger.: "In der Freizeit das ist vielleicht gern Freizeit mache.")
Ex.: Do you have a hobby? (Ger.: "Haben Sie ein Hobby?")
AP: A hobby? Oh well that I actually have no leisure time I cannot hm hm yes hm (Ger.: "Ein Hobby↗. Na ja, das habe ich eigentlich – keine Freizeit. Das kann ich nicht hm. hm.. ja.. hm. hm.")

Further excerpts of conversational speech are given in Appendix B.

AP's spontaneous speech gave the impression of "temporary barrel-organisms" (term coined by W. T. Gairdner) which were played over and over again barrel-organ-like until something new was perseverated, i.e., played on the barrel organ (see Buckingham, 1985; Hughlings Jackson, 1880; Wallesch, 1990). This process continued until the same phrases were continually repeated and the discourse was broken off. This behaviour was also observed in the various subtests. In particular, AP's utterances in the sentence-naming task of the AAT predominantly consisted of perseverated utterances.

Another brief conversation before the second testing session began was communicatively adequate. In response to how she was doing on that day, AP responded as follows:

AP: Oh well, I am doing rather well. Yes. (Ger.: "Na ja, es geht ganz gut. Ja")
Ex.: What do you think about the weather? (Ger.: "Was sagen Sie zum Wetter?") [note: It had rained that morning.]
AP: Oh well, the weather is// it-it has rained a little bit. That should be finished – the the rainy weather [and then AP laughs].uh hm. (Ger.: "Na ja, das Wetter ist// es es hat ein bisserl geregnet. Das soll wieder fertig werden das – das Regenwetter . uh hm")

During a break between subtests before AP was asked to read aloud words and sentences, the examiner asked AP whether she had reading glasses. (Note: We were told that she did not have eyeglasses.) This conversation took place after she had repeated sentences:

Ex.: Do you need eyeglasses to read? (Ger.: "Brauchen Sie eine Brille zu lesen?")

AP: Yes, I need eyeglasses to peel. Yes, I need// (Ger.: "Ja, ich brauche eine Brille abzuschälen. Ja, ich brauch//")
Ex.: Do you have your eyeglasses here in the hospital? (Ger.: "Haben Sie Ihre Brille hier im Spital?")
AP: Yes, I have a [pair of] eyeglasses [in order] to peel – to darken (Ger.: "Ja, ich habe eine Brille abzuschälen – abzuhellen")
Ex.: Where are your eyeglasses? (Ger.: "Wo ist Ihre Brille?")
AP: Oh well, I have eyeglasses - I do not have them to off// I have the eyeglasses to abzuhellen [nonword: Ger.: "auf-hellen"; Engl.: "to lighten"; ab- = from, thus the possible translation "to darken"] (Ger.: "Na ja, ich habe eine Brille - die habe ich nicht ab- [separable verb particle] // ich habe die Brille abzuhellen")
Ex.: Where are your eyeglasses? (Ger.: "Wo ist Ihre Brille?")
AP: Yes, the eyeglasses, I have them in ~ // I have the eyeglasses . I have them to pick up (Ger.: "Ja, die Brille, die habe ich in der ~ // ich habe die Brille, die habe ich abzuholen")

In this exchange, the perseverations from the sentence repetition subtest of the AAT are clearly evident. There is no direct source for the production of "abzuschälen", which is a real word, and "abzuhellen", which is a potential German word based on its structure—in analogy with the German word "aufhellen" (Engl.: "to lighten" or "to illuminate")—and could be translated as "to darken". However, the next production "abzuholen" (Ger.: "to pick up") is a clear case of perseveration and the two previously produced "verbs" can be assumed to derive from the blending of several verbs either in the stimulus sentences presented to AP to be repeated, or else they stem from AP's previous utterances and perseverative responses, e.g., the "sch-" from "ab*sch*neiden" (Ger.: "to cut off") or the "-hellen" from the incorrectly produced "abzust*ellen*" (Engl.: "to stop" or "to shut down", etc.).

A week following the initial interview and the above-mentioned conversational passages, a brief conversation at the beginning of the third testing session illustrates the echolalic nature of her spontaneous speech. AP was asked how she was doing and whether she had already had her breakfast, etc.:

Ex.: How are you doing today? Are you feeling better? (Ger.: "Wie geht's Ihnen heute? Geht's Ihnen besser?")
AP: Oh well, everything is all right. (Ger.: "Na ja, es geht ganz gut") (She appears to be subdued.)
Ex.: Did you already have breakfast? (Ger.: "Haben Sie schon gefrühstückt?")
AP: Yes, everything is OK. Yes! Yes! Yes! Yes! (Ger.: Ja, es geht ganz gut. Ja! Ja! Ja! Ja!)
Ex.: Did you have breakfast? (Ger.: "Haben Sie gefrühstückt?")
AP: Yes, there was~// Did you already have [Have you already had] breakfast? (Ger.: "Ja, hats~// Haben Sie schon gefrühstückt?") (AP nods yes.)
Ex.: And what did you eat? (Question asked twice) (Ger.: Und was haben Sie gegessen?)
AP: Well, Did you have [Have you had] breakfast? (Ger.: Na, Haben Sie gegefrühstückt?)

AP continued to perseverate the phrase: "did you have breakfast?" and then only the words "had breakfast" followed by "Please" (Ger.: "Bitte") and then after a few repetitions, she only produced "Yes! Yes! Yes! ..."

Language repetition

Examples of perseveration in the language repetition subtests

In the repetition subtests AP perseverated phonemes and whole words or she produced blends consisting of two perseverated items. The following examples[7] of perseveration were produced by AP:

Item 1. Ast (Engl.: "branch") ⇒ +
Item 2. Floh (Engl.: "flea") ⇒ +
Item 3. Mund (Engl.: "mouth") ⇒ +
Item 4. Glas (Engl.: "glass") ⇒ ***Ast***
Item 4. (item repeated) Glas ⇒ Gl**as*t***
....
Item 8. Knirps (Engl.: "little one" or name and also brand name of a foldable tote umbrella) ⇒ +
Item 9. Zwist (Engl.: "dispute") ⇒ ***Knir***st, ***K***wist, ***Kwist***

The blend perseverations usually result in nonwords, but they adhere to the phonotactic rules of German.

The repetition of foreign or loan words resulted in the following perseverative responses:

1. Kur (Engl.: "spa cure") ⇒ +
2. Kanu (Engl.: "canoe") ⇒ +
3. Püree (Engl.: "purée", "mashed potatoes") ⇒ ***K***üree, then self-correction +
4. Pilot (Engl.: "pilot") ⇒ *Pilo* (2x), then + (intonation and syllable structure of previous item is perseverated: cv-cvc ⇒ cv-cv)
5. Stern (Engl.: "star") ⇒ +
6. Fürst (Engl.: "prince") ⇒ +
7. Spruch (Engl.: "slogan") ⇒ +
8. Moderator (Engl.: "moderator") ⇒ +
9. Hepatitis (Engl.: "hepatitis") ⇒ **H*oterator***
9. second attempt: Hepatitis ⇒ H***o**taritis*, H***e**taritis*, ***Hetaritis***
10. Liliputaner (Engl.: "lilliputian", "midget") ⇒ +

Repetition of stimulus item: 4. Pilot ⇒ **P*itis***, +

For the subtest repetition of compound items, AP produced numerous perseverations, which are given in Appendix B.

Apart from phonemes, other language units were also perseverated in the word repetition subtests: syllables, morphemes, and word intonation patterns. The more complex stimuli resulted in jargon responses. For item 7, the examiner only repeated the derivational suffix morpheme: "-keit"; however, AP repeated the whole stimulus

[7] Those parts of the target that are perseverated are written in italics and in the case of single phonemes and parts of words, they are also in bold print. In the text examples the symbol "~" is used for an unrecognisable sound and the symbol "⇒" is used for "is produced as". The arrow is also used to denote the beginning of an additional response by AP to a single item. A correct response is marked by "+". The notation "-" is used for a brief interruption and a continuation, and "//" denotes a break-off with a new start ("//"). Squared brackets "[..]" are used for reconstruction of possible omitted words or comments to the transcript or text.

correctly. This indicates that she auditorily processed or "held on to" the first morphemes, and thus was able to repeat the whole word correctly.

As of the fourth item of the subtest, repetition of sentences of increasing length, AP's attempts to repeat items from the sentence repetition subtest resulted in predominantly semantic jargon due to perseveration. Phonemic paraphasias and phonemic jargon were also produced to a lesser extent. For the items 6 to 10, parts of several stimuli are entangled and perseverated.

Due to the length of the passages, AP's responses for the sentence repetition task (AAT) are given in Appendix B. For the first presentation and also for the second presentation of items 5 to 10, analysis of the perseveratory errors for the sentence repetition task reveals several systematic errors, for example:

(a) Although such errors are less frequent in occurrence, phonological errors affecting a single phoneme are self-corrected.
(b) Perseveratory responses consisting of parts of several stimulus items that are semantically inadequate are not corrected.
(c) Particular phrases are perseverated over and over again, although slight variations consisting of morphosyntactic errors appear to be unnoticed and/or are not self-corrected, e.g., "kein" Geld ⇒ keine and keinen Geld.
(d) Certain syntactic formations affecting the verb infinitive, which result in incorrect utterances, are perseverated and are also not corrected, e.g.: "abzuschneiden", "abzustellen", and "abzuholen".

Written language

Examples of perseveration in the reading aloud task

The first four items as well as the fifth item were read correctly. For the fifth item, AP produced the following response:

> 5. Eitelkeit (Engl: "vanity") ⇒ + "Eitelkeit schade dass ich nicht dich ab- abholen" (Engl.: "Vanity sorry that I do not pick you up – up")

That is, after she correctly read the stimulus word "Eitelkeit", AP spontaneously continued with part of a sentence she had not correctly repeated in the previous subtest. The word "abholen" (Engl.: "to pick up") (verb) could possibly have been perseverated from two former stimuli from the sentence repetition items 4 or 8:

> 4. Wir werden von ihm abgeholt (Engl.: "We will be picked up by him")
> 8. Er holte seine Mutter mit einem neuen Auto vom Bahnhof ab (Engl.: "He picked up his mother in a new car from the train station")

In the second task, assessing written language, AP was able to match the plastic letters and words to the correct positions on the test sheets and also to assemble the first four words out of the correct letters. While trying to compose words or sentences from the plastic letters, she repeated the target words and perseverated parts of words (syllables and morphemes) over and over again. As of the seventh item ("KAMEL-HAAR-MANTEL") (Engl.: "CAMEL-HAIR-COAT"), AP orally produced, i.e., blended, parts of the compound: "Kamel - Haar- Kar - Kar - Mantel -

Haar- Kar-Karmantelhaar - Karmantelhaar" ... Karmar - Karmar - Karmar mantel haar". The eighth item was repeated correctly and produced several times; however, she composed the sentence in the opposite order on the work space in front of her: "ER HAT SEIN BUCH" ⇒ "BUCH SEIN HAT ER". When asked if she had positioned the words in the correct order, she responded in the affirmative. After correctly assembling the ninth item, she failed at the last item. Her accompanying oral productions consisted of the correct question to be composed and perseverations consisting of variations of that question.

Examples of perseveration in the writing to dictation subtest

The two pages of the test booklet used for writing down the patient's responses are reproduced in Figures 5a and 5b.

In the writing to dictation subtest, the degree of perseveration increased with the complexity of the item to be written down. Before dictating the test items, the examiner asked AP to write down her name, which she did correctly.[8] After writing down the first item correctly, she wrote her name a second time without being asked to do so. In general, while attempting to write down each dictated item, AP continually spoke each stimulus item out loud. For the first item she repeated the stimulus word 7 times, and the number of repetitions of parts of the stimulus word or the entire word or phrase increased to 67 productions.

For the fourth item "Künstler" (Engl.: "artist"), she perseverated the whole previous word ("Schlucht") and repeated the correct target item out loud five times. Then she wrote down the word "Schlucht". Based on her behaviour, AP was apparently unaware of the discrepancy between the presented stimulus word and the word she wrote down. For the fifth item, "Montage" (Engl.: "installation", "montage", "assembly"), she began writing down the target word and managed to write down the first syllable correctly, but then she perseverated two letters from the last perseverated word (i.e., "Schlucht") and other errors were made, consisting of perseveration of single letters of the target word and the previously perseverated word. The sixth item was written correctly (i.e., "Heiterkeit", Engl.: "cheeriness"). The first five letters of the seventh item target—a compound with three morphemes "Leichtmetalleiter" (Engl.: "light metal ladder")—were correct, and then she began to perseverate: "Leich-" (Engl.: "light"). The first three letters of the second component ("-metal") were written correctly, and then she perseverated either the first four letters of the last item "Heit", or she may have perseverated the last morpheme of the previous target item "keit" incorrectly by writing "heit". In a second attempt at writing the target word, she once again wrote the first five letters correctly, but then left out the final "-t" of the first part of the compound "Leicht", and continued with the second compound component "metal" perseverating the "t" resulting in "metat-" instead of "metal". For the next item she wrote down the sentence, which she incorrectly repeated by changing "his" to "my" for the target sentence "She will become his wife" (Ger.: "Sie wird seine Frau"). Another error was also made "seine ⇒ meine ⇒ meine**r**, where the accusative is wrongly substituted by the genitive/dative. For the next item (number 9), instead of writing "heiter" (Engl.: "cheerful" or "jovial") she perseverated the incorrect word from the last sentence "meiner" (instead of "seine"), which consists of the same number of letters as the

[8] Her name is erased in Figure 5a for reasons of data protection.

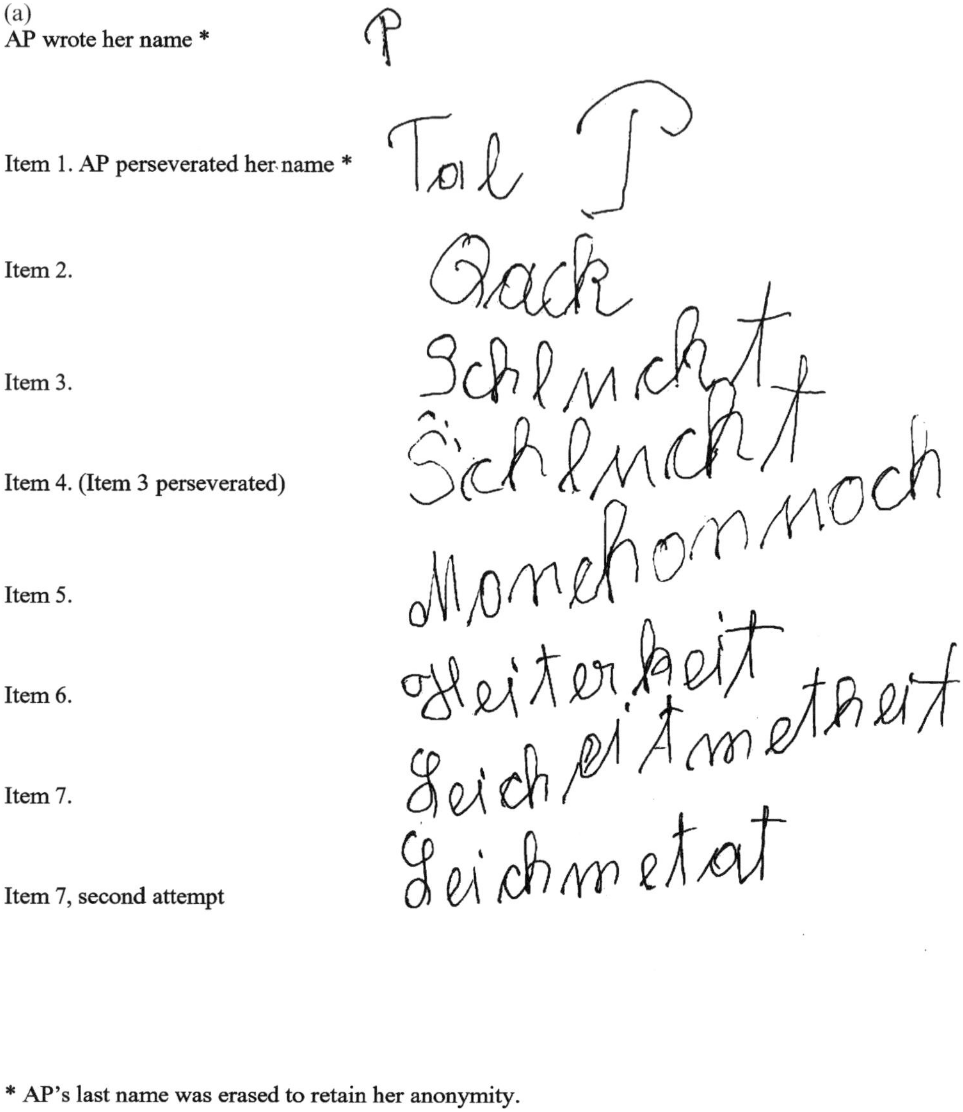

Figure 5. (a), (b): AP's protocols for the AAT subtest, writing to dictation.

target and has the same overall graphemic structure. NB: For the test item number 6, she correctly wrote the word "Heiter-keit" (Engl.: "cheeri-ness" or "jovial-ity"). While attempting to write item number 9, AP verbally repeated the incorrect sentence from item number 8 several times. She never correctly repeated the target sentence for item number 9 while attempting to respond to that target item. Although the stimulus sentence was presented orally several times, she continually perseverated the previous sentence.

Although she managed to write down the complete sentence for the final item, AP perseverated the first word of the sentence eight times in varying misspellings. The examiner had to read the stimulus sentence several times. AP finally was able to break away from the perseverated word "where" (Ger.: "wohin") and could

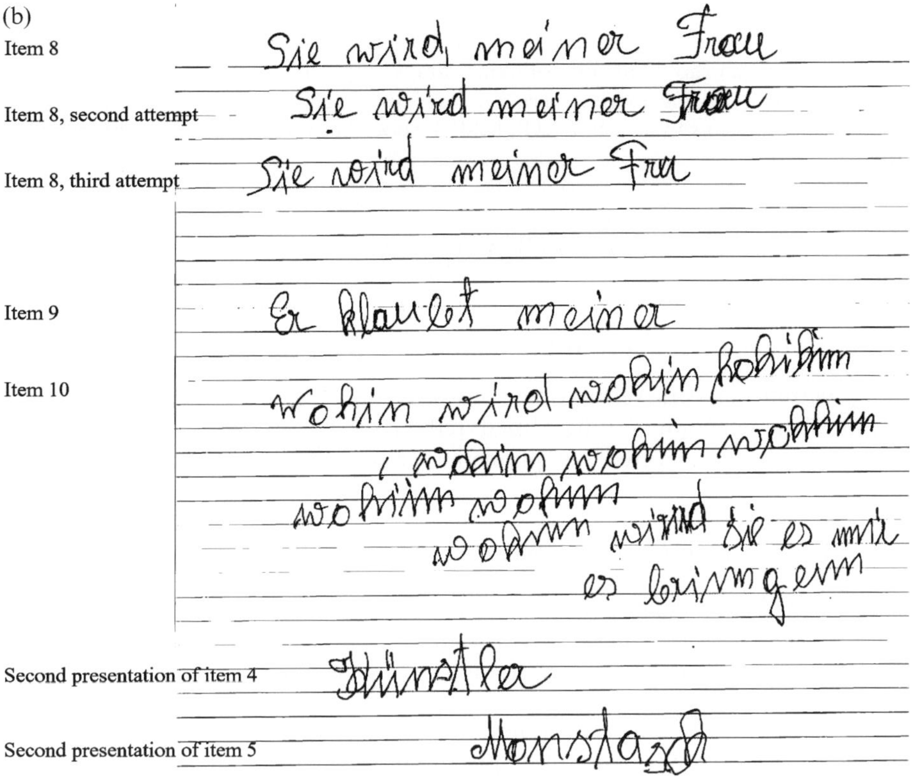

Figure 5. (a), (b): Continued.

complete the whole dictated question: "Where will she bring it to me?" Following the first presentation of this item, AP repeated the whole question correctly. She then produced either the first word, the first two words, or parts of the first word ("wo", "hin") for a total of 67 spoken productions.

Following the presentation of the 10 items in this subtest, 2 of the items were presented a second time: "Künstler" and "Montage". In the first case AP correctly wrote down the target, and in the second case the first three letters were again correct, but then she perseverated the next two letters from the previous item "st"—possibly because the same letters (-nst-) are in both words. She then wrote down the equivalent sound of the next letters instead of the actual spelling for this loan word, i.e., sch- instead of g- (pronounced as /ʃ/ when spoken out loud) and stopped writing the word.

Oral confrontation naming

Examples of perseveration from the naming of objects subtest

For the subtest naming drawings of objects (simple nouns), AP correctly named the first four items by saying "That is an X". For the fifth item she correctly named the object, but used a less common term (Ger.: "Riemen"). This is a possible target word for the more usual German word for "belt" ("Gürtel"). As of item 6, AP produced the following perseveratory responses:

5. belt ⇒ + (Ger.: "Riemen")
6. cigar ⇒ And that should be a *belt*(= "Riemen") (Ex.: "*What else could it be*?") That *could* also ... (pause) should also be smoking. Smoking it should also be// could be
7. nail ⇒ .. *It could also be a* ***rain*** *... a* ***rain*** *it could also be* (NB: Before the naming task was performed, the examiner and AP held a short conversation about the rainy weather.)
8. candle ⇒ +
9. scale ⇒ *It could also be a* ***candle***
10. bulldozer ⇒ *It could also be a* ***candle*** (Ger.: "Raupe") (a simple noun)

Examples of perseveration in the subtest on naming of colours

Embedded within her perseverative responses, AP produced correct colour names for five out of the ten colours to be named: red, green, yellow, brown, and grey, and for one item she self-corrected her phonemic error and produced a sixth correct colour, i.e., blue.

1. red ⇒ And here *it could also be a* ***candle*** (Ex.: "What colour is it?") AP: That is a red *colour*
2. white ⇒ *That could also be a red colour* – been; it also have been
3. green ⇒ And *that could also be a green* ***candle***
4. black ⇒ *And that could also be* a brown (Ger.: "braune") ***candle***
5. yellow ⇒ + That is a yellow colour
6. blue ⇒ *That could have been* a blueme// blue *colour* (Ger.: "blau**m**e- blaue Farbe") (This is a self-correction of a phonemic error; this production could be a perseveration of the incorrect response for item 4: "braune".)
7. brown ⇒ *And that could be a* brown *colour* +
8. grey ⇒ *And that could have been a* grey *colour* +
9. violet ⇒ vila (blend of "violet + lila")
10. orange ⇒ vila – vila . And *that could have* a- a- a- vila *colour could have been also* a vila colour

Examples of perseveration from the object-naming subtest on compound nouns

1. vacuum cleaner ⇒ Uh hm. And that could have very well been a- a vila colour could have been (Ger.: "Uh hm. Und das hätt's gern eine vila Farbe hätt's gewesen sein- hätt's gern gewesen sein)
2. refrigerator ⇒ And that could have – could have a- a vila – vila colour could have been necessary. Could have like to have been (Ex.: What do you need it for?) (Ger.: "Wozu braucht man das?") .. Das hätt's notwendig gebraucht . so notwendig gebraucht (Engl.: "That she(?) would have needed necessary . needed so necessary")

For items 2–10, AP perseverated syntactic phrases and colour names from the previous task such as "...could have been" and "vila". She also perseverated parts of interposed questions of the examiner. For example, in trying to break through the perseveration in order to obtain an answer, the examiner asked AP about how a particular object could be used or what it is needed for. This phrase and others were perseverated for the remaining eight items. The responses are interspersed with semantic jargon, which is also perseverated: For example, for the item "flashlight" or "torch" (Ger.: "Taschenlampe") she responded with the sentence: "This rascal did not come home". For item 10, "rollerskate" (Ger.: "Rollschuh"), AP produced the word "children" in her perseveratory response.

Examples of perseveration from the naming subtest of depicted activities in sentence form

For this subtest AP continued to perseverate a mixture of phrases she had already perseverated in the previous subtest, and she also incorporated fragments of the examiner's instructions and questions into her responses. None of the responses was an adequate description of the activity depicted in the stimulus drawing. However, among the repeated perseverative responses she occasionally managed to produce a word or phrase that could be considered relevant to the presented stimulus picture. Other than the adequate words: man, hat (Item 1) – dog (Item 3) – boot (Item 4) – tree, Indian (Item 6) – school, teacher (Item 9) – pipe (Item 10), AP initiated and aborted many sentences (which are marked by // in the transcribed texts). Her attempts at sentence naming consist of semantic paraphasias, jargon, and perseveratory responses. Due to the length of AP's responses, examples from the sentence-naming task are given in Appendix B (English translation and the original German responses). These examples demonstrate the carryover of perseverated phrases and utterances from one item to the next.

Comprehension subtests of the AAT

AP responded correctly to a few word-level items in this multiple-choice picture-pointing task. Her main error was that she perseverated the position to which she pointed. AP continually pointed to the same position on the page regardless of what was depicted in that particular position, i.e., one of the three foils.

Token Test

AP repeated the items several times but did not point to the tokens in the first four parts. However, she did manipulate the tokens in the fifth part of this task.

Perseveration in other language tasks

Picture description

"Cookie Theft" from the BDAE (Goodglass & Kaplan, 1983) (third test session). Text production was not possible. AP perseverated the instruction and her responses were produced in a slowed down manner: (Examiner: "What is happening in this picture?) AP: "What here is happening in the – is happening - please - is happening. In the is happening – please - yes in the is happening – is happening ("passiert" ⇒ passelt (twice))." Following an intervention by the examiner asking her who is depicted(= a woman drying a plate), she produced an utterance that consisted of semantic jargon and then perseverated that sentence several times: "Here the – the – the (= nominative case, masculine) Vierbauer (? A name of someone, which when translated into English means "four farmer") – the Vierbauer – the – the Vierbauer – Here is the – the Vierbauer – here is …".

Fluency

AP understood the task instructions and initially responded adequately, however, she perseverated animal names as demonstrated by the following examples from her protocol:

> AP: There are many animals... there are cows, there are, there are cattle (Ger.: "Rinder"; equivalent in English: cattle or bovine animals (plural form)), and there are calves, calves and so. ... There are calves so calves and so there are very, very much liked the calves hm hm ....
> (Ex.: What other animals are there?)
> AP: Oh, there are many animals..... Yes, yes, there are elephants and cattle (plural noun) there are so many - so many cattle (plural form) there are . yes, yes There are so many cattle (plural form), yes

AP continued to perseverate the animal names: cattle, calves, elephants and at one point she changed the syntactic structure into which the perseverated animal names were embedded: "You wanted many cattle (plural form) ... you wanted to have many cattle (plural form)". The word order was changed and topicalised versions of the same sentence were produced several times.

Word repetition

(Third test session, 1 week following the first repetition tasks): Another list of words was presented to AP consisting of 30 one- and two-syllable words of varying phonemic complexity. In total, 18 out of the 30 items were correctly repeated. However, two to three presentations of the target word were necessary for several of the items before a response was generated. The first six items were repeated correctly. In response to the seventh item—Ger.: "Spruch" (Engl.: "slogan")—AP responded with "Yes, yes", and after the third presentation she correctly repeated the stimulus word. This response was perseverated for the next item and it was produced again after an interval of eight presentations (including repetitions of stimuli) to which AP either responded correctly ($n = 4$) or only produced "yes, yes" ($n = 4$). This word ("Spruch") was perseverated for two more items with a correct response to an item in between. That is, the item "Spruch" was non-contiguously perseverated for three items over a span of eight items.

For the next four items, AP responded with "Yes, yes", and then the next three items were repeated correctly. For the item "Schlich" (Engl.: "dodge") (noun) her perseverative response consisted of parts from the last item "Schutt" and "Schlich" itself (-ch): ("Schutt" ⇒ +; "Schlich" ⇒ "Sch***u***ch***t***" which is a nonword). Thus, she perseverated the first two phonemes and the final one and inserted the phoneme /-ch/ from the stimulus item. For the next item, AP perseverated only the final –t: "Fass" (Engl.: "barrel") ⇒ "fast", the result of which is also another word in German (Engl.: "almost"). The next item was correctly repeated: "Dach" (Engl.: "roof"). However, for the next item "Rumpf" (Engl: "torso"), AP produced: "Jacht" which consists of parts perseverated from the items "Dach" and "Schutt": " ***–ach*** + *t*". However, the initial phoneme is from the liquid family (l, r, j). The next item was correctly repeated: "Fleisch" (Engl.: "meat") and for the following item: "Messer" (Engl.: "knife") the final phoneme "–sch" from "Fleisch" was perseverated:

"Messer" ⇒ "Me*sch*" (nonword) and the second syllable was not produced. To the last three items AP responded with "Yes, yes".

In summary, the following perseverations were produced:

"Spruch" +
"Taft" ⇒ "***Spruch***"
....
"Rache" ⇒ "***Spruch***", then +
"Schacht" +
"Sprache" ⇒ "***Spruch***"
....
"Schutt" +
"Schlich" ⇒ Sch***u***ch***t*** (produced twice)
"Fass" ⇒ "fas***t***"
"Dach" ⇒+
"Rumpf" ⇒ "J***acht***"
"Fleisch" (three times) +
"Messer" ⇒ Me***sch***

Boston Naming Test

(Third test session, a week later): After presentation of the first five items to which AP responded with echolalic phrases from the initial greeting and conversation with the examiner (Ex.: "How are you doing today?), she did manage to respond correctly to several items. After a long pause, AP responded to the first three items with the following production: "... doing – doing - today – doing today" (Ger.: geht – geht - heute – geht heute**n**"). The sixth to eighth items were correctly named, then AP perseverated the correct response from item six: "Schere" (Engl.: "scissors") for the items 9 through 13. After a self-correction of a phonological error, item 14 was correctly produced: "Schwammerl" ⇒ "Stammel", then "Schwammerl" (Engl.: "mushroom"). This response was perseverated for the next six items and the test was discontinued.

Automatised sequences

Days of the week[9]

After the examiner provided the first two days of the week (Sunday, Monday, ..), AP correctly repeated Monday and continued until Thursday, and then perseverated part of Tuesday, which begins with the same letter "D" in German: "Montag, Dienstag, Mittwoch, Donnerstag, ***Dien***erstag, Donnerstag, Freitag, Mittwoch, Fiertag, Mittwoch". AP repeated Thursday and produced Friday, followed by Wednesday, and then "Fiertag" which is not a word in German. AP continued to produce the days out of order and she also produced nonwords consisting of perseverations of previously cited days of the week: "Meitag", "Teitag".

[9] In German, the days of the week beginning with Sunday are: Sonntag, Montag, Dienstag, Mittwoch, Donnerstag, Freitag, Samstag.

Months[10]

Following the days of the week, AP was asked to recite the months of the year, which she began with "Monday". Attempts to get AP to produce the months of the year resulted in a mixture of months and days including distortions of both, for example: "Februar, Donnerstag .... Minter, Mintag, Freitag, Montag [Ex.: January, February, ...] AP: "Sentag, Sentag, Sentag, Sonntag".

However, following these perseverative and jargon responses, AP was able to repeat single months correctly one at a time. Asked once again to recite the months by herself, she began with a blend of the perseveration of December, September, or November and the correct initial phoneme: "Jotember" (Januar/Jänner and Dezember, September or November).

Numbers (Counting from one to ten)

For this task she produced the first three numbers correctly and perseverated the number three. Additional attempts resulted in sequences such as: ... 5- 6- 7- 8- 6- 7- 8- 6- 8- 7- 8- 9- 8- count- count- count- 10- 10-. NB: Ger.: "Zählen" (Engl.: "to count") and Ger.: "zehn" (Engl.: "ten"): The similarity between the two words may be playing a role here.

Sentence completion

AP did not complete sentences for which a particular single-word response was highly expected, for example: "I am thirsty. I would like something to ____ (drink)". (Ger.: "Ich bin durstig. Ich möchte etwas ____ (trinken)".) For the sentence: "Heute scheint die____" (Engl.: "Today is shining the ___"), AP perseverated the number eight from the previous task of counting from one to ten: "Er scheint acht- acht" (Engl.: "he is shining eight- eight"). In German the correct word order is: "Heute scheint die _____" (Sonne). In another attempt she produced the verb "scheint" and continued with the following: "scheint – scheint mir ernst - ganz ernst – ganz ernst..." (Engl.: "appears - appears to me serious – very serious – very serious"). The produced verb form has a different meaning here: "scheint" also means "appears" and "scheint mir" is equivalent in English to "[it] seems or appears to me".

DISCUSSION

In a recent publication, Sowman et al. (2006) report on a case of probable sporadic CJD exhibiting rapid progressive deterioration of speech and language. Comparing the language pattern observed in AP to the case discussed by Sowman et al. (2006), and other case studies reported in the literature on CJD, we find several parallels in clinical features and language performance including the regression to a global language impairment ending in mutism. Relevant case study reports are summarised in Table 5. Larger epidemiological studies also report on a percentage of cases exhibiting language impairments in the initial stages of the disease. These studies are

[10] In German, the months of the year are: Januar or Jänner, Februar or Feber, März, April, Mai, Juni, Juli, August, September, Oktober, November, Dezember.

TABLE 5
Parallel symptoms and differences observed in selected case studies of patients presenting with CJD (probable and autopsy-confirmed cases)

Initial symptom	*Parallels in language performance: Similarities with (and differences from) present case*	*Reference*
Wernicke's aphasia	Aphasia type: perseveration; paraphasia; progressive, fluent aphasia; repetition of phrases, long sentences and multi-syllabic words was paraphasic and perseverative; written language: perseverative (other than signature and overlearned phrases) (Differences: longer duration of illness)	Mandell et al. (1989)
Wernicke's aphasia secondary to non-convulsive status epilepticus	Aphasia type: fluent paragrammatic output with empty quality; perseveration; impaired confrontation naming; single words could be repeated, however, difficulty repeating sentences; multiple paraphasic errors (Differences: unable to read and comprehend written language)	Cohen et al. (2004)
Aphasia-like language disturbance	Progressive language disturbance and mild memory difficulties; language disturbance affecting mainly semantic ability and comprehension, perseverated words, sentences, and themes with practical no meaning or coherence; word-finding difficulties; similarities in sentence completion, word fluency and repetition; compromised self-monitoring; mild dysarthric signs; 1 month history of progressive language impairment, rapid deterioration in language functions within 1 week: progression to global language impairment (WAB*: AQ = 63.1 versus AAT: Wernicke's aphasia moderate to severe degree of impairment, except for written language) (Differences: functional automatic speech intact; auditory verbal comprehension less impaired [57/60 on WAB]; naming less impaired; reading more impaired)	Sowman et al. (2006)
Language deficits: Pure word deafness and severe anomia	AHG: Severe anomia; language impairment progressed to a global impairment; mild right facial palsy (Difference: pure word deafness) (NB: Two cases were reported on; the second [RGN] presented with progressive left neglect)	Hillis & Selnes (1999)
Progressive aphasia; Nonfluent aphasia; Transcortical motor aphasia	Confrontation naming moderately impaired; speech somewhat dysarthric (Differences: perseveration not observed or cited; nonfluent, effortful spontaneous speech; difficulty initiating spontaneous speech; comprehension of spoken and written language and repetition were normal)	Shuttleworth et al. (1985)
Aphasia; Motor aphasia	Aphasia; some difficulty with comprehension; very rapid deterioration of language functions (Difference: motor aphasia; right hemiparesis)	Yamanouchi et al. (1986)
Agraphia; Aphasia	Rapid progression of aphasia to loss of all verbal functions ending in mutism (Written language better preserved in AP; case study emphasises neuropsychological, i.e., cognitive deficits)	Pachalska et al. (2001)

* WAB=Western Aphasia Battery (Kertesz, 1982).

not included in Table 5 (see Bernoulli, Masters, Gajdusek, Gibbs, & Harris, 1979; Brown, Cathala, Sadowsky, & Gajdusek, 1979; Tsuji & Kuroiwa, 1983, among others).

The cases described as presenting with fluent aphasia, in particular Wernicke's aphasia, prevail. In the reports on anomic and fluent paragrammatic patients, perseveration is also observed (see Hier, Hagenlocker, & Shindler, 1985; Shindler et al., 1984). More interesting is the pattern of performance, for example in the context of word-finding difficulties or repeating words, phrases, and sentences: The more complex the target word, phrase, or sentence, the greater the probability that

TABLE 6
Haiganoosh Whitaker's neurolinguistic framework of levels of language functioning

Level I	Accurate auditory perception Accurate verbal production	SPEECH
↕	Intact phonological organization (phonemic patterns, stress, and intonation, etc.);	↕
Level II	Over-learned aspects of grammatical organization which become automatic (late rules of syntactic agreement, function words, etc.);	LANGUAGE (automatic, non-volitional)
↕	Probably certain semantic features of lexical items in addition to phonological ones and certain over-learned phrases and verbal automatisms.	↕
Level III	Cognition, intellectual functions, and creative aspects of language	LANGUAGE (creative, volitional)

Whitaker, 1976, p. 51.

the response will be paraphasic and perseverative. The patient described in Sowman et al. (2006) produced perseverative output in response to the interviewer's questions and also to the stimuli for sentence completion and repetition tasks (p. 586), which is similar to AP's output. The pattern of perseveration is similar in both patients, e.g., the perseverative phrases are changed somewhat in the course of being repeated.

Whitaker's (1976) comprehensive discussion of a case of the isolation of the language function in terms of a tripartite neurolinguistic framework provides a basis for discussing AP's language data and the process of language deterioration in progressive disease in general. The three levels summarised in Table 6 are: Level I = overt speech, Level II = automatic language, and Level III = cognition. Applying this framework, Whitaker demonstrated in great detail how Level III was severely affected in her patient (HCEM). In particular, high-level grammatical rules of both syntactic and semantic nature, which underlie creative aspects of language, showed the most impairment.

With regard to Whitaker's (1976) framework, analysis of AP's language performance reveals the following: At the time of the first two language test sessions, AP was functioning predominantly at Level I, and even at that level her verbal output was accurate only in so far as she did not perseverate. AP's self-corrections provide evidence for accurate auditory perception. In the repetition and naming tasks she corrected errors that were phonological in nature and which affected only a single phoneme in an otherwise correct production. However, even one- and two-syllable nouns revealed perseverative errors that, with increasing structural complexity, resulted in phonemic jargon. Perseverative errors also affected the stress pattern of individual items. Attempts at correcting complex errors were not observed.

Level II features were partially functioning, in particular with regard to phonological organisation. Although numerous responses and utterances consist of neologisms, semantic and phonological, AP does not violate phonotactic rules of the German language. Late rules of syntactic agreement were affected; that is, in her perseverative repetitions AP produced the wrong case markers (gender and number). These errors were not corrected. (Morpho-) syntactic ability is compromised, particularly when perseveration can be considered to be the source of the error.

AP's perseverative utterances are often ungrammatical. Kempler, Curtis, and Jackson's (1987) finding that syntactic ability is relatively preserved in Alzheimer's disease in the context of impaired semantic processing cannot be upheld for this case of CJD. Sentences could not be completed in which the missing word(s) were highly constrained and anticipated as automatic responses. Even very overlearned sequences were not possible (days of the week, months of the year).

Level III was notably affected at all test times. In the contextual situation, AP understood more than her actual test results in the AAT comprehension subtests reveal. Again her perseverative behaviour was the main source of her errors. She understood the instructions for the various subtests. However, her momentary state was the determining factor in whether she would perseverate or be able to respond to the actual task type or task item. She answered several questions correctly; she named a number of common everyday objects and colours intermittently; she also responded to the fluency task with accurate animal names and stayed within the semantic category. However, based on AP's language data, monitoring and processing of semantic features were absent, as judged by the non-existence of corrections or attempts at repairing her semantically inadequate verbal output. Thus, Level III creative functions, which require adequate semantic processing, were noticeably missing.

The main errors observed in spontaneous speech and on the various language tasks and levels are perseverative (cf. Tables 2 to 5). Overall, the majority of AP's errors were perseverative in nature. On the AAT subtests perseveration accounts for 87% of the repetition errors, 71% of the errors in written language tasks, 97% of the errors in the naming tasks, and 97% of the errors in the language comprehension tasks. In some instances, e.g., object and colour naming, a correct response was embedded in a perseveration. What can be deduced from AP's overall language performance? Moreover, what do these errors tell us with respect to the mechanisms of perseveration? Allison's (1966a, 1966b) dichotomy of perseveration as a sign of diffuse and focal brain damage finds application in the interpretation of AP's behaviour. Initially, it can be assumed that AP started out with perseverative behaviour that reflected a more circumscribed language disorder (Type 1: sign of focal damage). This rapidly progressed to a severe impairment of language production and comprehension with semantic and phonemic jargon output (Type 2: sign of diffuse brain damage) with perseverative responses in all language tasks—intra-task and inter-task. Therefore, Stark's (1984) account of perseverative responses as Type 2 (Yates, 1966) or Type b (Teuber & Weinstein, 1955) effects of brain damage, which mirror the specific language-processing difficulties, also holds for AP's perseverative behaviour: the types and extent of verbal perseveration observed in AP reflect the severity and magnitude of her language impairment, which at the time of the first three language test sessions was so pervasive that the initial specific, i.e., more circumscribed, processing difficulties were no longer pronounced. The pattern of perseverative responses observed in individual aphasic patients presenting with various specific language-processing disorders resulting from focal lesions due to a single stroke differs from that observed in AP due to the progressive overall breakdown in linguistic processing.

Although the deterioration of her language processing had advanced rapidly, it was in a transitional state at the time of testing. It had evolved from an initial inability to retrieve lexical items and it ended in an akinetic mute state with no functional language. Evidence for the assumption of AP's processing system being in a state of flux can be found in the pattern of language performance. In each subtest of the AAT and in other language tests, the first three to five items were correctly produced, then processing broke down. Responses were perseverated or were contaminated by perseveration. Even after producing perseverative responses, AP was still able to produce a correct response, i.e., repeat a word or name an object. The intricate linguistic entanglements or blends as perseverations observed, particularly in response to the more complex stimuli, provide evidence for a severely impaired yet dynamic system. The complex input resulting in the perseverative verbal output exhibited by AP reflects a major problem in inhibiting or suppressing the irrelevant information available in various modalities for the particular response (see Dempster, 1991). At the time of testing we observed a patient whose language processing was in an almost permanent state of being overtaxed by the task demands and in all verbal communicative situations. Her decay rate for previously produced responses and utterances was very slow, if it functioned at all. This situation, in combination with her severe primary language impairment consisting of word-finding difficulties and concurrent difficulties monitoring her verbal output for semantic adequacy and syntactic well-formedness, results in the clinical symptoms present in AP. Shindler et al.'s (1984) four-stage process account of intrusions applies for interpreting AP's perseverative[11] responses. However, the description of the second stage, i.e., "he/she then *selects* from short-term memory a recently heard word or phrase" implies a voluntary action, which in the case of the perseverative responses produced by AP is questionable. It is rather the case that, due to permanent overactivation and little or no suppression of irrelevant information, those items are produced which have remained highly activated.

In terms of the accounts of perseveration discussed in Stark (2007 this issue) and descriptions in the literature on perseverative responses in dementia, AP's pervasive and complex pattern of perseverative behaviour demonstrates the intricacy of the phenomena to be accounted for. In terms of the classical accounts discussed in Stark (2007 this issue), we assume that in the context of a severe primary lexical retrieval deficit (Heilbronner, 1906; Lissauer, 1890) resulting in a permanent overtaxing of AP's language-processing system ("cognitive overload"), von Sölder"s (1899) overactivation account of perseveration captures her verbal perseverative behaviour at the time of the language testing for this report. In the case of AP, the gap caused by the initial primary deficit widened, which rapidly and progressively evolved into a global language impairment with perseverative responses mirroring the increasingly more severe breakdown in language and cognitive processing, until no functional language was possible at all.

REFERENCES

Allison, R. S. (1966a). Perseveration as a sign of diffuse and focal brain damage – I. *British Medical Journal*, *2*, 1027–1032.

[11] We consider the "intrusions" as defined by Shindler et al. (1984) to be examples of perseveration. In our data from AP, we have only one explicit example of an intrusion. "For no apparent reason" she suddenly spoke of children in a very negative manner (Ger.: "Gefraster") in a sentence that was not perseverated.

Allison, R. S. (1966b). Perseveration as a sign of diffuse and focal brain damage – II. *British Medical Journal*, *2*, 1095–1101.

Bayles, K. A., Tomoeda, C., Kasniak, A. W., Stern, L. S., & Eagans, K. K. (1985). Verbal perseveration of dementia patients. *Brain and Language*, *25*, 102–116.

Bernoulli, C., Masters, C. L., Gajdusek, D. C., Gibbs, C. J., & Harris, J. O. (1979). Early clinical features of Creutzfeldt-Jakob disease (subacute spongiform encephalopathy). In S. B. Prusiner & W. J. Hadlow (Eds.), *Slow transmissible diseases of the nervous system, Vol. 1* (pp. 229–251). New York: Academic Press.

Boller, F., Boller, M., Denes, G., Timberlake, W. H., Zieper, I., & Albert, M. (1973). Familial palilalia. *Neurology*, *23*, 1117–1125.

Brown, P., Cathala, F., Sadowsky, D., & Gajdusek, D. C. (1979). Creutzfeldt-Jakob disease in France: II. Clinical characteristics of 124 consecutive verified cases during the decade 1968–1977. *Annals of Neurology*, *6*, 430–437.

Buckingham, H. (1985). Perseveration in aphasia. In S. Newman & R. Epstein (Eds.), *Current perspectives in dysphasia* (pp. 113–154). Edinburgh, UK: Churchill Livingstone.

Cohen, D., Kutluay, E., Edwards, J., Peltier, A., & Beydoun, A. (2004). Sporadic Creutzfeldt-Jakob disease presenting with nonconvulsive status epilepticus. *Epilepsy & Behavior*, *5*(5), 792–796.

Critchley, M. (1927–1928). On palilalia. *Journal of Neurology and Psychopathology*, *7*, 23–32.

Dempster, F. N. (1991). Inhibitory processes: A neglected dimension of intelligence. *Intelligence*, *15*, 157–173.

Gálvez, S., Dörr-Zegers, O., & Cartier, L. (1982). Zur Klinik, Neuropathologie und Pathogenese der Creutzfeldt-Jakobschen Krankheit anhand von 40 gesicherten Fällen. *Nervenarzt*, *53*, 132–140.

Goodglass, H., & Kaplan, E. (1983). *Boston Diagnostic Aphasia Exam*. Philadelphia: Lea & Febiger.

Heilbronner, K. (1906). Über Haftenbleiben und Stereotypie. *Ergänzungsheft der Monatsschrift für Psychiatrie*, *18*, 293–371.

Hier, D. B., Hagenlocker, K., & Shindler, A. G. (1985). Language disintegration in dementia: Effects of etiology and severity. *Brain and Language*, *25*, 117–133.

Hillis, A. E., & Selnes, O. (1999). Cases of aphasia or neglect due to Creutzfeld-Jakob disease. *Aphasiology*, *13*(9), 743–754.

Huber, W., Poeck, K., Weniger, D., & Willmes, K. (1983). *Der Aachener Aphasie Test (AAT)*. Göttingen: Hogrefe.

Hughlings Jackson, J. (1880). On affections of speech from disease of the brain. *Brain*, *2*, 323–356.

Kaplan, E., Goodglass, H., & Weintraub, S. (1983). *Boston Naming Test*. Philadelphia: Lea & Febiger.

Kempler, D., Curtiss, S., & Jackson, C. (1987). Syntactic preservation in Alzheimer's disease. *Journal of Speech and Hearing Research*, *30*, 343–350.

Kertesz, A. (1982). *Western Aphasia Battery*. New York: Grune & Stratton.

Kirshner, H. S., Webb, W. G., Kelly, M. P., & Wells, C. E. (1984). Language disturbance: An initial symptom of cortical degenerations and dementia. *Archives of Neurology*, *41*, 491–496.

Kleist, K. (1934). *Gehirnpathologie vornehmlich auf Grund der Kriegserfahrungen*. Berlin: Karger.

Lebrun, Y. (1993). Repetitive phenomena in aphasia. In G. Blanken, J. Dittmann, H. Grimm, J. C. Marshall, & C-W. Wallesch (Eds.), *Linguistic disorders and pathologies: An international handbook* (pp. 225–238). Berlin: Walter de Gruyter.

Lissauer, H. (1890). Ein Fall von Seelenblindheit nebst einem Beitrage zur Theorie derselben. *Archiv für Psychiatrie und Nervenkrankheiten*, *21*, 222–270.

Mandell, A. M., Alexander, M. P., & Carpenter, S. (1989). Creutzfeldt-Jakob disease presenting as isolated aphasia. *Neurology*, *39*, 55–58.

Matthews, W. B. (1985). Creutzfeldt-Jakob disease. In J. A. M. Frederiks (Ed.), *Handbook of clinical neurology* (Vol. 46, pp. 289–299). Amsterdam: Elsevier.

Moen, I. (1993). Perseveration in the speech of a patient with fluent anomic aphasia. *Clinical Linguistics and Phonetics*, *7*(1), 1–17.

Nagahama, Y., Okina, T., Nabatome, H., & Matsuda, M. (2006). The cerebral correlates of different types of perseveration in the Wisconsin Card Sorting Test. *Journal of Neurology, Neurosurgery and Psychiatry*, *76*, 169–175.

Pachalska, M., Kurzbauer, H., MacQueen, B. D., Forminslka-Kapuscik, M., & Herman-Sucharska, I. (2001). Neuropsychological features of rapidly progressive dementia in a patient with an untypical presentation of Creutzfeldt-Jakob disease. *Medical Science Monitor*, *7*(6), 1307–1315.

Possin, K. L., Filoteo, J. V., Roesch, S. C., Zizak, V., Rilling, L. M., & Davis, J. D. (2005). Is a perseveration a perseveration? An evaluation of cognitive error types in patients with subcortical pathology. *Journal of Clinical and Experimental Neuropsychology*, *27*, 953–966.

Rosenberg, M. (1912). Über gewisse Regelmäßigkeiten der Perseveration. *Zeitschrift für die gesamte Neurologie und Psychiatrie*, *8*, 123–132.

Shindler, A. G., Caplan, L. R., & Hier, D. B. (1984). Intrusions and perseverations. *Brain and Language*, *23*, 148–158.

Shuttleworth, E. C., Yates, A. J., & Paltan-Ortiz, J. D. (1985). Creutzfeldt-Jakob disease presenting as progressive aphasia. *Journal of the National Medical Association*, *77*(8), 649–656.

Sowman, R., Robinson, D., O'Riordan, R., Connolly, S., & O'Neill, D. (2006). Rapidly deteriorating speech and language in a case of probable sporadic Creutzfeldt-Jakob disease. *Aphasiology*, *20*(6), 579–592.

Stark, J. (1984). *Verbale Perseveration bei Aphasie. Ein neurolinguistischer Ansatz*. Unpublished doctoral thesis, University of Vienna.

Stark, J. (2007). A review of classical accounts of verbal perseveration and their modern-day relevance. *Aphasiology*, *21*, 928–959.

Teuber, H. L., & Weinstein, S. (1955). General and specific effects of cerebral lesions. *The American Psychologist*, *10*, 408–409.

Tsuji, S., & Kuroiwa, Y. (1983). Creutzfeldt-Jakob disease in Japan. *Neurology*, *33*, 1503–1506.

von Sölder, F. (1899). Über Perseveration, eine formale Störung im Vorstellungsablaufe. *Jahrbücher für Psychiatrie und Neurologie*, *18*, 479–525.

Wallesch, C-W. (1990). Repetitive verbal behaviour: Functional and neurological considerations. *Aphasiology*, *4*(2), 133–154.

Wechsler, A. (1977). Presenile dementia presenting as aphasia. *Journal of Neurology, Neurosurgery, and Psychiatry*, *40*, 303–305.

Whitaker, H. (1976). A case of the isolation of the language function. In H. Whitaker & H. A. Whitaker (Eds.), *Studies in neurolinguistics, Volume 2* (pp. 1–58). New York: Academic Press.

Yamanouchi, H., Budka, H., & Vass, K. (1986). Unilateral Creutzfeldt-Jakob disease. *Neurology*, *36*, 1517–1520.

Yates, A. L. (1966). Psychological deficit. *Annual Review of Psychology*, *17*, 111–144.

APPENDIX A: AACHEN APHASIA TEST RESULTS

AATP für Windows

Auswertungsprogramm für den Aachener Aphasie Test

Routineklassifikation

(Spontansprache, Token Test, Nachsprechen, Spontansprache, Schriftsprache, Benennen, Sprachverständnis)

Patient:	A P		
Adresse:	Vienna		
Patienten-ID:	1	**Geburtsdatum:**	06.01.1931
Untersuchung:	1	**Alter (T/M/J):**	11 / 09 / 56
		Beginn der Aphasie:	01.10.19--
		Dauer (T/M/J):	16 / 00 / 00
Untersucher:	SYSADMIN	**Testdatum:**	17.10.19--

Ergebnisse der Untertests

	Punktwerte	Prozentränge	Schweregrad allgemein	Schweregrad Syndrom
Spontansprache (Profil)	1 4 2 3 5 3	-----	-----	
Token Test (alterskorr.)	40	28	S* M*	* S*
Nachsprechen	96	38	* M*	* M*
Schriftsprache	62	63	* M* L	* L*
Benennen	37	30	* S* M	* S* M
Sprachverständnis	28	7	* S*	* S*

MI:Minimal
L: Leicht
M: Mittel
S: Schwer

Diagnose

(X) **Aphasie**
( ) **keine Aph./Restsympt.**
( ) **nicht-klass. Aphasie**

( ) **Globale Aphasie**
(X) **Wernicke Aphasie**
( ) **Broca Aphasie**
( ) **Amnestische Aphasie**

( ) **Leitungsaphasie**
( ) **transkortikale Aph.**

( ) **Alexie ohne Agraphie**
( ) **Alexie mit Agraphie**
( ) **Agraphie**
( ) **Dysarthrie**
( ) **Sprechapraxie**

ALLOC-KLASSIFIKATION:

Aphasie(A):	100.0%	**keine Aphasie(NA):**	0.0%
Global Aphasie(GL):	0.0%	**Wernicke Aphasie(WE):**	100.0%
Broca Aphasie(BR):	0.0%	**Amnestische Aphasie(AM):**	0.0%

Sortierte T-Werte:

SV	TT	BEN	NACH	SCHRIFT
35	44	45	47	53

SIGNIFIKANT:(GES.-ALPHA=10%)

TT - SCHR.
TT - SV
NACH - SCHR
NACH - SV
SCHR. - BEN
SCHR. - SV
BEN - SV

TT:	Token Test
NACH:	Nachsprechen
SCHR:	Schriftsprache
BEN:	Benennen
SV:	Sprachverständnis

Sonstiges:

Figure 6. Overall AAT results and classification of AP's language disorder as Wernicke's aphasia.

AATP Für Windows

Auswertungsprogramm für den Aachener Aphasie Test

T-Wert Profil der Untertests

Patient:	A P		
Adresse:	Vienna		
Patienten-ID:	1	**Geburtsdatum:**	06.01.1931
Untersuchung:	1	**Alter (T/M/J):**	11 / 09 / 56
		Beginn der Aphasie:	01.10.19--
		Dauer (T/M/J):	16 / 00 / 00
Untersucher:	SYSADMIN	**Vergleichsdatum:**	17.10.19--

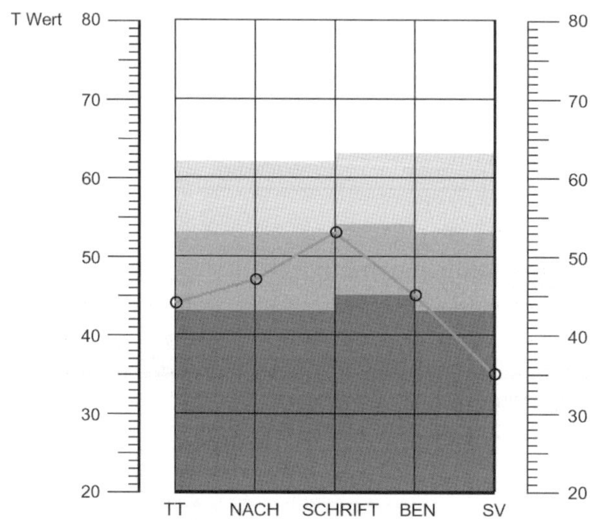

schwer   mittel   leicht   minimal/keine Störung

Einzelfalldiagnostische Ergebnisse:

SV	TT	BEN	NACH	SCHRIFT
(35)	(44)	(45)	(47)	(53)

Figure 7. Aphasia profile for AP.

APPENDIX B: EXCERPTS FROM VARIOUS LANGUAGE TASKS

Key:

Bold: words written in bold print indicate relevant, new information.
Bold and italics: words, phrases, and utterances perseverated from one item to the next.
"//" indicates a break-off followed by a new start.
"-" indicates a repetition of the last word or phrase.
"[...]" denotes an interposed question.
When several responses were produced in a row without a pause, these are marked by an arrow.

Excerpts from a semi-standardised interview, i.e., conversational speech

Test session one:

Ex.: "Do you have little time?" (Ger.: "Haben Sie wenig Zeit?")
AP: "Little time" (Ger.: "Wenig Zeit?")
Ex.: "At home do you have little time for your hobbies?" (Ger.: "Zu Hause haben Sie wenig Zeit für Ihre Hobbies?")
AP: "Oh well, . I . leisure time – [in] the leisure time uh hm that I [in] the leisure time have" (Ger.: "Na ja, . ich . Freizeit – [in] der (dative case) Freizeit uh hm dass ich [in] der (dative case) Freizeit habe?")
Ex.: Do you like to go walking? (Ger.: "Gehen Sie gern spazieren?")
AP: Walking that I like to do very-very much (Ger.: "Spazieren gehe ich schon ganz-ganz gern")
Ex.: Where do you go walking? (Ger.: "Wo gehen Sie spazieren?")
AP: Oh well, already. In the garden I like to walk very, very much (Ger.: "Na ja, schon. Im Garten gehe ich schon ganz-ganz gern spazieren.")
Ex.: Do you have a garden? (Ger.: "Haben Sie einen Garten")
AP: I do have a garden uh hm ... (Ger.: "Ein[en] Garten habe ich schon uh hm")
Ex.: What do you have in the garden: flowers or vegetables? (Ger.: "Was haben Sie im Garten – Blumen oder Gemüse?")
AP: Yes, in the garden I do like flowers very very much and so ... yes. (Ger.: "Ja, im Garten habe ich schon ganz ganz gern Blumen und so. Ja!")
......
Ex.: Do you like listening to the radio? (Ger.: "Hören Sie gern Radio?")
AP: Oh well, ... from the radio. from the radio one can very very well// in the TV one can very very well // one can very very well in the TV // one can very very well . one can very well ... (Ger.: "Na ja, . vom Radio . vom Radio kann man ganz ganz gern // im Fernsehen kann man ganz ganz gern // kann man ganz gern im Fernsehen // kann man ganz ganz gern ganz gern kann man ganz gern")

Excerpts from the word repetition task (AAT)

1. Verbot (Engl.: "prohibition", "ban") ⇒ +
2. Haustür (Engl.: "house door") ⇒ +

3. Umleitung (Engl.: "detour") ⇒ +
4. Handschuhfach (Engl.: "glove compartment" or "glove box") ⇒ Handschuhfach +
5. Vormundschaftsgericht (Engl.: "guardian court") ⇒ ***hantschua:tutst*** ⇒ Vor***schu****mants* ⇒ Vormundsch***ants***gericht
6. Kraftfahrzeugschein (Engl.: "motor vehicle registration certificate") ⇒ Kraft***schu****s*choint- tsuruft ⇒ Kraft***schuh***schein
7. Unverhältnismässigkeit (Engl.: "disproportionalness" or "disproportionality") ⇒ Unverhältnis-; second attempt ⇒ +
8. Farbfernsehgeräteverkauf (Engl.: "selling of colour television units") ⇒ fartsummere.*sich* "***knesigkeit***; second attempt ⇒ Fansense-***sich***-ke-***karesichkeit***
9. Verantwortungslosigkeit (Engl. "irresponsibility") ⇒ Verantwortungs***mässigkeit***; second attempt ⇒ Verantwortungs***mässigkeit***
10. Hallenhandballweltmeisterschaft (Engl.: "indoor handball world championship") ⇒ Handeb-***beltnis- mech– moechtig – moechtnsi- mechtigkeit***; second attempt ⇒ Hand***fer***-pes- mich- ***heit- knoesmichkeit*** (perseveration of part of the compound: "-mässigkeit" (Eng.: "-moderation", "mediocracy")

Excerpts from the sentence repetition task (AAT)

1. Der Hund bellt (Engl.: "The dog is barking") ⇒ +
2. Die Kleine läuft schon (Engl.: "The little one is already walking") ⇒ +
3. Wir werden von ihm abgeholt (Engl.: "We will be picked up by him") ⇒ +
4. Sie leiht ihm kein Geld mehr (Engl.: "She is lending him no more money") ⇒ *Wir werd// von ihm* keine . *abgeholt*; second attempt ⇒ + (Engl.: "*We will be (werden ⇒ werd) by him* no one/nothing ("keine") . *picked up*") (perseveration of item 3 with insertion of "keine" from item 4, albeit in a changed form)
5. Fritz lässt sich ungern die Haare schneiden (Engl.: "Fritz does not like to get his hair cut") ⇒ als der Welz *keinek Geld mehr* (Engl.: "as the Welz no (*kein ⇒ keinek) money more*") ⇒ *keine Geld mehr* (Engl.: "no (*kein ⇒ keine) money more(= no more money)*") ⇒ het die Haare lässt sie *kein Geld mehr* (Engl.: "has the hairs let her *no more money*") ⇒ Er *leiht ihm kein Geld mehr* (Engl.: "He is lending him *no more money*"; she ⇒ he) (repeated perseveration of the phrase "no more money" and the complete stimulus sentence item 4, except for a change in gender **she** ⇒ **he**; several words i.e. productions are distorted.)
6. Er versprach mir heute noch vorbeizukommen (Engl.: "He promised me to still come by today") ⇒ heults ihm .. *hein Geld// wir lassen kein Geld mehr* (Engl.: "today (phonologically distorted) *him no* (*perseveration of /h-/ from heute "today) money// we are letting/leaving no more money*") (Parts of item 3 ("no more money") and item 5 (let = lassen") are perseverated.)
7. Sie ist nicht leicht zufrieden zu stellen (Engl.: "She is not easy to please") ⇒ *Er lässt ihm kein Geld mehr* (Engl.: "*He is leaving/allowing him no more money*") (Parts of items 4, 5 and 6 are perseverated.)
8. Er holte seine Mutter mit einem neuen Auto vom Bahnhof ab (Engl.: "He picked up his mother in a new car from the train station") ⇒ *Er leiht ihm von kein Geld mehr* (Engl.: "hm *he is lending him from no more money*") and then without any pause AP continues: ⇒ *Er leiht ihm kein Geld mehr* (Engl.: "hm *he is lending him no more money*") (Parts of items 4 and 6 are perseverated.)
9. Es wurde gesagt, dass immer mehr Menschen Hunger leiden (Engl.: "It has been said that more and more persons are starving/suffering from hunger") ⇒ *Er leiht ihm kein Geld mehr* (Engl.: "*He is lending him no more money*") and then without any pause AP continues and repeats the perseverated utterance twice: ⇒ *Er leiht ihm kein***en*** Geld mehr*

(Engl.: "*He is lending him no* (incorrect case marking: kein ⇒ keinen) *more money*") ⇒ Er leiht ihm von Gel// kein Geld mehr ab- ab (Engl.: "*He is lending him from money// no more money up- up*" (verb particle from item 8)) (Parts of items 4, 6 and 8 are perseverated)
10. Der Mann, der unser Auto kaufte, ist seit gestern verheiratet (Engl.: "The man, who bought our car, is married since yesterday") ⇒ Uh hm *er leiht ihm keine Geld mehr ab* (Engl.: "*He is lending him no* (incorrect case marking: kein ⇒ keine) *more money*") Ex. repeats stimulus sentence: ⇒ *Er* ~ *von Geld mehr abholt* (Engl.: "*He* ~ *from money more is picking up*") and then without any pause AP continues: ⇒ Es konnt *ihm kein Geld mehr ab-ab hal// holt* (Engl.: "It could *him no money more up- up picking// picking*" (phonological error which is immediately self-corrected: holt ⇒ hal-; the word order in German for "picking up" is "up+picking")) (Parts of items 4, 6 and 8 are perseverated).
Items 5 to 10 were presented again to AP, however they were not included in the test scoring:
5. ⇒ *Er* lässt sie für *Geld mehr* die –die hel-// hab// gerne die Haare *ab*schneiden" (Engl.: "*He* is letting her for *money more* the- the hel- (? Geld = money)// have// very much to cut *off* the hair") (Parts of items 3 or 8 ("ab"), 4 and 5 are perseverated.)
6. ⇒ *Er lässt sie ihm* ~ *keine Geld mehr abzuschneiden* bitte (Engl.: "*He is letting her (to) him* ~ *no* (incorrect case marking: kein ⇒ keine) *money more* to *cut off* please") (Parts of items 4 and 5 are perseverated.)
7. ⇒ *Er lässt nichts sich die Geld mehr abzu*stellen uh hm (Engl.: "*He is letting nothing himself the money more* to switch *off*" (incorrect gender for the article for money: "Geld" requires the neuter gender ("das") not the feminine ("die").)
8. ⇒ *Er lässt sie vom Bahnhof abzuholen* (Engl.: "*He is letting her from the train station topick up*") (Parts of 5 and 6 or 7 ("zu") are perseverated.)
9. ⇒ Es kommen immer mehr- *kein Geld mehr abholen* (Engl.: "There are coming always more *no money more (to) pick up*") (Parts of items 3 or 8 and 5 are perseverated.)
10. ⇒ *Er hat das// Er hat sich immer mehr – das Geld abholen* (Engl.: "*He has that/the// He has himself always more- the money (to) pick up*") (Parts of items 4, 8 and 9 are perseverated.)

Excerpts from the sentence naming task

Before going through the test items, the examiner wants to make sure of AP's visual acuity and asks her whether she needs eyeglasses to look at the stimuli. AP responds: "If I here - If I had eyeglasses, then I could read the ***children*** – I could the ***children*** – I could the children read (in German, the verb-final position of the verb is correct). (Note: The nurses reported that AP did not have eyeglasses. The word "children" is perseverated from the last item of the previous task.)

In extracts, the perseverative responses for the 10 items in the sentence naming task include:

Example:
1. Target: "The man is begging" or "the man is holding out his hat for alms"
AP: "Ah, that is the **man**// there I could – I could a- a- a- ***eyegla***// I could it/the (fem.) // here ***I could the (fem.) read. Could I the – the – the*** (fem.) **hat** ***I could let read- let read.*** (Note: The word "hat" requires the masculine form of the article, "der" in German.). ***The man could- could let the eyeglasses read//***"
(Ger.: "Aha, das ist der **Herr**// da könnte ich – könnte ich eine-eine- eine ***Bril***// konnte ich die // da ***könnte ich die lesen – konnte ich die- die- die*** **Hut** ***konnte ich lesen lassen- lesen lassen. Der Herr könnt- könnte die Brille lesen lassen//***")

2. Target: The woman is drying/cleaning a coffee pot /teapot (with a dish towel)"
AP: "Uh hm. What it . ***the eyeglasses - the eyeglasses leg-*** (second self-correction of a phonemic error: "lesen" ⇒ "leg-" which is immediately corrected ⇒ lesen) ***let read*** . ***What*** he already // ***eyeglasses already read – read*** uh hm ***eyeglasses already*** a read uh hm" [Ex.: "What is happening here?"] "***The eyeglasses already let*** go – ***already let go***" (Ger.: "Uh hm. Was es . ***die Brille – die Brille leg-// lesen lässt***. ***Was*** er schon// ***Brille schon lesen- lesen*** uh hm. ***Brille schon-*** eine Lese uh hm." [Ex.: "Was geschieht hier?"] "***Die Brille schon*** los ***lässt- schon los lässt***")

3. Target: "The boy is playing with the dog" *or* "The boy is feeding the dog"
AP: "Ah! That// Here is the **dog** – the ***dog – the – the uh hm could already – already ... he could read already*** still. Here is ***already*** then the-the donkey. ***The donkey could already*** necessary ***already // already necessarily read***"
(Ger.: "Aha! Das// Da ist der **Hund** – der ***Hund - der – der uh hm könnt schon- schon . könnte er schon*** noch ***lesen***. Da ist ***schon*** dann der-der Esel. ***Der Esel könnt schon-*** notwendig ***schon // schon notwendig lesen***.")

4. Target: "The man has caught a boot (with a/his fishing rod)"
AP: "***He could already necessarily read ↗. He could so necessarily read***." (AP repeats the utterance three more times) [Ex.: "What is that called?"] "That is a **boot** – a **buskin**" [Ex.: "What is happening here?"] "***He so necessary(il)y – he already so necessar(il)y- he could already necessarily*** **the buskin/boot**"
(Ger.: "***Der könnte schon notwendig lesen ↗. Der könnte schon notwendig lesen***" (AP repeats the utterance three more times)) [Ex.: "Wie nennt man das?] "Das ist ein **Stiefel**. – ein **Halbstiefel**" [Ex.: "Was passiert da?"] "Der so ***notwendig - der schon so notwendig- der könnte schon notwendig*** **den Halbstiefel**")

5. Target: "The boy has broken a glass"
AP: "Here uh hm . uh hm . yes . ***could already*** uh hm yes uh hm ***he could already*** take down ..." [Ex.: "What is happening here?"] "***Here one cannot take dow// down . It one cannot take down*** (repeated three times) from the – ***the dog***. It/Him ***one cannot take down***. That I have had. It is not possible. ..."
(Ger.: "Hier uh hm . uh hm . ja. ***könnt schon*** uh hm ja uh hm ***der könnte schon*** herunternehmen ..." [Ex.: "Was geschieht hier?"] "Da kann man nicht her- ***herunternehmen*** . Den ***kann man nicht herunternehmen- den kann man*** nichts ***herunternehmen*** von den – ***den Hund. Den kann man nicht hinunternehmen.*** Das habe ich gehabt. Das geht nicht. ...")

6. Target: "Father and son are playing Indians"
AP: "Ah! He is that// That is a **tree** ***down// Here one may not take down.// may not take anything down*** [Ex.: "What is happening here?"] "***He is . taking down***. Tied down" (Ger.: "herunter gebunden" (Engl.: "tied or bound down"). "***That/He may not take down*** . [One] may not do that. .. ***take that down*** ..." [Ex.: "But what's happening here?"] "That is like an **Indian**. So one ***may not take – take anything down***."
(Ger.: "Ah! Der ist das// Das ist ein **Baum** ***runter// Da darf man nicht hinunternehmen! Darf man nichts herunternehmen***" [Ex.: "Was geschieht da?"] "Der ist . ***runter nehmen*** herunter gebunden. ***Das darf*** [man] ***nicht herunternehmen"*** [Ex.: "Was geschieht aber da?"] "Das ist wie ein **Indianer** so derer – so derer ***darf*** man ***nichts herunternehmen – nehmen***")

7. Target: "The policeman is arresting a criminal"
AP: "***That is like an Indian. One may not take that***" [Ex.: "What is happening here?"] "***That is like an Indian. Here one may not take down***" (utterance repeated two more

times) [Ex.: What is going on?] "Ah! ***He-he may not*** the – the (feminine gender) // ***one may not take down-one may not take down***"
(Ger.: "***Das ist wie ein Indianer. Das darf man nicht nehmen.***" [Ex.: "Was geschieht da?"] "***Das ist wie ein Indianer. Da darf man nicht herunternehmen- darf man nicht herunternehmen – darf man nicht herunternehmen***" [Ex.: "Was geschieht da?"] "***Ah! Der-der darf*** die-die // ***darf man nicht herunternehmen- darf man nicht herunternehmen***")

8. Target: "Both of them are fighting" or "They are fighting with each other"
AP: "***Take down one may not ... one may not take*** ..uh hm ***one may down not take down***, she's said. ***That she may take. That she may not – that she [may] not do"*** [Ex.: "And what is happening here?"] "***Here one may not take down, she has said- she has said und that she can not// may she- she may take down, she has said*** uh hm".
(Ger.: "***Herunter nehmen darf man nicht... darf man nicht nehmen*** uh hm ***darf man herunter nicht herunternehmen*** .. hat's gesagt. ***Das darf sie nehmen Das darf sie nicht- das [darf] sie nicht machen"*** [Ex.: "Und was geschieht da?"] "***Da darf man nicht herunternehmen, hat sie gesagt – hat sie gesagt und das kann sie nicht// darf sie- darf sie herunternehmen, hat sie gesagt*** uh hm.")

9. Target: "The teacher is explaining something to the girl on the blackboard" or "The teacher is writing something on the blackboard for the girl"
AP: "What is here? That is like she's – like her/she in the **school**, ***she has said, in the school she has said and that she may// ... school . she may not// that she may take down, she has said***" [Ex.: "What is happening?"] "That is like a **Mrs. teacher** and ***one may take*** up//***down, she has said.***"
(Ger.: "Was ist da? Das ist wie's- wie die in die **Schule**, ***hat sie gesagt, in die Schule, hat sie gesagt und das darf sie// ... Schule . darf sie nicht// das darf sie herunternehmen, hat sie gesagt***" [Ex.: "Was geschieht da?"] "Das ist wie eine **Frau Lehrer**[in] und ***darf man*** herauf// ***herunternehmen, hat sie gesagt***")

10. Target: "The man is lying on a couch, reading a newspaper and smoking a pipe"
AP: "***That one may not take down, she has said. Can she take down, she has said*** uh hm . uh hm. ." [Ex.: "What is happening here?"] "That is like... like a // that ***one cannot take down . she has said.// what she can take down.*** I know - do not know, ***what she [can] take down.*** [Ex.: "What is going on here?"] "ah that- ***that she may take*** out – ***down*** // That one can .. like a – like a a- a- a- - a **pipe** ***one can take down*** uh hm."
(Ger.: "***Das darf man nicht herunternehmen, hat sie gesagt. Kann sie herunternehmen, hat sie gesagt*** uh hm . uh hm ." [Ex.: "Was geschieht da?"] "Das ist wie ...wie eine// das ***kann man nicht herunternehmen, hat sie gesagt// was sie herunternehmen [kann].*** Das weiß ich- weiß nicht, ***was herunternehmen***" [Ex.: "Was geschieht da?"] "Ah das- ***das darf*** sie heraus- ***herunternehmen//*** Das kann man .. wie ein – wie eine ... eine ... eine ... eine **Pfeife** ***darf man herunternehmen*** uh hm.")

APHASIOLOGY, 2007, 21 (10/11), 1114–1142

Psychology Press
Taylor & Francis Group

Syntax detached from semantics: Qualitative analysis of examples of verbal perseveration from a transcortical sensory aphasic patient

Jacqueline Stark

Austrian Academy of Sciences, Vienna

Background: An individual showing an intricate pattern of errors as a consequence of brain damage affords the clinician an opportunity to analyse language data, the *exact* pattern of which would be impossible to generate. This situation is particularly valuable when the phenomenon to be investigated is unique. This is the case with verbal perseveration. It does not always occur in aphasia. However, when it does, qualitative analysis of the perseveratory errors sheds light on the individual's underlying disorder(s).
Aims: In this paper verbal perseverative errors produced by a client with transcortical sensory aphasia during routine language testing are analysed. The aim of this study is to characterise the types of perseverative responses and related phenomena and to arrive at an understanding of the mechanisms of the underlying disorders on the various linguistic levels.
Methods & Procedures: Client MH, clinically diagnosed as having transcortical sensory aphasia, was administered several language tests. The language data were transcribed and a qualitative analysis of her oral language production was performed with particular emphasis on perseverative and paraphasic responses of the semantic, syntactic, and ideational error types.
Outcomes & Results: Verbal perseveration is the most prominent symptom in client MH's language data. The perseveratory errors display a complex development within a task (interstimuli), across tasks and task types and they extend over 2 days. The produced perseverations in the different tasks vary in their linguistic complexity from word-level to text-level responses. Analysis of MH's perseverative errors within the framework of Levelt's (1993) model of language production and comprehension with modifications from Dietrich (2002) reveals impairment to several processing components of the conceptualiser: monitoring, discourse processing, message generation, and lexical/semantic aspects of the lexicon.
Conclusions: The pattern of perseveratory errors in client MH lends support to the relative preservation of grammatical encoding, phonological encoding, and articulation. She produced well-articulated, grammatically correct utterances. However, her responses were semantically inadequate and she showed word retrieval deficits. Pre- and post-production monitoring was impaired for semantic aspects of the utterances. Few phonological errors were made, and they were immediately corrected by MH. Self-corrections were not observed for semantically inadequate and contradictory responses.

Address correspondence to: Jacqueline Stark PhD, Department of Linguistics and Communication Research, Austrian Academy of Sciences, Kegelgasse 27 / 3rd Floor, A - 1030 Vienna, Austria. E-mail: jacqueline-ann.stark@univie.ac.at

The language data reported on in this paper are discussed in detail in German in my unpublished PhD thesis (Stark, 1984). I would like to express special thanks to Karin Geisler, Leena Martin, Christiane Pons, and Heinz Karl Stark for their constructive comments and assistance on versions of this paper. I would also like to thank the reviewers of this paper for their valuable critique and suggestions.

http://www.psypress.com/aphasiology DOI: 10.1080/02687030701198429

This case report focuses on a characterisation of complex interactions among perseveratory responses produced by an individual with transcortical sensory aphasia (TSA). Intricate examples of verbal perseveration—semantic perseverations, perseverations of syntactic form, and ideational perseverations—are discussed with reference to how some linguistic "levels" can be affected (semantic) while others are intact in language production (phonological, syntactic). Analysis of the examples reveals that, although utterances are semantically inadequate, they are syntactically well formed.

Various studies have explored the dissociations or disconnection of different domains of language such as syntax, phonology, and semantics, in aphasic clients. In this regard, the research on agrammatism illustrates how analysis of qualitative language data and results from experimental studies has refined the accounts of agrammatism. Based on language data from agrammatic clients, relevant associations and dissociations among the symptoms have led to a better understanding of the agrammatic patient's processing difficulties and better-preserved language functions. Dissociations across modalities—e.g., spontaneous speech and language comprehension—and dissociations between morphology and syntax are two areas of intense investigation.

With regard to possible dissociations among language domains, another area of aphasia research that has drawn a great deal of attention concerns transcortical sensory aphasia (TSA). A dissociation between syntactic and semantic abilities has been posited by several authors for TSA.

TRANSCORTICAL SENSORY APHASIA OR ECHOLALIC APHASIA

Preserved or relatively intact repetition of language stimuli varying in complexity is the hallmark symptom of TSA. Good performance on repetition tasks contrasts with impairment on other tasks. Other clinical features of TSA include fluent, paraphasic, and empty spontaneous speech, impaired auditory comprehension, and impaired naming. Two symptoms related to perseveration have also been cited to occur in TSA, namely echolalia and completion phenomenon. Echolalia is "the repetition of the investigator's utterances with or without mild changes in position and choice of words" (Huber, Poeck, & Weniger, 1982, p. 80), and the completion phenomenon is an almost automatic provision of the end of an utterance initiated by the investigator. For the modalities reading and writing, the abilities of clients with TSA can vary within and across these modalities. According to Benson (1979), reading aloud can be preserved. (See Berthier, 1999; Branch Coslett, Roeltgen, Gonzalez-Rothi, & Heilman, 1987; Cimini-Knight, Hollingsworth, & Gonzalez-Rothi, 2005; Gonzalez-Rothi, 1997, for comprehensive descriptions of transcortical aphasias.)

Regarding how TSA comes about, numerous researchers—starting with Wernicke (1874) and Lichtheim (1885)—have put forward explanations. Rubens and Kertesz (1983) postulate "a plausible disconnection between the auditory input and the semantic processes that was postulated by Lichtheim" (p. 264). In the face of severely impaired language comprehension in TSA, "phonological and syntactic processing is not affected and repetition is very good. These behavioural features correlated with the relatively well-preserved temporoparietal, perisylvian connections necessary for syntactic and phonological function and repetition, and involvement of the posterior association areas important for comprehension" (Rubens & Kertesz, 1983, p. 264).

Branch Coslett et al. (1987) provide evidence for two subtypes of transcortical sensory aphasia.[1] Characterisation of these subtypes is based on the assumption that repetition is accomplished by at least two mechanisms: (a) a lexical repetition mechanism and (b) a direct, nonlexical repetition mechanism. The lexical processes involve "those processes mediating visual or auditory recognition and production that involve the recognition and subsequent activation of stored word representations" (Branch Coslett et al., 1987, p. 363). The direct, nonlexical repetition processes—which do not depend on the recognition of stored word representations—refer to "auditory analysis, phonologic decoding, and 'direct' phonologic encoding from immediate memory" (p. 363). The two subtypes are (I) TSA with lexical repetition and (II) TSA with nonlexical repetition. For this discussion, the relevant point is the type of errors that are postulated by damage to each mechanism. Clients with type I TSA with lexical repetition produce verbal paraphasias, whereas clients with type II TSA with nonlexical repetition produce verbal and phonemic paraphasias.

SELECTED STUDIES ON DISSOCIATIONS IN TSA

Berndt, Basili, and Caramazza (1987) discuss a case of TSA showing dissociation between intact syntactic and phonological processing and impaired semantic processing. Their client's spontaneous sentence production is characterised as being syntactically well formed but empty, and as containing semantic errors and few phonemic errors. Surface syntax was intact in both sentence repetition and sentence completion tasks.

In the study by Branch Coslett et al. (1987), patients classified as Group I (TSA with lexical repetition) showed a dissociation of semantics from the lexical system. When reading sentences aloud they showed evidence of automatic syntactic processing: syntactically incorrect sentences were recognised as incorrect. However, the patients in Group I performed differently on the task of correcting the errors in the sentences. In contrast, patients in Group II (TSA with nonlexical repetition) did not show evidence of automatic, online syntactic processing (see also Berthier, 1991). This illustrates that the patients in Group II not only showed a dissociation of semantics from linguistic input, "they also had an impairment of lexical and syntactic processing mechanisms. This impairment was manifested in their production of literal and verbal paraphasias" (Branch Coslett et al., 1987, p. 374).

Dogil, Haider, Schaner-Wolles, and Husmann (1995) present a case study of an individual with transcortical sensory aphasia who showed preserved competence in the area of core syntax, but exhibited problems accessing the semantically controlled parts of the lexical entries. The authors discuss their client's corrective repetitions of sentences as demonstrating "his sensitivity to *syntactically autonomous, obligatory dependency relations* that typically occur with antecedent-governed agreement relations" (p. 577). (The features gender, number, and person are considered typical

[1] Goldstein (1915) also postulated two types of transcortical sensory aphasia in his monograph on the transcortical aphasias.

agreement features.) The authors concluded that "this provides evidence for the modular processing of information stored with a lexical item. Categorical and morphosyntactic properties are accessible, while access to other components of the lexical entries (argument- structure, sub-categorization and conceptual structure) is impaired" (p. 595).

Studies based on different clinical populations (dementia: Kempler, Curtiss, & Jackson, 1987; Whitaker, 1976) have also emphasised the relative preservation of syntactic ability in the context of impaired semantic functions. In this regard, Whitaker's (1976) patient also revealed perseveratory responses and related phenomena including echolalia and completion phenomena.

In summary, although the TSA clients discussed in the aforementioned studies demonstrate dissociation between syntactic and semantic abilities in the context of relatively preserved repetition, their language performance differs in certain respects from case to case. For this reason, each additional case report adds to our knowledge base and is valuable in arriving at a comprehensive understanding of the underlying mechanisms. The particular feature that makes this case stand out is the prominence of the phenomenon of perseveration.

ASSUMPTIONS ON MH'S LANGUAGE-PROCESSING DEFICITS WITHIN THE FRAMEWORK OF A LANGUAGE-PROCESSING MODEL

Before discussing the assumptions with regard to MH's language-processing difficulties, a brief summary will be given of the structure of the speech-processing system as described by Levelt (1993). Figure 1 provides the schematic representation of the subcomponents of the speech-processing system with minor modifications based on the model put forward in Dietrich (2002). The modification to Levelt's model is the inclusion of *concepts* in the lexicon with a link to the conceptualiser. In Dietrich's schematic representation, a bidirectional arrow links concepts—which are considered to be part of the lexicon system as a store of knowledge—to a part of the conceptualiser that he describes as being responsible for micro-planning including: selection, propositional structuring, and determination of topic/focus (Dietrich, 2002, p. 124).

Levelt (1993) postulates as highest processing level the conceptualiser, which contains the three subcomponents: message generation, monitoring, and discourse processing. The function of the conceptualiser is manifold:

(a) It subserves the micro- and macro-planning of a communicative intention (quaestio), selecting the relevant information to be expressed.
(b) It is responsible for generating a preverbal message.
(c) It is responsible for monitoring the input from the parser and discourse processing and for controlling the state of the message generation process (feed-forward and feed-backwards).

The output of the conceptualiser is a preverbal message.

Based on the information coming from the conceptualiser, grammatical encoding is performed. A syntactic structure is built up in interaction with the lexicon (lemmas). The resulting surface structure is the input for the phonological encoding component which, based on information from the lexicon (lexemes), builds a phonetic articulatory plan for the articulator. The articulator maps the phonetic

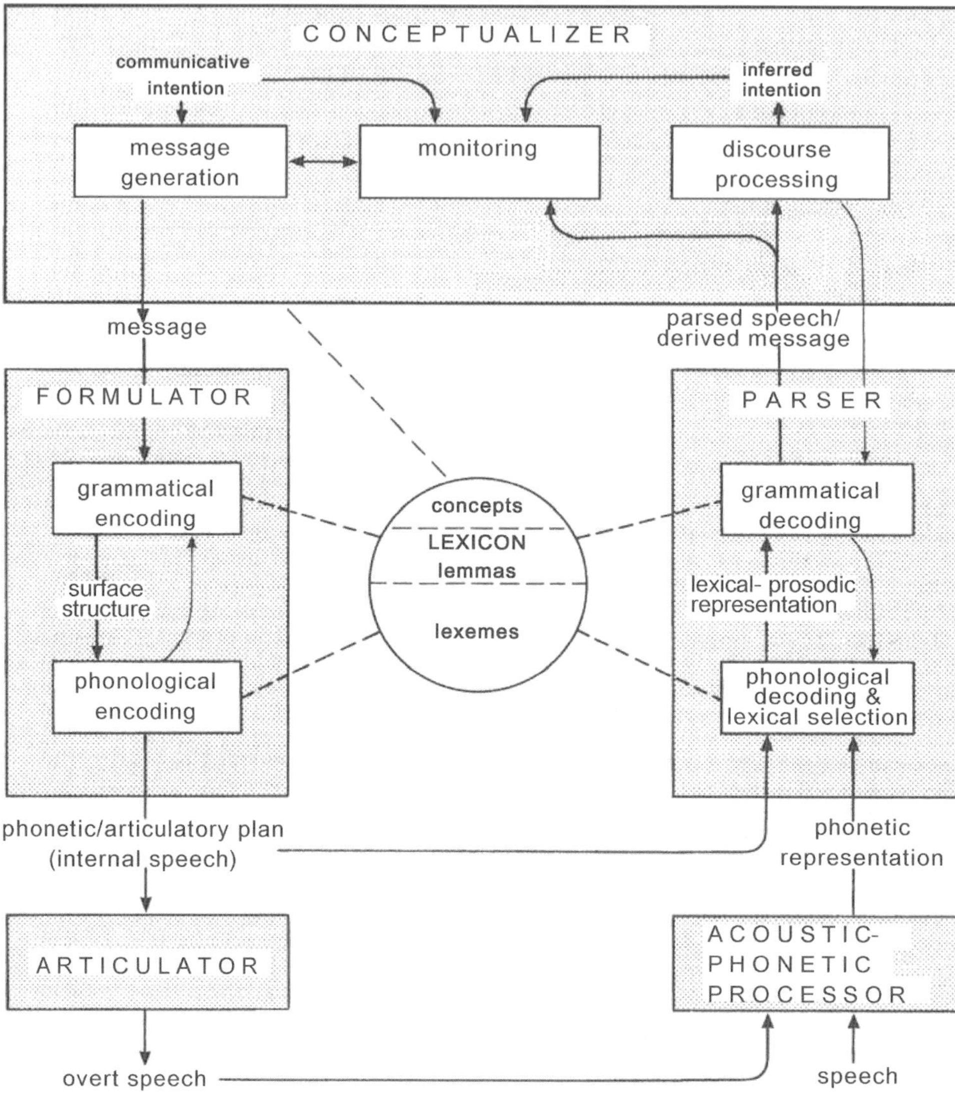

Figure 1. A modified version of Levelt's (1993) model of the processing components involved in spoken language use with minor adaptations by Dietrich (2002).

information onto programs of motor control. The output of the articulator is overt speech.

On the comprehension side, overt speech is analysed by the acoustic phonetic processor. In the parser component, phonological decoding as well as grammatical decoding of the input (internal and overt speech of the speaker, also speech from other speakers) is carried out. The derived message or the parsed speech is the output of the parser and is fed into the discourse-processing component of the conceptualiser and to the monitoring component.

The following assumptions will be evaluated based on the framework of Levelt's (1993) model of language production and comprehension and Dietrich's (2002) adapted model when interpreting qualitative aspects of MH's language performance:

1. If *phonological encoding* and *articulation* are intact, auditory analysis and phonological processing should be preserved.
2. Under the assumption that the lexicon contains concepts, lemmas, and lexemes (see
3. Dietrich, 2002), if *semantic processing* is intact, retrieval of semantically adequate lemmas from the lexicon should be intact for the building up of the *syntactic structures* by the *grammatical encoding* of the formulator.
4. If *grammatical encoding* is intact, syntactic processing should be preserved, i.e., the surface structures of the produced utterances should be syntactically correct, i.e., well formed.
5. If the *message generator* is intact, it will send conceptually correct messages to the formulator.
6. If *monitoring* is intact, the speaker should be able to repair, prepair, and/or verbally reject syntactically incorrect and/or semantically inadequate utterances as incorrect or anomalous.

PATIENT INFORMATION

MH is a right-handed, 42-year-old female high-school graduate who, following a left carotid angiography, developed global aphasia and right hemiplegia. The incident is assumed to be due to incompatibility with the contrast agent used. Her hemiplegia subsided quickly, as did her clouding of consciousness. The results from an EEG examination were abnormal, with a focus in the left parieto-temporal area. A radioisotope scan performed 1 week post aphasia onset showed an uptake in the left fronto-parietal area.

At 4 weeks post onset, MH was alert and fully oriented. With regard to her language production, MH produced fluent paraphasic speech. Her speed of language production was at times slow; otherwise her prosody and articulation were normal. Her auditory comprehension was moderately impaired. Overall, the most striking features of MH's oral language production were verbal perseverative and echolalic responses.

Follow-up information provided by her husband at 1 year post onset revealed that MH had recovered almost completely from her aphasia. Her family noted that she had minimal and infrequent word-finding difficulties.

METHOD

Language testing was done 4 weeks post onset on three consecutive days. The language parameters tested encompassed:

- *Spontaneous speech*: interview.
- *Narrative speech*: picture descriptions (Cookie Theft from the BDAE, Goodglass & Kaplan, 1983; three pictures from Norden, 1953).
- *Auditory comprehension*: Yes–No questions; Story Completion Test (SCT) (Goodglass, Berko Gleason, Bernholtz, & Hyde, 1972).
- *Naming*: visual confrontation naming (coloured drawings).
- *Repetition*: words, sentences.
- *Fluency*: animals, letter "m".

All tasks were tape recorded and transcribed by the examiner.[2] The corpus of this paper is an interlinear transcription of the transcribed test data consisting of 1816 words produced by MH resulting in a 478-line transcription, which is broken into an interlinear transcription consisting of MH's original German responses and an English translation. This transcription includes all productions of the client and the examiner.

Types of perseveration analysed

A *perseveration* is the unintentional production of a linguistic unit—phoneme, word, phrase, sentence, or concept—which, based on contextual information, has been previously produced by the speaker, read by the speaker, heard or seen by the speaker (auditorily or visually perceived, i.e., "picked up" when the speaker is not actively attending to speech) (see Stark, 2007 this issue, the historical review of perseveration). Crucial for deciding whether it is a perseveration is that it must be possible to establish a relationship between the previous production of the particular unit and the actual production.

Furthermore, the perseverative response is usually inappropriate in the context in which it is repeated. A repetition of a word *anywhere* in the corpus is not a perseveration.

The following perseverative error types are differentiated:

- *Verbal perseveration*: In this case the perseverated unit is a single word that shows no clear direct semantic relationship to the expected target word.
- *Semantic perseveration*: In the case of a semantic perseveration, a single word is perseverated which shows a semantic relation or a semantic feature to the expected target word.
- *Perseverations of syntactic form* refer to the perseveration of previously produced types of syntactic construction, which can be appropriate or not in the subsequent utterances. For example, the imperative syntactic structure construction is perseverated and produced in place of an active declarative target sentence.
- *Semanto-syntactic perseverations* are a variant of the syntactic perseverations. In this type of error it is the perseveration of the meaning of a syntactic unit, i.e., a "syntagma", which is perseverated as a *unit* and not individual words of the phrase, e.g.: "to be unhappy (about something)" ("copula + adjective phrase (+ prepositional phrase").

An *ideational perseveration* constitutes a more complex error, which usually shows a longer history of development. The essence of an ideational perseveration is that the concept or idea of an earlier response is carried over to subsequent responses and, in the process of being perseverated, the resulting utterance becomes semantically anomalous or even contradictory in the new context, e.g., "to be unhappy about something " → "to be happy about something". In ideational perseverations, concepts and thoughts are perseverated over several task items or from one task or text to another. (See the historical survey by Stark, 2007 this issue. See also Pick, 1906.) It must be stressed that several perseverative responses require a multiple classification: a previously produced verbal or semantic paraphasia, a

[2] MH was transferred to a hospital nearer to her home. For this reason testing could not be continued.

semantic perseveration, syntactic perseveration of form and/or semanto-syntactic perseveration can be part of an ideational perseveration.

RESULTS

The emphasis in this paper is on qualitative aspects of the perseverative responses produced by MH. However, before discussing these selected distinctive aspects of MH's intricate pattern of verbal perseveratory responses, a summary of the results for speech production, naming, repetition, and the SCT will be given.

Quantitative analysis of MH's spoken utterances reveals that out of the 1816 words constituting her language corpus, 385 words (21%) were produced in the context of perseverative responses and 440 words (24 %) of the corpus were echolalic responses. Taken together, these two symptoms make up almost half of her productions. For the repetition of single words ($n = 40$) she correctly repeated the words, with 100% accuracy. The results for naming and for the SCT are given in Table 1 and Table 2, respectively. Tables 3 to 6 provide an overview of the various errors for the corpus as a whole.

A total of 70% of the objects were named correctly and 15% of the responses were recurrent perseverations with an interstimulus interval ranging from two to eight items. In contrast, MH's responses to the more complex SCT test stimuli—this task requires that the subject understands the story to be completed and produces a semantically adequate response—show an decrease in number of correct responses (43%), as well as an increase in the number of responses characterised as perseverations (47%). For both tasks, additional perseveration and echolalia accompanied the responses.

Phonology

MH's performance with regard to phonological processing is intact: auditory analysis, phonemic decoding, activation of the output auditory word form, and phonemic encoding.

MH's repetition of words and sentences is intact. The word repetition lists, with which MH had no difficulties, consisted of linguistically structured items comprising one to six syllables. They ranged from monomorphemic to compound words consisting of several morphemes and the phonemic structure of the items increased in complexity from, e.g., "Leicht" (Engl.: "light") to "Leicht+gläub+ig+keit" (Engl.: "gullibility"), or "Soldat" (Engl.: "soldier") to "Beruf+s+soldat+en+stand" (Engl.: "professional soldier guild").

TABLE 1
Object naming of coloured drawings two ($n = 40$)

	Correct	*Incorrect*	*Semantic paraphasia*	*Perseverative*	***Perseveration produced after other response was given ****
Sample 1 ($n = 20$)	14/20	–	2/20	4/20	3 cases
Sample 2 ($n = 20$)	14/20	2/20	2/20	2/20	7 cases
Total sample ($n = 40$)	28/40 (70%)	2/40 (5%)	4/40 (10%)	6/40 (15%)	10 cases

TABLE 2
Error pattern for the Story Completion Test (Goodglass et al., 1972)

	Correct response	*Incorrect*	*Perseverative response*	*Plus accompanying echolalia**	*Plus accompanying perseveration***
Sample 1(1a–8b) (*n* = 16 items)	7/16	1/16	8/16	5	2
Sample 2 (8a–14b) (*n* = 14 items)	6/14	214	6/14	7	1
Total	13/30 (43%)	3/30 (10%)	14/30 (47%)	12	3

* In addition to a response that was correct, incorrect, or perseverative, echolalia accompanied her response. ** In addition to a response that was correct, incorrect, or perseverative, MH's response was accompanied by perseveration.

In the entire corpus, only three phonemic errors were observed and immediately self-corrected. In three further examples that were not self-corrected, lexical interference played a role, i.e., the errors could be due to a perseverative blend of two forms or interference due to the similarity of the two forms:

1. (several items earlier MH could only repeat the word "Netz" (Engl.: "net")) Nets (Engl.: "net") is produced for "Nest" and;
2. a response later: "Nets"(Engl.: "net") is produced instead of Nest (Engl.: "nest") (produced twice);

TABLE 3
Verbal/lexical perseverations produced by MH

Target	*Perseveration*	*Task*	*Linguistic span*
the Mr.[Smith] G.: der Herr[Schmidt]	the dog G.: der Hund	SCT	intertextual, inter-item
the mother G.: die Mutter	the dog G.: der Hund	SCT	intertextual, intertextual
net G.: Netz	airplane G.: Flieger	N	intersentential, inter-item
balls G.: Bälle	watch G.: Uhr	N	intersentential (4 items in-between)
girl G.: Mädchen	doll G.: Puppe, dann (+)	N	intersentential (intratextual)
zoo G.: Zoo	nest G.: Nest	N	intersentential, inter-item
soldier G.: Soldat	son G.: Sohn	SCT	intertextual (1 text in-between)
bitten G.: gebissen	run over G.: überfahren	SCT	intertextual, inter-item
the boy G.: der Bub	the dog G.: der Hund	SCT	intertextual, inter-item
house G.: Haus	car G.: Auto	SCT	intertextual, inter-item

G: original German response; SCT: story completion test; N: naming task.

TABLE 4
Semantic paraphasias produced by MH

Target (reconstructed)	*Paraphasia*	*Task*	*Relation between target and paraphasia*	*Differences between paraphasia and target*
pipe	cigarette G.: Zigarette	SCT	- same category	(− smoking utensil)
cat	mouse G.: Maus	PS	- same category - polarity - associate / situative	
squirrel	rabbit G.: Hase	N	- same category - visual similarity	(− bushy tail; multiple)
(shopping) bag	pail G.: Kübel	N	- same category - visual similarity	(number of handles) pail: 1 handle bag: 2 handles
ball (s)	balloon G.: (Luft)ballon	N	- same category - visual similarity	(+opening) (+string)
scallywag	brat G.:Zornpinkel	Binet P.	- character labelling - negative	(+angry)
open	closed G.: geschlossen	N	- antonym	(− open)
turn on	turn off G.: abschalten	SCT	- antonym	(− function)
hides	holes up G.: verkriecht	Binet P.	- to keep hidden: to make oneself invisible, result, activity	(+hidden)
cries	carries on G.: bitzelt	Binet P.	- expression of emotion	(+angry)
overflows	falls over G.: umstürzt	CTP	- change of position	
warns (frightens)	frightens off G.: abschreckt	CTP	to draw attention to (signal)	(+intense)
wipe up (turn off)	slow down G.: bremsen	CTP	to put an end to an activity (brake: for mechanical objects: change the speed	
expressive	articulated G: artikulierte	N	form of expression: visible – gesticulate	
carrot	red beet root G.: rote Rübe	N	same category	(+round) (− long)
different colours	various colour names	N	same category	

SCT: story completion test; PS: picture story; N: Naming; Binet P.: Binet picture description; CTP: Cookie Theft picture.

3. knabbern (Engl.: "nibble on") (previously produced: "Das Eichhörnchen knabbert" (Engl.: "The squirrel is nibbling") // schnappen (Engl.:"snap") → "Der Fisch *schnappert" (Engl.: "The fish is *snapping(?)).

Morphology

MH's performance with respect to morphology is affected only when she perseverates a morpheme. Once again, these perseverations are observed during episodes of word-finding difficulty. Two neologisms were produced in the whole

TABLE 5
Semantic perseverations produced by MH

Target	*Perseveration*	*Source of error*	*Semantic relation (between context or target and perseveration)*	*Linguistic span*
grass G.: Rasen/Gras	lawn mower G.: Rasenmäher	SCT: lawn mower	situative object instrument	Intersentential (intratext.)
Johanna	Hans	SCT: Hans	(− fem)	Intertextual (1 SCT item in-between.)
to want, to take G.: wollen, nehmen	to fall G.: stürzen	Cookie Theft Picture: falls over	similar activity movement umfallen, stürzen	(intratextual)
does not pay attention G.: passt nicht auf	is startled G.: erschrickt	"abschreckt" = semantic paraphasia	(+become attentive)	intratextual.
to not let G.: (nicht) lassen	to not hold G.: (nicht) halten	picture description: slow down = semantic paraphasia	context and perseveration similar activity	intratextual
to wipe up G.: aufwischen	to crash G.: abstürzen **	picture description: water "umstürzt" = semantic paraphasia	context and perseveration similar activity	intratextual
cat G.: Katze	mouse G.: Maus	picture story: mouse = semantic paraphasia	same situative and associative category	intratextual.
door G.: Tür	table G.: Tisch	naming: table	same category, material composition: made out of wood	intersentential (3 items in-between)
stronger G.: stärker	taller G.: größer	SCT: larger (größer)	similar attributes	intertextual, inter-item
red feet G.: rote Füsse	red boots G.: rote Stiefel	naming: red boots	same colour (on the drawing to be named); visual similarity	intersentential, inter-item
woman G.: Frau	aunt, sister in law G.: Tante, Schwägerin	Kinship terms were tested on a previous day (several semantic paraphasias)	(+animate, +fem.)	intertextual, inter-item

corpus. The first example "*schnappert" has already been cited, and the second example derives from a perseveration of an inseparable prefix "*ent-*"(English meaning: "establishment or entry into a new state or abandonment of an old state"): "**ent*-zürnt" for "*er*-zürnt" (Engl.: "angry"). The history of this production—which can also be classified as a semanto-syntactic perseveration—is:

Example 1: "*ent*-rüstet" (Engl.: "indignant")
"*ent*-fällt" (produced twice) (Engl.: "escape", "something escapes him"))
"*ent*-rüstet" (Engl.: "indignant")
"**ent*-zürnt" (Engl.: "*angry")
"**ent*-zürnt" (Engl.: "*angry")
"*ent*-rüstet" (Engl.: "indignant")
"*er*-staunt" (Engl.: "amazed", "taken aback")

TABLE 6
Ideational perseverations produced by MH

Type I Contradictions	*Type II a Real world*	*Type II b Association*	*Task*	*Type of original perseveration*	*Simple (S) or complex (C) origin*
X			Spont. Sp.	semanto-syntact. pers.	S
X	X		PD	semanto-syntact. pers.	C
	X		PD	syntactic pers. form	C
	X		SCT	syntactic pers. form	C
		X	SCT	semantically anomalous	S
	X		SCT	semantically anomalous	S
X	X		SCT	lexical, syntactic pers. (semantically anomalous)	C
	X		SCT	syntactic pers. form	C
		X	PD	morphological (multiple)	C
	X		PD	semantic (multiple)	C
X			PD	semantic paraphasia semantic (multiple)	C
X	X	X	PS	semantic (multiple)	C
	X		N	lexical, semanto-syntactic pers.	S?
	X		N	lexical (multiple)	S
	X	X	SCT	semantically anomalous	C
	X	(X)	SCT	(enumerating) lexical semanto-syntact. pers.	C
X	(X)		SCT	(comprehension difficulties) multiple	C
	X		SCT	semanto-syntact. pers. multiple	C
		X	SCT	lexical (multiple)	C
X	X	(X)	SCT	lexical (multiple)	C
	X	(X)	N	semantic	S

Spont.Sp.: Spontaneous speech; SCT: Story Completion Test; PD: picture description; PS: picture story.

This sequence extends over two picture descriptions.

Another example requiring a faceted/multiple classification in a naming task is:

Example 2: MH: “Und das ist eine *Puppe*, und das ist ein *Püppchen* (‘Mädchen’) und das Mädchen spielt mit der Puppe” (Engl.: “And that is a *doll* and that is a *little doll* (‘girl’) and the girl is playing with the doll”)

This perseverative response could stem from a perseveration of a morpheme (that correctly receives an umlaut “u” when combined with the diminutive suffix “-chen”) or it is a lexical error.[3]

Perseverative responses affecting other morphological categories were observed for the plural forms, both for nouns and verb inflections, gender, and comparative “–er”. In all of these cases the errors resulted from word-finding difficulties and also when MH was experiencing difficulties understanding the investigator. The

[3] The word “Püppchen” is also a negative reference to a woman who wants to look like a girl.

perseverations resulted in semantically inadequate or contradictory utterances when they were produced as part of a larger perseverative episode.

Syntax

The surface structures of MH's utterances were syntactically well formed. Her use of various sentence types was not restricted. She produced simple and complex sentences with a length of up to 13 words. Moreover, she completed sentences that were begun by the investigator (completion phenomenon); she broke off sentences as soon as a syntactic error was made and she corrected them spontaneously. Two examples are:

Example 3: "Die Tochter/: f-// Der Tochter fällt etwas hinunter" (Engl.: "The daughter (nominative case) f-// The daughter (dative case (= correct) something is falling down on/from her"

Example 4: "Der Mann pass// hörte den Zug nicht. Es passierte … Es passierte mit ihm, dass er sich nicht beruhigen konnte" (Engl.: "The man happ// did not hear the train. It happened… It happened with him that he could not calm himself down" (Target: The man was run over by the train)

In both examples, the dative case is required: "der Tochter" and "dem Mann". In the first case MH corrected the case error and in the second example she produced another verb that matched the case of the produced noun phrase. Examples affecting morphosyntactic aspects are included in the morphology section.

Although MH produced grammatically correct utterances, she also produced intricate syntactic perseverations, which are classified as perseverations of syntactic form (i.e., syntactic constructions). Exemplars of this error type can also make up part of an ideational perseveration when their history of origins is considered.

Perseveration of syntactic form

(a) Perseveration of the imperative construction (from Picture description and SCT):

Example 5: Picture description

MH: "***Die Mutter sagt***: ***Pass auf, dass dir nichts*** // ***verl*** : ***umfällt***// ::"
(Engl.: "The mother says: Be careful / that nothing / ver // : falls over on you::"
Target: Ger.: "Kinder passt auf, dass euch nichts passiert!"
Engl.: "Children be careful that nothing happens to you!"

SCT
MH: "***Pass auf, damit dir nichts geschieht***!" (Engl.: "Be careful so that nothing happens to you!")
SCT Target: Ger.: "Setz dich nieder!"
Engl.: "Sit (yourself) down!"

MH: "***Pass auf, damit dir nichts passiert***." (Engl.: "Be careful so that nothing happens to you!")

SCT Target: Ger.: "Komm herein!"
Engl.: "Come in!"

MH: "***Folge mir, damit dir nichts passiert***!" (Engl.: "Follow me so that nothing happens to you!" (repetition of the item)
SCT Target: Ger.: "Komm herein!"
Engl.: "Come in!"

MH: "***Trink sie, damit // damit / du gesund bleibst***!" (Engl.: "Drink it so that // so that / you stay healthy!")
SCT Target: Ger.: "Trink die/deine Milch!"
Engl.: "Drink the/your milk!"

MH: "***Schneide den Rasenmäher, damit dir nichts passiert***!" (Engl.: "Cut the lawnmover so that nothing happens to you!)
SCT Target: Ger.: "Schneide den Rasen/das Gras!"
Engl.: "Cut the lawn /the grass!"

MH: "***Spiele nicht mit dem Spielzeug, sonst passiert dir etwas***!" (Engl.: "Do not play with the toy or else something will happen to you!)
SCT Target: Ger.: "Es (= das Baby) wird weinen"
Engl.: "It (Ger. Neuter gender = the baby) will cry".

In Example 5, the first response was produced as part of a picture description: "Blind man's bluff" and was not semantically adequate, because the dishes had already fallen off the table.

Minimally altered, the second response is perseverated from that picture description in response to the first item of the Story Completion Test. Several items are in between. The target construction for the next five SCT examples is an imperative construction. However, the expected imperative target form is different in each case. "Drink your milk, ..." is even a semantically adequate response. The additional phrase "so that nothing happens to you" is also perseverated from its first occurrence in a picture description and is carried over to each response and adapted in each story, until its form and meaning are changed in the last part of Example 5 to: "or else something will happen to you!". In the last occurrence, a simple declarative sentence construction is the target structure, however MH produced an adapted imperative construction. The negation "nothing" is now moved to the imperative clause and the second clause takes on a new semantically anomalous meaning for that item.

(b) Perseveration of several syntactic constructions: The next example of syntactic perseveration of form encompasses several syntactic constructions from the SCT, which are perseverated over several task items. The complexity of this example requires that several utterances are provided. Excerpts from the responses are provided below, although it must be stressed that Example 6 has an even longer perseverative history:

Example 6: Th.: "Johann ist in seinem Zimmer. Er glaubt, er höre seine Mutter rufen. Er geht die Treppen hinunter, um festzustellen, ob sie ihn gerufen hat/ und er fragt, was?" (Engl.: Th: "John is in his room. He thinks he hears his mother calling. He goes down the stairs to see if she has called him/ and he asks, what?")

MH: "***Er fragt, hast du mich gerufen***?" (Engl.: "He asks, ***Did you call me***?" (correct response to SCT item 6a)

MH: "***Hast Du deine Zähne wirklich geputzt***?" (Engl.: "***Have you really brushed your teeth***?") (correct response to SCT item 6b) Th.: "Johanna kann ihre Schuhe nicht finden. Ihre Mutter hat das Zimmer gerade aufgeräumt. Sie weiß, dass ihre Mutter sie irgendwo hingestellt hat. Also, fragt sie? Was?) (Engl.: "Jane cannot find her shoes. Her mother has just cleaned up the room. She knows that her mother has put them somewhere. So she asks, What?") (SCT item 7a)

MH: ***Hast du deine Schuhe*** irgendwo hingestellt? (Engl.: "***Have you put your shoes*** somewhere?"
Target Ger.: "***Wo hast du meine Schuhe hingestellt***?"
Engl.: "***Where have you put my shoes***?"

Th: "Und wenn sie genau wissen möchte wohin sie gestellt // gesteckt worden sind. Dann fragt man? (Engl.: Th.: "And if she would like to know exactly where they were put // placed? Then one asks?")

MH: "worden sind". Th: "Dann fragt man?" MH: "Dann fragt sie?.Hast du deine Schuhe // ::" (long pause) MH: "Hast du deine Schuhe") (Engl.: "Been put" Th.: Then one asks MH.: "then she asks? Have you your shoes // Have you your shoes :"
Target Ger.: "*Wo hast du meine Schuhe hingestellt?*"
Engl.: "***Where have you put my shoes***?"

Th.: "Der Vater hat das Spielzeug zerbrochen und er konnte es auch nicht reparieren. Aber sein Sohn reparierte es und der Vater wunderte sich wie. Daher fragte er? Was?") (Engl.: Th.: "The father broke the toy and he could not repair it. But his son repaired it and the father wondered how. And he asks, What?")

MH: "***Wie hast du das Spielzeug repariert?***" (Engl.: "How did you repair it?") (correct response for SCT item 7b)

Th: "Peter arbeitet jeden Samstag. Er arbeitete letzten Samstag auch. Und nächsten Samstag? Was?" (Engl.: "Peter works every Saturday. He worked last Saturday too. And next Saturday? What?")

MH: "Fragt er :: w***o hast Du Peters Spielzeug hingestellt?***" (Engl.: "He asks :: where have you put Peter's toy?")
Target Ger.: "***Er wird wieder arbeiten***."
Engl.: "***He will work again***"

(Examiner repeats SCT item 8a)

MH: "***Da wird sein dass er Peter frägt : Wo hast Du das Spielzeug von Peter hingestellt?***" (Engl.: "***It will be that he asks*** (present indicative with an overgeneralised umlaut) ***Peter : Where have you put Peter's toy***?")

MH: "***Wo hast Du Deine Zigarette geraucht?***" (Engl.: "***Where have you smoked your cigarette?***"
Target Ger.: "***Er wird seine Pfeife (wieder) rauchen.***"
Engl.: "***He will smoke his pipe (again).***"

This example requires multiple classification. Numerous error types are present, ranging from semantic paraphasias to several perseverations of the syntactic constructions. It also demonstrates that correct and incorrect responses alternate in an intricate manner:

SCT item 6a: correct response
SCT item 6b: correct response
SCT item 7a: perseveration of Yes-No question
Repetition of item 7a: inclusion of a phrase regarding questioning, perseveration of Yes–No question
SCT item 7b: correct response
SCT item 8a : ***Where have you Peter's toy put***?
SCT item 7a, 8a, 7b, 7a
Repetition of item 8a: same perseveration, even more complex
SCT item 8b: perseveration of WH-question

Semanto-syntactic perseverations

Nine examples of semanto-syntactic perseverations were found in MH's corpus extending over two (one response in between or interaction by the examiner) to several items in between, i.e., several conversational turns and utterances both by the examiner and MH. That part of each response perseverated in each response in the example of a perseveration of a syntactic construction "so that nothing happens to you" could additionally be classified as a semanto-syntactic perseveration. Another example of a semanto-syntactic perseveration is the previously discussed example including the neologism "*ent-zürnt" extending from one picture description to another one. This example is also part of a semanto-syntactic perseveration (and an ideational perseveration) for the semanto-syntactic unit or syntagma: "to be __X__ (X = some *feeling* expression) about something". In addition to the utterances (lines 44 to 60), the following utterances constitute this example:

Example 7: Syntactic form: (Conj.) NP Copula Adj Adv:
MH: "Die Mutter ist ***unglücklich*** darüber ..." (Engl.: "The mother is unhappy about ...")
MH: "Die Mutter ist ***unglücklich*** darüber ..." (Engl.: "The mother is unhappy about ...")
MH: "Der Mutter// die **freut** sich darüber, dass die Tochter ***unglücklich*** ist" (Engl.: "The mother (dative case)// she is happy about it, that the daughter is *unhappy*")
MH: "... die Mutter ist ***zornig*** darüber..." (Engl.: "The mother is angry about it")

The change from "happy" to "unhappy" in this example results in an ideational perseveration. The utterance "the mother is *happy*, that the daughter is *unhappy*" does not coincide with what is depicted in the picture to be described. MH's utterance is semantically anomalous. In the last case, the combination "zornig+ darüber" is less adequate. Another example in this category from the Story Completion Test is "to be run over by X" or "to be injured by X":

Example 8: (Th.: Der Zug...) MH: "... wird ihn ***überfahren*** haben" (Engl.: "The train ... ") MH: "will have run him over"

MH: "Sie ist von dem bösen Hund ... ertrun// nein nicht ertrunken[4] Sie ist ***von dem bösen Hund überfahren worden***." (Engl.: "She is by the mean dog ... drow// no not drowned. She has been ***run over by the mean dog***") (Target: **The girl is bitten by a dog**)

This example was very difficult for MH to understand and she responded with echolalia several times, before she produced a response. Other syntagmas which are perseverated refer to the following semanto-syntactic "chunks", e.g., "to listen to X", "to like X", "to play with X", "to tell/have the time on X", "to have an article of clothing/hat on", "to be injured by X", "to owe someone X".

Semantics

In this category, the errors relate to single word responses and they are classified either as verbal paraphasias, verbal/ lexical perseverations, semantic paraphasias, or semantic perseverations.

Verbal paraphasias

Only two paraphasias were produced by MH which showed a minimal or no relation at all to the target word.

Verbal/lexical perseverations

With respect to perseveratory lexical errors, MH produced 10 verbal or lexical perseverations. These are given in Table 3. With regard to the linguistic extent, they range from intersentential to intertextual over several task stimuli and/or conversational turns. In all but one case, a noun is perseverated. The one example affecting a verb can be classified as a syntactic perseveration of content or also a semantic perseveration (i.e., association). On closer examination, for most of the examples in Table 3, a loose semantic relation or association holds between the perseveration and the target word.

Semantic paraphasias

MH produced 16 semantic paraphasias and an additional 4 paraphasias of colour names. The grammatical categories are nouns, adjectives, and verbs. They are given in Table 4 with additional information including the task, description of the relations

[4] This is one of two examples in the entire corpus where it is not possible to rule out the possibility that MH repaired her error based on lexical and/or semantic processing of the phonological form. The other example is the rejection of an activity she performs in her spare time: "fris// nicht frisieren" ("to do//not to do one"s hair")

that hold between the target, and the paraphasia. The main relationship between the target and the paraphasia is same semantic category, e.g., cat and mouse are animals.

Semantic perseverations

A total of 12 examples of semantic perseverations were produced by MH. These examples are summarised in Table 5. The context, semantic relations, and linguistic interval are given for each of the examples in Table 5.

Text

Discourse production is secondarily impaired in MH due to her word retrieval difficulties, impaired monitoring of semantic information, and the various perseverative responses, in particular the syntactic perseverations of form. These errors necessarily result in violations of the criteria of textuality as proposed by de Beaugrande and Dressler (1981).

The following examples from conversational speech (Example 9) and a picture story task (Example 10) exemplify the impact of MH's semantic processing deficits on her discourse production:

Example 9: Th.: "Schauen Sie gerne Fernsehen an?" (Engl.: "Do you like to watch television?")
MH: "Ja, aber nicht sehr gerne" (Engl.: "Yes, but not very much")
Th.: Können Sie sich an ein Programm erinnern, das Ihnen besonders gefallen hat?") ("Can you recall a programme that you really liked?")
MH: "Ja schon. Ich schaue gerne fern. Dann sehe ich mir Sachen an") (Engl.: "Yes all right. I like to watch TV. Then I watch things"

The conversation continues with answers such as in Example 9.

Example 10: Content of the story: A girl watches a sleeping cat. The girl pulls the cat's tail and wakes it up. The cat jumps up and scratches the girl. In the last picture one sees the girl crying.

MH calls the "cat" a "mouse" several times and she does not respond to the questions adequately, which are asked for clarification purposes:

(a) The girl cries because she pulls the cat by the tail;
(b) The girl begins to cry
(c) The girl will scratch the cat
(d) (Who scratches?) The girl
(e) In response to why the girl is crying at the end, MH states, because she was disturbed.

This type of response is observed for the SCT (see Example 20): For the target sentence: *Peter will work again*, MH replies that he will *visit his sister*. Following repeated presentation of the stimulus by the examiner, stressing that Peter does not have time off from work, she replies that he *will* be off from work. After the examiner supplies the correct response, namely, "*Peter will work again*" MH continues by stating, but then he must *visit his sister*. For the target sentence of the next item: *Father will smoke his pipe*, she responds that "*his sister has off*". After repeating the story once again, MH answers: "*He will examine his son*" followed by: "*and he will do it, that he smokes in spite of it*". Examples from the various tasks reveal MH's comprehension difficulties.

Ideational perseverations

Several of the examples already discussed can also be classified as ideational perseverations. A total of 21 examples of ideational perseveration can be discerned in MH's corpus. This number is possibly greater since in some cases an ideational perseveration is embedded in a more extended example. The ideational perseverations are enumerated in Table 6. These examples are also described with regard to their history of origins as being simple or versus complex.

Three types have been differentiated:

1. Type 1: Contradictory statements
2. Type IIa: Real world
3. Type IIb: Associations

Several of the ideational perseveration examples require a multiple classification.

Type 1: Contradictory statements. The truth of the utterances is relevant for inclusion in this category. This category refers to examples in which contradictory statements are produced that derive from perseverations. Seven of the ideational perseverations include contradictory statements. For example, the previously discussed productions of the phrase "to be happy about something" turned into "to be unhappy about something" in the repeated productions.

Type Iia: Real world. In this type of ideational perseveration the resulting utterance deviates from real-world norms. A total of 15 (possibly 16) of MH's ideational perseverations include statements that deviate from real-world norms and world knowledge. For example, in the real world a clock or watch is used to tell the time and not a table or an aeroplane:

Example 11: MH: "Das ist eine Uhr." Th: "Wie spät ist es?" MH: "Es ist darauf :: zwölf Uhr. Das ist ein Tisch." Th: "Und was ist damit?" MH: "***Mit dem Tisch : : da ist es zwölf Uhr dreißig.***" (Engl.: MH: "That is a watch." Th: "How late is it?" MH: "On it it is :: twelve o"clock. That is a table." Th: "And what about it? MH: "***With the table – here it is :: twelve thirty***")
MH: "Das ist ein Flieger." Th:"Ja" MH: "***Aber ich weiß es nicht, wie spät es darauf ist***" (Engl.: MH: "That is an aeroplane." Th: "Yes" MH: "***But I do not know it – what time it is on it.***" (immediate spontaneous continuation of her production after the examiner says "yes")

Type IIb: Associations. In MH's corpus five examples of this type of ideational perseveration were documented (and three borderline cases). This type of ideational perseveration is set off by an association, for example a possibly dangerous situation. Another example from the SCT exemplifies this. This example was discussed under the subheading Semanto-syntactic perseverations of content: The association with a dangerous situation "to be run over/hit by a train" or "to drown". This associative connection also applies for the following example from the Cookie Theft picture description (Goodglass & Kaplan, 1983). Several possible situations could be triggered by the production "*umstürzt*" (Engl.: "fall" or "tumble over"). In this example, the situation could be associated with an impending accident, e.g., slipping on the overflowing/spilled water or falling off the stool and hurting oneself:

Example 12: MH: "... Das ist das Wasser, das um/ umfällt / um***stürzt***". (Engl.: MH: "...That is the water, that over/ falls over / *tumbles over*." MH: "Die Kinder machen :: machen :: Die Kinder *stürzen*." Th: "Ja, aber was tun die Kinder? Was wollen die Kinder?" MH: "Die Kinder wollen, dass es im Haus : ***nicht brennt***." (Engl.: MH: "The children are doing : doing :: The children are *falling*." Th: "Yes, but what are the children doing? What do the children want?" MH: "The children want, that the house ***does not catch fire***."

Several triggers could be posited to characterise MH's ideational perseverations of the associational subtype.

Echolalia

An analysis of MH's echolalic responses revealed that when MH only produced an echolalic response, her syntax was correct. She produced numerous examples of unmitigated and mitigated echolalic responses. In episodes of echolalia, MH's responses showed correctly adapted pronominal and verb forms:

Example 13: In response to a question about her hobbies she replied: "In der Freizeit was ich da mache ..." (Engl.: "In my spare time what I do then ...")

Example 14: Th: "... Was werde *ich* sagen?" (Engl.: "... What will *I* say?")
MH: "... Was werden *Sie* sagen?" Engl.: "... What will *you* say?")

In Example 13, MH changed the word order to produce a grammatical utterance that requires verb final. In Example 14 she produced the correct forms and maintains the correct word order (verb second position) for German:

Example 15: "In welcher Schule ich war ..." (Engl.: "in which school I was...")

As soon as echolalia is affected by perseveration, MH perseverated pronouns among other forms, e.g.:

Example 16: Th.: "***Sie*** möchten, dass ***ich mich*** niedersetze" (Engl.: "***You*** would like that ***I myself*** (reflexive) sit down")
MH: "***Sie*** möchten, dass ***Sie sich*** niedersetzen" (Engl.: "***You*** would like that ***you yourself*** (reflexive) sit down")
Target: Ger.: "***Ich*** möchte, dass ***Sie sich*** niedersetzen"
Engl.: "***I*** would like ***you*** to sit down"

Example 17: MH: "Pass auf, damit Dir nichts passiert" (Engl.: "Be careful, that nothing happens to you ") (Target: Setz Dich nieder! (Engl.: "Sit yourself down!") (= Perseveration from a picture description administered earlier in the session))

In Example 16, the first occurrence of the pronoun "Sie" is perseverated in her echolalic response. In Example 17, the perseveration is more complex; it stems from a picture description, which is a perseveration from an earlier picture description. This interaction of (1) echolalia with (2) perseveration is often observed in the corpus. The *degree* to which difficulties in word finding and/or MH's difficulties understanding the examiner interact and play a role is difficult to discern. In several cases it was possible to "break through" the echolalia and also to break through echolalia and/or perseveration with a question from the examiner or repetition of the stimulus item.

Related to echolalia is the question whether MH's tendency to enumerate, i.e., to recite a whole list once she has started to give a response, is induced by a question from the examiner. Out of a total of 12 examples of producing a list of responses, in 8 cases (66%) the examiner's question triggered the list recitation, and in 4 cases (33%) MH spontaneously produced a list, e.g.:

Example 18: Th: "What does he (= snowman) have on (its head)"?
MH: "*Einen Hut und Schnee s t i e f e l und Arme hat er und einen ..*"
(Engl.: "A hat and snow b o o t s (produced slowly) and arms he has and a ...")
(NB: the snowman does not have snow boots)

Pause distribution and slowing of speech tempo

Three pause lengths were differentiated in the transcription of MH's utterances: a short, an intermediate, and a long pause. Regarding the distribution of pauses, the following points are relevant. Short and long pauses were observed:

(a) preceding and following echolalia (more often subsequent to it);
(b) when she was enumerating;
(c) preceding and following various types of perseverative responses;
(d) before and after a semantic paraphasia;
(e) before she broke off an utterance;
(f) after a question was posed by the examiner;
(g) before and after she spoke more slowly.

There are three examples in the corpus where no pause was found before the production of an error. A finer analysis of the pauses is necessary; however it appears that the pauses are an indication not only of word-finding difficulties, but mainly of difficulties understanding the test items or understanding the examiner. This is based on MH's facial expressions and other reactions.

A momentary slowing down of her speech tempo is observed in combination with a pause, echolalia, enumerating things she was presently talking about ("list"), when she produced a continuation of a response after it was considered by the examiner to be complete.

Spurious continuation of an utterance

Six examples of spurious continuation of an utterance were analysed in the corpus. These continuations appear to be triggered by some word in the utterance. In examples 19 to 21, for three items of the SCT, she produced the following continuations:

> Example 19: MH: "Der Hund jagt die Katze" Th.: "Gut" MH: "***und beisst die Maus***"
> (Engl.: MH: "The dog chases the cat" Th.: "Good!"
> MH: "***and bites the mouse***")

This continuation is semantically inadequate for the completion of the story: "Peter wird wieder arbeiten" (Engl.: "Peter will work again"):

> Example 20: MH: "wird er wieder arbeiten ***aber dann : muss er seine Schwester besuchen***!" (Engl.: MH: "he will work again ***but then he will visit his sister***!")

In this case, the additional response was produced with a slower speech tempo and has nothing to do with the story to be completed.

> Example 21: MH: "So hat sie das Glas aufgemacht ***und die Frau war größer als Hans***"
> (Engl.: "Thus she opened the jar ***and the woman was bigger than Hans.***"

In Example 21, not only did MH produce a semantically anomalous response to the story, since her *husband,* and not she, was able to open the jar, she also continued the utterance with the response from the last item in an adapted form: the sister in the last story was able to take the cookies down from a shelf for her brother, Hans, because *she* was taller than Hans.

In Example 22, upon naming an object we observe this continuation of a response even though only an object is to be named:

> Example 22: MH: "Das ist ein Flieger" Th.: "Ja" MH: "Aber ich weiss es nicht wie spät es darauf ist" (Engl.: MH.: That is an aeroplane" Th.: "Yes" MH: "But I do not know it, what time it is on it"

This addition to her response was perseverated from naming the picture of a watch.

Although these aspects of language production are interrelated and complex to analyse, they provide additional information on MH's semantic processing difficulties.

DESCRIPTIVE SUMMARY OF MH'S LANGUAGE PERFORMANCE

In summary, the client discussed in this paper, MH, can be characterised as having Type I TSA based on her language performance, i.e., the error pattern that has been described in the previous sections. The spontaneous sentence production observed in Berndt et al.'s client (1987) bears resemblance to MH's language performance. However, the salient feature of verbal perseveration observed in MH distinguishes them. MH produced numerous examples of verbal paraphasia, semantic paraphasia, semantic perseverations, perseverations of syntactic form, and ideational perseverations.

Echolalia was a prominent feature of MH's productions for all of the administered tasks. Two other striking symptoms were her completion of utterances begun by the examiner without any hesitation and an occasional spurious continuation of an utterance or press of speech, after she had completed her utterance. With regard to perseveration, MH perseverated right from the start of a session and, since no test was longer than half an hour, fatigue could not be considered to play a crucial role. Also, interspersed among the perseveratory responses MH provided correct responses. In some cases a correct response was produced after the investigator repeated the question or task stimulus. Examples in MH's data show that she perseverated from the previous day, e.g., the kinship terms that she had produced on the previous day were repeated in her picture description on the next day. In terms of the duration of a perseveration within a session, she perseverated over several stimuli, i.e., from one text (picture description) to the next and through five stories (SCT). With regard to the task complexity, MH perseverated on simple stimuli as well as on more complex stimuli, although her comprehension difficulties were more apparent in the story completion test and in describing a picture or telling a story to several pictures. For several perseverative responses a multiple classification of the error is necessary, e.g.: (1) a semantic perseveration, and (2) part of an ideational perseveration. MH's naming ability for single words is less impaired. A prominent feature is that for the majority of the items to be named MH perseverated, e.g., either a semantic feature (colour) or a syntagma, after she provided an adequate name for the depicted object.

GENERAL DISCUSSION

Verbal perseveration is not observed in every case of aphasia. However when it is, the pattern of occurrence provides valuable information with regard to the origin of the deficits at hand. That is, the verbal perseverative responses are considered to mirror an aphasic person's underlying language-processing difficulties (cf. Stark, 1984). Thus, when the primary deficits are directly treated, or when the symptoms spontaneously recover, perseverative responses will decrease in number (see Buckingham, 2007 this issue; see also Basso, 2004).

Analysis of MH's verbal perseverations lends support to this account of perseveration. Her perseverative responses do not reflect across the board impairment of all components of her processing system. The clinical features observed in MH include a word retrieval problem coupled with auditory comprehension deficits and also severely impaired monitoring of her own oral language production with regard to its semantic content and semantic adequacy. In terms of indicators of impaired functioning in brain-damaged clients, perseveration is often considered to take an intermediate stand between: highly specific, selective, local, focal, or localising symptoms; *and* non-specific, diffuse, general, non-focal, or non-localising symptoms. According to Teuber and Weinstein's (1955) and Yates' (1966) tripartite differentiation of the effects of brain damage, perseveration reflects Teuber and Weinstein's (1955) type-b, or Yates' (1966) type-2 effects; namely systematic differential effects, depending on the location and extent of the damage. These changes are in contrast to type-c or type-1 general deterioration affecting all aspects of functioning, or type-a or type-3 highly specific effects such as agrammatic sentence production in Broca's aphasia or paragrammatic sentence production in Wernicke's aphasia.

In the case of MH, several interrelated deficits can be discerned. Her perseverative responses reflect these processing deficits. Based on the language parameters tested, at least four prominent features stand out. These are related to the hypotheses put forward in this paper with respect to the occurrence of perseveration:

1. MH produced syntactically, i.e., grammatically, correct utterances, which were semantically anomalous.
2. MH spontaneously produced phonologically correct utterances and she repeated words and sentences accurately phonologically.
3. MH did not correct her semantically anomalous utterances.
4. MH showed naming and comprehension deficits, as also judged by her echolalic expressions, the speed of her language production and the distribution of her pauses.

Regarding MH's language performance and, in particular, the occurrence of perseveration, the five previously cited assumptions can now be addressed:

- *Assumption (1) is correct*: Auditory analysis and phonological processing are preserved in MH, therefore *phonological encoding* and *articulation* can be assumed to be intact.
- *Assumption (2) is not correct*: Under the assumption that the lexicon contains, concepts, lemmas, and lexemes (see Dietrich, 2002), if *semantic processing* is intact, MH will be able to retrieve semantically adequate lemmas from the lexicon for the building up of the *syntactic structures* by the *grammatical encoding* of the formulator. Based on analysis of her produced utterances, it is not the case that she produced semantically adequate responses.
- *Assumption (3) is correct*: *Grammatical encoding* is intact. This is based on the fact that the surface structures of MH's utterances are syntactically correct, i.e., well formed.
- *Assumption (4) is not correct*: The *message generator* appears to be impaired. Based on MH's productions, it is assumed that conceptually correct messages are *not* being sent to the formulator.
- *Assumption (5) is not correct*: *Monitoring* is not intact; syntactically incorrect and/or semantically inadequate utterances that should be repaired, prepaired, or verbally rejected as incorrect or anomalous are *not repaired, prepaired, or verbally rejected*.

Based on the test results and her completion phenomena, spurious continuations of utterances, and her perseverative and echolalic behaviour, assumptions (4) and (5) best describe MH's processing difficulties.

With regard to models of sentence production, Garrett (1975, p. 136) addresses "stages" or "levels" and distinct linguistic types:

> It would, for example, be important to know whether there were "stages" or levels in the processing which correspond to the distinct linguistic types characteristic of semantic, syntactic, and phonetic descriptions of sentences. It is entirely consonant with our acceptance of structural descriptions as constraints on translation models, that there should be *no* stage in the processing at which the "decisions" are primarily syntactic or semantic.

In this context, an important question arises: what happens when the scope of one of the stages (e.g., lexical and/or semantic processing) is severely affected as a consequence of brain dysfunction or brain damage? For example, does the syntactic component run through its procedures "automatically"? Based on the language data, in MH's case, the answer appears to be yes. Whatever information is "fed" to the formulator, it is encoded adequately—syntactically and phonologically. The result is that MH produces semantically incorrect and inadequate utterances in the various contexts. In this context, van Lancker (2001) draws attention to the ramifications of semantic versus syntactic processing deficits and emphasises the negative impact of semantic deficits on an aphasic individual's ability to participate in verbal communicative interactions. In contrast to syntactic deficits, van Lancker stresses that "lack of meaning (or semantic ability) DOES render people incapable of communicating" (p. 398). With regard to MH, her semantically anomalous productions had severe effects on her communicative interactions: She contradicted herself and produced semantically incorrect utterances—also in conflict with world knowledge. This is assumed to be the result of her inability to generate adequate messages. They were not filtered and the result was perseverative responses of varying complexity.

If we address MH's language-processing difficulties with reference to Levelt's (1993) model, several loci can be posited for her impairment. Figure 2 is a modified version of Levelt's (1993) model, with minor adaptations taken over from the model discussed in Dietrich (2002), depicting Example 6 from the text.

Since concepts are part of our knowledge store, the proposed connection between the conceptualiser and concepts in the lexicon system is suggested, although the presence of words in the message generator is not accurate. However, they were placed there to symbolise MH's assumed semantic, conceptual difficulties in message generation. Based on qualitative analysis of MH's language performance, the main processing difficulties observed in MH are located in the conceptualiser: (a) message generation and (b) monitoring. MH's macro-planning and micro-planning are impaired. Another possible locus is the lexicon. Based on a qualitative analysis of her responses in the naming versus story completion test, her word retrieval is not as severely impaired as her production of semantically anomalous utterances. However, due to her lexical retrieval problems, adequate lemmas are also not forwarded to the formulator for grammatical encoding and phonological encoding. Already activated information from past test items—spontaneous speech, naming, picture description—which is still available, i.e., activated, is sent from the message generation component to the formulator. The interactions between the message generation device and the monitoring component are defective, so that the semantic adequacy of the information passed on to the formulator is not controlled. Already produced utterances are only monitored for syntactic and phonological adequacy. Aside from minimal attempts at self-correcting her utterances, which possibly could be attributed to processing of semantic information, MH does not show any repair behaviour regarding the semantic adequacy of her productions. The degree to which MH's impaired language comprehension plays a role is masked by the perseveratory responses. Does the over-activation of the previously produced lexical items predominate although she understands more? If that were the case, we would expect repair behaviour related to the semantic aspects of her utterances. This is not observed. The only repairs and even fewer examples of prepair relate to examples of self-correction of the phonological structure of a word and in another few cases the syntactic structure. In the latter cases the utterance is broken off after an incorrect case has been produced. Two examples in the whole corpus are ambiguous with regard to the exact nature of the repair; i.e., in two cases it cannot be ruled out that

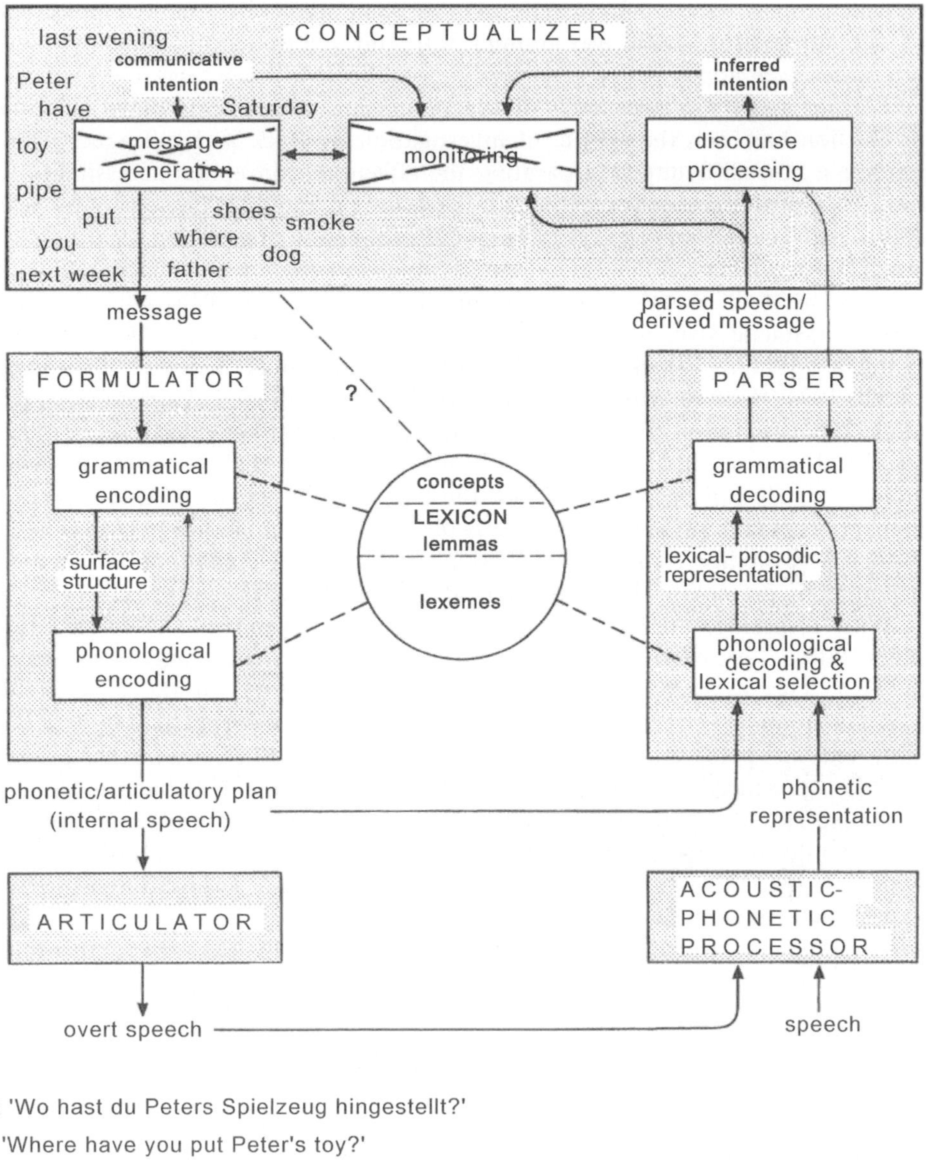

Figure 2. A modified version of Levelt's (1993) model of the processing components involved in spoken language use with minor adaptations by Dietrich (2002) showing MH's assumed processing deficits.

MH performed *only* phonologically decoding. The pervasive nature of the semantic deficit is even observed in perseverations of other linguistic units, e.g., on the morphological level of plural forms or comparatives ("-er"). In addition to being syntactically processed, these morphological aspects also require semantic processing: the concepts of plurality, or concept of comparison, e.g., something being larger than something else.

Other symptoms observed in MH's language data, including echolalia, completion phenomena, and the uncontrolled, automatic continuation of an utterance, provide support for the selective impairment or in other word selective preservation of the formulator, both for grammatical and phonological encoding. Several utterances even appear to be generated automatically.

Teasing apart the roles each of the processing components plays in sentence production has been the subject of investigation by Bock and colleagues over the years, e.g., the difficulty of separating the effects of conceptual accessibility from those of lexical accessibility. From this literature on language processing by healthy control subjects, several aspects of language production are striking regarding MH's language performance. The main aspects relate to the effects of accessibility and availability of information (e.g., the influence of conceptual accessibility on the surface syntactic structure, the accessibility of word forms) and the priming of syntactic structures (Bock, 1982, 1986, 1987; see also Bock & Irwin, 1980; Bock & Levelt, 1994; Bock & Warren, 1985). According to Bock and Warren (1985, p. 63), under the assumption that "a conceptual representation activates a set of possible structural realizations, one of which may be more highly activated than its alternatives. It can be proposed that the most highly activated realization is one maps conceptual representations directly onto surface grammatical relations in terms of their accessibility". Thus, conceptual accessibility is assumed to influence directly or indirectly grammatical role assignments and word order.

With respect to MH's language performance, several effects related to the accessibility of conceptual information and lexical information may be exacerbated in MH. This exacerbation is due to her impairment(s) in the conceptualiser component and/or concepts in the lexicon: Those limited forms that are still highly activated, i.e., perseverated from one production to another, are further processed and then produced in semantically anomalous sentences. The given information, i.e., perseverated information precedes new information, because in numerous cases the new information cannot be activated. A disruption in coordinating word forms with syntactic plans is observed as perseveration of several linguistic units. Conceptual accessibility is severely affected in MH as judged by her intricate perseverations in which those items that are conceptually accessible and produced are also perseverated. The impaired monitoring, i.e., control mechanisms, also fail to prevent MH from producing semantically inadequate utterances and to repair them after they are produced. Thus, syntax detached from semantics is at work in MH.

Summary

Naturally occurring incidents affecting language processing in clients with brain dysfunction and/or brain damage provide the clinician or researcher with language data actually produced—in contrast to hypothetical simulation of error patterns. These data constitute the basis for addressing the underlying cause(s) of the impaired language-processing system or components thereof, which have to be accounted for. In this case, the intricate pattern of verbal perseveratory responses provides the investigator with data demonstrating the selective nature of MH's difficulties responding to the language tasks administered. The data are limited; however, the systematic nature of the pattern of perseveratory errors observed in MH's language corpus provides relevant information for understanding her language impairment.

REFERENCES

Basso, A. (2004). Perseveration or the Tower of Babel. *Seminars in Speech and Language, 25*(4), 375–389.

Benson, D. F. (1979). *Aphasia, alexia and agraphia*. New York: Churchill Livingstone.

Berndt, R. S., Basili, A., & Caramazza, A. (1987). Dissociation of functions in a case of transcortical sensory aphasia. *Cognitive Neuropsychology, 4*(1), 79–107.

Berthier, M. L. (1999). *Transcortical aphasias*. Hove, UK: Psychology Press.

Norden, I. (1953). *Binetarium (Intelligenzprüfung nach Binet-Bobertag)*. Göttingen: Hogrefe.

Bock, J. K. (1982). Toward a cognitive psychology of syntax: Information processing contributions to sentence formulation. *Psychological Review, 89*, 1–47.

Bock, J. K. (1986). Syntactic persistence in language production. *Cognitive Psychology, 18*, 355–387.

Bock, J. K. (1987). An effect of the accessibility of word forms on sentence production. *Journal of Memory and Language, 26*, 119–137.

Bock, J. K., & Irwin, D. E. (1987). Syntactic effect of information availability in sentence production. *Journal of Verbal Learning and Verbal Behavior, 19*, 467–484.

Bock, J. K., & Levelt, W. J. M. (1994). Language production grammatical encoding. In M. A. Gernsbacher (Ed.), *Handbook of psycholinguistics* (pp. 945–984). San Diego: Academic Press.

Bock, J. K., & Warren, R. K. (1985). Conceptual accessibility and syntactic structure in sentence formulation. *Cognition, 21*, 47–67.

Branch Coslett, H., Roeltgen, D. P., Gonzalez-Rothi, L., & Heilman, K. M. (1987). Transcortical Sensory Aphasia: Evidence for Subtypes. *Brain and Language, 32*, 362–378.

Buckingham, H. W. (2007). Introductory essay: Perseveration happens! *Aphasiology, 21*, 916–927.

Cimino-Knight, A. M., Hollingswoorth, A. L., & Gonzalez-Rothi, L. J. (2005). The transcortical aphasias. In L. LaPointe (Ed.), *Aphasia and related neurogenic language disorders* (pp. 169–185). New York: Thieme.

de Beaugrande, R., & Dressler, W. U. (1981). *Einführung in die Textlinguistik*. Tübingen: Niemeyer.

Dietrich, R. (2002). *Psycholinguistik*. Stuttgart: Metzler Verlag.

Dogil, G., Haider, H., Schaner-Wolles, C., & Husmann, R. (1995). Radical autonomy of syntax: Evidence from transcortical sensory aphasia. *Aphasiology, 9*(6), 577–602.

Garrett, M. F. (1975). The analysis of sentence production. In G. Bower (Ed.), *Psychology of learning and motivation: Volume 9*. New York: Academic Press.

Goldstein, K. (1915). *Die transkortikalen Aphasien*. Jena: Gustav Fischer.

Gonzalez-Rothi, L. J. (1997). Transcortical motor, sensory and mixed aphasias. In L. LaPointe (Ed.), *Aphasia and related neurogenic language disorders* (2nd ed., pp. 91–111). Stuttgart: Thieme Verlag.

Goodglass, H., Berko Gleason, J., Bernholtz, N. A., & Hyde, M. R. (1972). Some linguistic structures in the speech of a Broca's aphasic . *Cortex, 8*, 191–212.

Goodglass, H., & Kaplan, E. (1983). *The assessment of aphasia and related disorders* (2nd ed.). Philadelphia, PA: Lea & Febiger.

Huber, W., Poeck, K., & Weniger, D. (1982). Klinisch-neuropsychologische Syndrome Aphasie. In K. Poeck (Ed.), *Klinische Neuropsychologie*. Stuttgart: Thieme.

Kempler, D., Curtiss, S., & Jackson, C. (1987). Syntactic preservation in Alzheimer's disease. *Journal of Speech and Hearing Research, 30*, 343–350.

Levelt, W. J. M. (1993). Language use in normal speakers and its disorders. In G. Blanken, J. Dittmann, H. Grimm, J. C. Marshall, & C-W. Wallesch (Eds.), *Linguistic disorders and pathologies: An international handbook* (pp. 1–15). Berlin: Walter de Gruyter.

Lichtheim, (1885). On aphasia. *Brain, 7*, 433–484.

Pick, A. (1906). Rückwirkung sprachlicher Perseveration auf den Assoziationsvorgang. *Zeitschrift für Psychologie und Physiologie der Sinnesorgane, 42*, 241–257.

Rubens, A. B., & Kertesz, A. (1983). The localization of lesions in transcortical aphasias. In A. Kertesz (Ed.), *Localization in neuropsychology* (pp. 245–268). New York: Academic Press.

Stark, J. (1984). *Verbale Perseveration bei Aphasie – Ein neurolinguistischer Ansatz*. Unpublished PhD Thesis, University of Vienna, Austria.

Stark, J. (2007). A review of classical accounts of verbal perseveration and their modern-day relevance. *Aphasiology, 21*, 928–959.

Teuber, H. L., & Weinstein, S. (1955). General and specific effects of cerebral lesions. *The American Psychologist, 10*, 408–409.

Van Lancker, D. (2001). Is your syntactic component really necessary? *Aphasiology, 15*(4), 343–360, and 396–406.

Wernicke, C. (1874). *Der aphasische Symptomencomplex*. Breslau: Cohn & Weigert.

Whitaker, H. (1976). A case of the isolation of the language function. In H. Whitaker & H. A. Whitaker (Eds.), *Studies in neurolinguistics, Volume 2* (pp. 1–58). New York: Academic Press.

Yates, A. L. (1966). Psychological deficit. *Annual Review of Psychology*, *17*, 111–144.

NEW FROM PSYCHOLOGY PRESS!

The Aphasia Therapy File

Volume 2

Edited by Sally Byng, Judith Duchan and Carole Pound

"ANOTHER EXCELLENT VOLUME IN WHAT WILL HOPEFULLY BE AN ONGOING SERIES RELATED TO CLINICAL APHASIOLOGY, THE BOOK PRESENTS AN ECLECTIC MIX OF APHASIA TREATMENT PROGRAMS, WITH AN OVER-ARCHING AND OBVIOUS INTEREST IN MATCHING TREATMENTS TO THE INDIVIDUAL NEEDS OF PEOPLE WITH APHASIA. THE CASE BASED NATURE OF THE CONTENT PROVIDES A RARE PERSPECTIVE IN AN APHASIA TEXT. IT IS INFORMATIVE AND CURRENT, UTILIZING BOTH IMPAIRMENT AND SOCIAL APPROACHES TO APHASIA THERAPY."
ELIZABETH ARMSTRONG, DEPARTMENT OF LINGUISTICS, MACQUARIE UNIVERSITY

The Aphasia Therapy Files represent a practical resource for people who work with individuals with aphasia, either as therapists or as researchers. An overview of issues associated with current practices is combined with a study of the practicalities of determining, designing and implementing therapies.

This second volume continues to explore the possibility of bridging the gap between therapy in a clinical setting and the practical issues faced by the person living with aphasia. Each author presents one or more of their clinical practices in order to share their therapy experiences and reasoning with others. These contributions provide an insight into the complex issues that face both the practitioner and the person with aphasia, including discussion of subjects such as:

- Revealing competence and rethinking identity for people with severe aphasia using drawing and a communication book
- Respecting the rights of a person with aphasia to their own life choices: a longitudinal therapy study
- A group approach to the long-term rehabilitation of people with acquired head injury within the community
- Lexical and functionally based treatment: effects on word retrieval and conversation.

While each of the chapters is of considerable interest on its own, the final chapter offers readers a method of describing and capturing what happens in therapy and why, to enable comparisons between therapies and application by readers themselves. Written by speech and language therapists working in clinical practice, the studies included in this unique resource reflect the realities of everyday practice and will appeal to therapists, students and researchers in aphasia.

PUBLISHED NOVEMBER 2006
HARDBACK BOOK • 246X189 • 304PP • £29.95 / $53.95
1-84169-270-0 • ISBN13: 978-1-84169-270-8

ORDER YOUR COPY ONLINE AT

www.languagedisordersarena.com

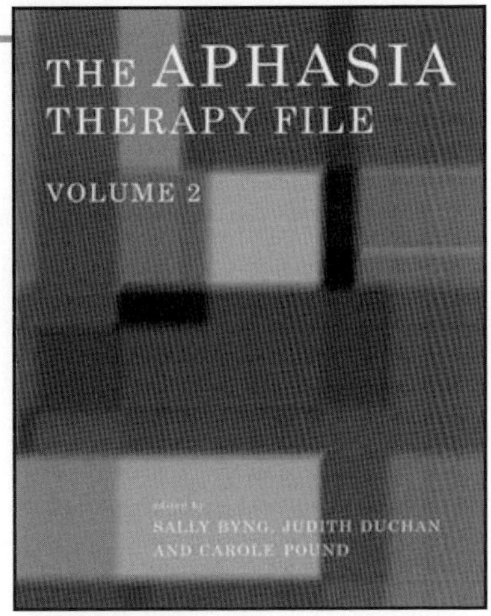

CONTENTS

Psychology Press
Taylor & Francis Group